Minimally Invasive Surgery in Cancer

Mallika Tewari
Editor

Minimally Invasive Surgery in Cancer

Techniques and Outcomes

Springer

Editor
Mallika Tewari
Department of Surgical Oncology
Inst. of Medl Scienc, Banaras Hindu Univ
Varanasi, Uttar Pradesh, India

ISBN 978-981-97-7058-8 ISBN 978-981-97-7059-5 (eBook)
https://doi.org/10.1007/978-981-97-7059-5

This Springer imprint is published by the registered company Springer Nature Singapore Pte Ltd.
The registered company address is: 152 Beach Road, #21-01/04 Gateway East, Singapore 189721, Singapore

Contents

About the Editor

Mallika Tewari MBBS, MS, M.Ch. (Surgical Oncology), MRCS.Ed. graduated from the Institute of Medical Sciences at Banaras Hindu University (BHU), India. She is Professor and Head of the Department of Surgical Oncology and Chief of the Hepato-Pancreatico-Biliary and Gastrointestinal Division at the Institute of Medical Sciences, BHU. She has been a pioneer in establishing minimally invasive surgery for cancer in her department. She has more than 100 peer-reviewed international/ national publications and has coordinated several symposiums and panel discussions, delivered orations, and organized guest lectures.

Dr. Tewari has had an outstanding career and graduated with 10 medals and 23 academic prizes from her medical school. She is the recipient of several prestigious international fellowships such as UICC ICRETT, International Guest Scholarship of the American College of Surgeons, and European Society of Surgical Oncology travelling fellowship. She is the executive member of the World Federation of Surgical Oncology Societies (WFSOS), Indian Association of Surgical Oncology (IASO), Association of Surgeons of India (ASI), and IHPBA amongst many others. She is a reviewer for several international scientific journals and Editor of *Indian Journal of Surgery*, the official publication of the ASI.

Her previous book "Surgery for Pancreatic and Periampullary Cancer; Principles and Practice" fetched over 40k accesses.

Expert Commentary: Minimally Invasive GI and HPB Surgical Oncology

1

David A. Kooby

1.1 Minimally Invasive Surgery in GI and HPB Oncology: Thoughtful Innovation

My interest in Medicine as a career began during doctor visit when I was young. I remember the pediatrician asking me to take deep breaths when he placed the stethoscope on my chest and back to listen to my heart and lungs. I could conceptualize what he was doing, and I wanted to understand it better. How did the stethoscope work, and who invented it? Later, I read about Rene Laënnec, the "father of clinical auscultation" and his early descriptions of thoracic and abdominal pathology with "mediate" (through a wooden tube) rather than "immediate" auscultation (placing one's ear directly on the patient) in the early 1800s [1]. It was a leap forward in medicine, and had we stopped there we would all carry blocks of wood in our lab coats and miss out on the tremendous diagnostic power of the modern stethoscope.

Surgical innovation is rarely adopted instantly. Surgical innovators, such as Joseph Lister (antisepsis), John H. Gibbon (heart-lung machine), and Thomas Starzl (liver transplantation), would attest to the challenges associated with getting a "practice changing" concept up and running. Each of these giants in their fields of surgery built their ideas off concepts developed by others, and they were not satisfied with the status quo. Their initial efforts were plagued by failure, poor outcomes, and ridicule, yet they modified their ideas, improved their designs through multiple iterations and attempts, leaving tremendous impacts on clinical medicine and humanity.

Minimally invasive abdominal surgery developed somewhat serendipitously through a combination of the techniques of inducing pneumoperitoneum to tamponade gastrointestinal hemorrhage (Jorge Kelling) with peritoneoscopy (Hans Jacobius) [2]. Progress was slow until the development of the three-chip camera allowed everyone in the operating theater to view the procedure simultaneously. Thereafter, it became a race to perform the first of each kind of laparoscopic resection possible. Early efforts at relatively easy laparoscopic surgery, such as cholecystectomy, often took two expert surgeons working together over several hours to complete successfully. Ultimately, the cynics accepted that minimally invasive surgery was beneficial, and minimally invasive approaches are standard for many operations.

Minimally invasive complex gastrointestinal surgery was another matter. The 1990s saw the early efforts at esophagectomy, gastrectomy, partial hepatectomy, and pancreatectomy. Focusing on distal pancreatectomy as an example, because it is an ideal operation for innovation given the

D. A. Kooby (✉)
Surgical Oncology/Winship Cancer Center, Emory Saint Joseph's Hospital, Atlanta, GA, USA
e-mail: dkooby@emory.edu

M. Tewari (ed.), *Minimally Invasive Surgery in Cancer*,
https://doi.org/10.1007/978-981-97-7059-5_1

challenges of getting to the left side of the pancreas due to its retroperitoneal location and associated nest of critical mesenteric vessels, it requires a sizeable incision when performed open, making the effort to approach this operation with minimally invasive approaches particularly worthwhile. Couple this with no necessity of any complex anastomotic steps, and the operation can still be accessible to surgeons with lesser experience.

The initial literature for laparoscopic distal pancreatectomy was replete with small series from various medical centers around the world demonstrating that these operations were feasible. In 2008, a multicenter study published from the Central Pancreas Consortium compared perioperative outcomes of 167 laparoscopic distal pancreatic resections to those of a matched cohort of 200 open cases and showed fewer wound complications and shorter hospital stays than seen with the open approach [3]. This report was widely cited as more surgeons took efforts to perform this operation and more patients sought this approach. Similar studies appeared for other foregut operations. Finally, 10 years after the CPC study, the Dutch Pancreatic Cancer Group published the LEOPARD-1 trial results that compared perioperative outcomes for 100 patients who underwent open versus 100 who underwent minimally invasive approach showing that perioperative outcomes for the laparoscopic distal pancreatic resection group were noninferior to those of the open group, thus completely taking us further along the cycle of innovation, which moves from "Innovators" to "Early Adopters" to "Early Majority" to "Late Majority" and finally Laggards [4].

For more complex procedures, such as pancreatoduodenectomy, innovation and adoption often take longer. In a subsequent randomized controlled trial of laparoscopic versus open pancreatoduodenectomy, safety concerns were raised without benefit for the laparoscopic approach [5]. Recent progress coincided with the development and widespread use of the surgical robotic platforms [6]. Today the surgical community is just approaching the "late majority" phase of the curve for minimally invasive pancreatoduodenectomy, as it is more widely adopted at various medical centers. Robotic surgery itself followed a similar innovation curve and is now commonly performed in most surgical disciplines for nearly all types of surgical procedures.

The cancer question is an important one. Many abdominal operations are performed for malignant indications. Initial enthusiasm for minimally invasive colectomy was tempered by a report of early recurrence due to concerns of pneumoperitoneal dissemination of cancer cells, and inadequate margin clearance and node dissection [7]. Here, an early randomized trial of laparoscopic versus open partial colectomy was performed, which allayed many of these concerns, lifting some of the initial hesitancy with minimally invasive resection of abdominal malignancies [8]. Today most complex foregut gastrointestinal cancer operations are performed using these minimally invasive approaches at many medical centers around the world, with excellent outcomes and true downstream benefits for many patients, much like development, innovation, and adoption of the original Laënnec stethoscope.

So, what is the future? Much of what is described above still requires a transabdominal approach to get to the organ in question. Endoscopic, transcatheter, and alternative energy-based approaches are available and being further developed for mucosal and submucosal tumor, and solid organ tumor ablation and resection, all with the promise of better accuracy and fewer complications. Artificial Intelligence provides the ability to process large datasets quickly to help surgeons learn in newer, more efficient ways [9]. These systems will have the ability to guide surgeons step-by-step to achieve the surgical goals more safely and efficiently. Likely, these systems can cross countries and cultures to provide better care for everyone, irrespective of geography and socioeconomic status. It is time to leave the wood block behind and move forward.

References

1. Jay V. The legacy of Laënnec. Arch Pathol Lab Med. 2000;124:1420–1.
2. Kooby DA. Laparoscopic surgery for cancer: historical, theoretical, and technical considerations. Oncology (Williston Park). 2006;20(8):917–27. PMID: 16922261
3. Kooby DA, Gillespie T, Bentrem D, et al. Left-sided pancreatectomy: a multicenter comparison of laparoscopic and open approaches. Ann Surg. 2008;248(3):438–46.
4. de Rooij T, van Hilst J, van Santvoort H, et al. Minimally invasive versus open distal pancreatectomy (LEOPARD): a multicenter patient-blinded randomized controlled trial. Ann Surg. 2019;269(1):2–9.
5. van Hilst J, de Rooij T, Bosscha K, et al. Laparoscopic versus open pancreatoduodenectomy for pancreatic or periampullary tumours (LEOPARD-2): a multicentre, patient-blinded, randomised controlled phase 2/3 trial. Lancet Gastroenterol Hepatol. 2019;4(3):199–207.
6. Zureikat AH, Postlewait LM, Liu Y, et al. A multi-institutional comparison of perioperative outcomes of robotic and open pancreaticoduodenectomy. Ann Surg. 2016;264(4):640–9.
7. Berends FJ, Kazemier G, Bonjer HJ, et al. Subcutaneous metastases after laparoscopic colectomy. Lancet. 1994;344:2.
8. Clinical Outcomes of Surgical Therapy Study Group. A comparison of laparoscopically assisted and open colectomy for colon cancer. N Engl J Med. 2004;350:2050–9.
9. Nathan J. Four ways artificial intelligence can benefit robotic surgery. Forbes. 15 Feb 2023.

2 History of Minimally Invasive Surgery in Cancer

Mallika Tewari and Manjot Kaur

Abstract

Large incisions were traditionally used for carrying out radical resections as the emphasis was on removal of the cancer and possible cure. A paradigm shift has occurred over a period of several decades now with technological advances enabling radical resections using smaller incisions that reduce the morbidity of radical open surgery while remaining oncologically safe. Introduction of minimally invasive surgery (MIS) has brought about a phenomenal change in the way surgery is performed by the surgeon. Although first developed for benign diseases, MIS has rapidly evolved in cancer surgery. It is associated with lower blood loss, smaller scar, shorter length of hospital stay (LOS) and improved overall quality of life (QOL) in most instances. MIS not only has a role in the diagnosis and staging of cancers but is also widely used for radical resections, most notably of esophageal, gastric, colon, and prostate cancer as well as for various palliative procedures. The introduction of robotics has further refined MIS, the benefit lies in crisp precision and 7° of freedom configuration, which enhances surgeon's dexterity and aids in performing complex surgeries even in a narrow pelvis. This chapter gives an outline of the evolution of MIS in cancer and its present status across some common cancers.

Keywords

Minimally invasive surgery · History · Cancer

2.1 Introduction

It was in 1986 that the term "minimally invasive" was first used, followed by John Wickham, a urologist, in 1989 who used the term "minimally invasive therapy" to describe various procedures through tiny incisions for treatment of ailments that traditionally would have been approached through large incisions [1].

Minimally invasive surgery (MIS) hence describes surgical procedures via small surgical incisions and result in less pain, early recovery, shorter length of hospital stay (LOS), infection, blood loss, and postoperative complications compared to the open technique [2]. Although, with frequent implementation of the "Enhanced Recovery After Surgery (ERAS)" protocols in surgical units, the apparent advantage of reduced LOS in the MIS group has become less relevant. The use of MIS techniques in radical cancer resections was initially slow due to concerns

M. Tewari (✉) · M. Kaur
Division of Hepatobiliary and Gastrointestinal Oncology, Department of Surgical Oncology, Institute of Medical Sciences, Banaras Hindu University, Varanasi, Uttar Pradesh, India

M. Tewari (ed.), *Minimally Invasive Surgery in Cancer*,
https://doi.org/10.1007/978-981-97-7059-5_2

regarding oncological outcomes vis-à-vis traditional open methods [3–5]. With ample data now available regarding feasibility and safety of MIS in various cancers, early gastric cancer, colon cancer, esophageal cancer, and various gynecological cancers are now frequently resected using MIS techniques and the scope is rapidly expanding to include other cancers [2, 4]. MIS is an important diagnostic and also a staging tool often complemented with a laparoscopic ultrasound (LUS) performed prior to definitive surgery either in the same or a separate setting.

Palliative procedures using MIS techniques also help advanced stage cancer patients achieve the desired goal obviating the need for a more invasive open surgery. We herein discuss in brief the history and evolution of MIS in oncology and its current status.

2.2 History of Minimally Invasive Surgery

The origin of MIS dates back to more than 200 years when in the year 1806 Phillip Bozzini came up with the idea of using an imaging system and a light source to visualize internal organs, which he called the "Lichtleiter (light conductor)" [2]. This prototype endoscope used a tube, candlelight, along with a system of mirrors and was used as a cystoscope and a vaginoscope. It was a revolutionary concept, but was not well accepted and he was ironically punished for this invention. However, various modifications evolved over time and the technique was popularized by a French surgeon Antoine Jean Desormeaux and Francis Cruise from Dublin in the mid-1800s using the scope for visualizing the rectum, uterus, auditory canal, pharynx, larynx, esophagus, and stomach. This was followed by a slew of developments in the field with immense clinical implications in diagnosing luminal cancer, for example, gastric cancer by Johann Mikulicz, a surgeon in Vienna in and around 1881 [2].

Until the early twentieth century, laparoscopy was in the experimental stage, with limited clinical utility. George Kelling, a German surgeon in 1901 first performed laparoscopy in dogs and coined the term *coelioskope* [4]. Hans Christian Jacobaeus, an internist from Stockholm, is credited to have first published his report in 1911 on laparoscopy and thoracoscopy in humans and termed it *laparothorakoskopie*. Early part of the twentieth century saw a gradual evolution of laparoscopy from a predominantly diagnostic modality to an increasingly utilized therapeutic modality in procedures such as cauterization, biopsies, and pneumolysis, the latter was used in tuberculosis patients before streptomycin was discovered.

Major technological breakthroughs included the discovery of fiber optics in 1952, "cold light source" by Max Fourestier in 1952, the Hopkins rod-lens system in 1953, and charged-coupled device (CCD) video imaging in 1985 [2].

Kurt Semm, a German gynecologist, introduced CO_2 insufflator for creating pneumoperitoneum and even performed the first laparoscopic appendectomy in 1981 [6]. Raoul Palmer in 1944 first published on diagnostic laparoscopy (who also monitored the intra-abdominal pressure during the procedures) and Kurt Semm, who practiced CO_2 hysteroscopy from mid-1970 [6]. By 1985, endoscopic procedures included cholecystectomy, which was first performed by a German Professor of Surgery, Erich Muhe [7]. P. Mouret (France) and J B McKernan and W. Saye (United States) reported successful results in 1987 and 1988, respectively.

Until the computer chip television camera was introduced, the surgeons used one hand to hold the laparoscope and had only one hand available to operate. The subsequent development of new instruments over the years has allowed complex oncologic procedures to be performed safely and efficiently via laparoscopy. The modern laparoscopic camera also available with a flexible tip allows automatic focus, 3-D images, ultrahigh definition images, in situ fluorescence imaging. A variety of devices are freely available allowing excellent tissue handling and hemostasis and includes graspers/retractors/dissectors/clamps, and laparoscopic clip applicators, staplers, and needle holders. Modern energy devices utilizing monopolar electrocautery, ultrasonic, and bipolar vessel sealers ensure good hemostasis and bloodless dissection in surgical planes.

2.3 Evolution of MIS in Cancer

The role of MIS in cancer was initially limited to diagnosis and staging of cancers. DeVita et al. in 1971 successfully carried out diagnostic staging peritoneoscopies under local anesthesia in 38 patients with Hodgkin's disease obviating the need for a laparotomy [8]. In this series, patients having liver and splenic involvement were upstaged and this had a significant clinical impact. In 1978, Cuschieri and colleagues published their experience on laparoscopy and found it to be useful in diagnosis (enabling tissue/cytological sampling), staging, and also exclusion of cancer [9, 10]. Laparoscopy was increasingly used initially in diagnosing and staging various other malignancies as well such as those arising from the colon, liver, or disseminated/metastatic spread [11, 12].

The introduction of laparoscopic ultrasound (LUS) examination in 1993 was a major milestone in the evolution of MIS as it significantly enhanced the accuracy of diagnostic laparoscopy [13, 14]. Liu et al. [14] found that LUS significantly enhanced the pickup diagnostic rate of liver tumors, 14 of 43 patients (33%), and also more accurately informed of their resectability status, 18 of 43 (42%), over laparoscopy alone. Similar superior results of the combined approach were reported for pancreatic cancer and Bemelman et al. [15] even found that 21 of 22 lesions deemed resectable at laparoscopy were actually surgically resectable.

2.3.1 MIS in Colorectal Cancer

Colon resections are commonly performed these days via laparoscopic approach [16]. One of the first procedures in 1990 was right hemicolectomy by M. Jacobs et al. using laparoscopic staplers [16], sigmoid colectomy by D. Fowler, colostomy closure by J. Uddo, and low anterior resection (LAR) by P. Leahy [16, 17]. These encouraging results led to frequent implementation of the laparoscopic approach for colorectal resections.

However, the acceptance for laparoscopic colectomy was slow unlike that for laparoscopic cholecystectomy. This primarily was owing to concerns regarding oncological equivalence to open technique, port site recurrences, difficult and steep learning curve, and paucity of evidence from randomized controlled trials (RCTs) [17]. It was only after publication of the COST (The Clinical Outcomes of Surgical Therapy Study Group) Trial that laparoscopic-assisted colectomy was deemed noninferior to open colectomy [16].

The COLOR (Colon Cancer Laparoscopic or Open Resection) [18] Trial was a multicenter study that recruited colon cancer patients from 1997 to 2002. Of 1248 patients, 627 were randomized to laparoscopic and 621 to open group, respectively. Although with the conversion rate of 17% and longer operating times, the laparoscopic group reported lower blood loss, quicker return of bowel function, reduced pain, and less LOS with no difference in radicality of resection or 28-day morbidity and mortality. This trial firmly established the feasibility and oncological safety of laparoscopic colon cancer resections.

The Medical Research Council (MRC) CLASICC (Conventional vs. Laparoscopic-Assisted Surgery in Colorectal Cancer) Trial was the very first RCT conducted between 1996 and 2002 [19] across 27 UK centers that randomized 794 colorectal cancer patients into laparoscopic ($n = 526$) and open ($n = 268$) resection group in 2:1 ratio. The results revealed higher complication rates in those with conversion and an overall conversion rate of 29%. The incidence of a circumferential resection margin (CRM) positivity was also higher after laparoscopic AR though not statistically significant. No difference was found in hospital mortality or quality of life (QOL) postoperatively. While this trial reiterated the safety of laparoscopic approach for colon cancer, its applicability for rectal cancer remained inconclusive owing to impaired short-term outcomes.

Abraham et al. [20] reported a meta-analysis of 12 RCTs up to 2002 with 2521 procedures laparoscopic vs. open for colorectal cancer. They found that although the laparoscopic approach took 30% longer, it resulted in lower morbidity, quicker return of bowel movement (33%), less pain (37%), and LOS (20%). The mortality and oncological outcomes were equivalent. The authors hence stated that laparoscopic colorectal cancer resection resulted in better short-term results without compromising on oncological safety parameters.

Jayne et al. [19] reported the 3-year follow-up results of the UK MRC CLASICC Trial Group wherein the 3-year overall survival (OS), disease free survival (DFS), local recurrence (despite higher positive CRM rates after laparoscopic AR), and QOL were not significantly different among the open and laparoscopic groups. These results supported laparoscopic surgery for colorectal cancer.

Several studies such as by Franklin et al. [21] and Lacy et al. [22] also reported favorable data for laparoscopic colon resection including equivalent lymph node harvest, resection margins, and OS and DFS. Other landmark trials reinforcing safety of laparoscopic colon resections were The COREAN (Comparison of open versus laparoscopic surgery for mid or low rectal cancer after neoadjuvant chemoradiotherapy) trial [23] wherein 340 patients were randomized on a 1:1 basis, and COLOR II (Colorectal cancer laparoscopic or open resection) trial where 1103 patients were randomized on a 2:1 basis [24]. Laparoscopic colon resections were deemed safe with equivalent oncological results such as quality of the resected specimen, CRM, lymph node yield, morbidity, and mortality although it was associated with longer operating time. Similarly, no significant difference was observed in DFS, OS, lymph node yield, and margin status among patients with colon cancer with at least 3 years of follow-up between open and laparoscopic groups in a pooled analysis of the Barcelona, COST, COLOR, CLASSIC, and ALCCaS (Australasian Laparoscopic Colon Cancer Study) trials [25].

2.3.1.1 MIS in Rectal Cancer

The laparoscopic resection for rectal cancer remains debatable. In a meta-analysis of prospective trials including 11 studies (4 randomized) and 1684 patients, Arezzo et al. [26] in 2013 reported lower mortality rate (1.2% vs. 2.3%) and overall complications (31.5% vs. 38.2%) in laparoscopic versus open groups, respectively. The Australasian Laparoscopic Cancer of the Rectum (AlaCaRT) [27] and ACOSOG Z6051 [28] RCTs in T1–T3 rectal cancers used a composite of oncologic factors indicating the adequacy of surgical resection, which included margin status (CRM, distal margin), and quality of total mesorectal excision (TME). However, both the RCTs failed to prove non-inferiority of the laparoscopic approach in rectal cancer with respect to pathological variables but worded caution for routine use of the laparoscopic resections pending long-term results.

Two important meta-analysis also reported no significant differences between laparoscopic and open rectal resections across the studies and RCTs included in the meta-analysis. The meta-analysis of four studies (2319 patients) by Creavin et al. [29] reported margin status and completeness of mesorectal resection were acceptable in both the groups. Milone et al. [30] in 2018 also reported no statistically significant differences between either group among 12 trials included in their meta-analysis.

Multiple other studies (Sara et al. [31], Boutros et al. [32], Penninckx et al. [33]) have reported comparable surgical outcomes for the laparoscopic approach with respect to status of CRM and distal margin, TME completeness, and lymph node retrieval. Similar long-term results and oncological safety for Laparoscopic-Assisted Rectal Resection (LARR) were reported by Feliciotti et al. [34]; no higher morbidity or mortality by Barlehner et al. [35]. Two meta-analyses [36, 37] did not find any difference in the oncologic outcomes between open versus laparoscopic groups. While similar wound infection rates, anastomotic dehiscence, mortality, longer operative times but lower morbidity were reported by Gao and co-workers [36] in their analysis of 11 studies, 285 patients (1995–2005) who underwent LARR, Aziz et al. [37] found early return of bowel movement, stoma function, and overall decreased LOS in 909 patients across 20 studies (1993–2004) who underwent laparoscopic resection versus 1162 open resection for rectal cancer.

In addition, laparoscopic Abdomino—Perineal Resection (APR) patients had lower requirement of parenteral analgesia and had less incidence of wound infections.

Colorectal cancer laparoscopic or open resection (COLOR II) trial [24] was a landmark prospective, phase III, RCT conducted by the American College of Surgeons Oncology Group (ACOSOG) (between January 2004 and May 2010). Patients with localized rectal cancer within 15 cm from the anal verge were randomized into the laparoscopic (n = 739) versus open (n = 364) groups. Of 1044 patients included in the final analysis, (699 and 345, respectively) it was found that the laparoscopic procedure took longer time but it had less blood loss, bowel function returned sooner, and LOS was shorter. Similar overall morbidity, mortality, and the macroscopic completeness of resection was reported in both the groups.

Pigazzi et al. in 2006 [38] first reported their data on robotic TME for rectal cancer wherein they confirmed the feasibility of robotic LAR with TME and autonomic nerve preservation. Baik et al. in 2007 [39] first reported robotic TME in Asia and also published results of the first prospective pilot RCT showing feasibility and safety of robotic LAR versus laparoscopic LAR (with 18 patients in either group) in 2008 [40].

The ROLARR trial [41] was a large, multicenter, randomized, unblended, parallel group trial conducted at 29 different hospitals in 10 countries with 40 experienced surgeons. 471 resectable rectal cancer patients were randomized in robotic-assisted versus standard laparoscopic surgery groups (n = 237 vs. 234, respectively). Robotic surgery group offered no significant advantage over the conventional laparoscopic technique vis-à-vis conversion rate, CRM positivity and eight other different intra-/postoperative complications studied.

2.3.1.2 Transanal Minimally Invasive Surgery (TAMIS)

Atallah et al. [42] first introduced TAMIS in 2010 wherein TME is performed in a "bottom up" approach by making an incision at or just above the dentate line using a variety of portals such as transanal endoscopic microsurgery (TEM) scope and a single port scope with assistance from the upper abdomen and finally a coloanal anastomosis is completed. Only a few case series exist on the topic of selected patients [43].

2.3.2 MIS in Esophageal Cancer

Esophageal cancer remains a difficult cancer to cure with surgery remaining the cornerstone of the treatment. The 5-year survival remains poor at 15–25% [44]. The approach to management is multimodality treatment with esophagectomy remaining the cornerstone for localized disease. Esophagectomy traditionally done via a thoracotomy was associated with significant morbidity and mortality. Minimally invasive esophagectomy (MIE), thoracoscopic and/or robotic-assisted, offers to remove the esophagus with the same radicality but less morbidity and has hence been quickly adopted across various centers.

In the year 1995, DePaula and colleagues [45] first reported favorable outcomes following laparoscopic Transhiatal Esophagectomy (THE) in 12 patients with esophageal disease, both benign and malignant. Postoperative complications and LOS were less in the MIS group. Shortly thereafter, in 1997, Swanstrom and Hansen [46] reported their data on laparoscopic THE in nine patients (six cancer, two dysplastic Barrett's esophagus, one peptic stricture). The results were again favorable with no anastomotic leaks, wound complications, conversions, or local recurrence in 13 months of follow-up. In 1998, Luketich and co-workers [47] from the University of Pittsburgh reported their data with MIE with mini-laparotomy/thoracotomy as needed for eight patients (five stage one cancer). The technique appeared feasible with no mortality and two major complications one cervical anastomotic leak and one delayed gastric emptying (DGE). The same group published their data on 1011 patients who underwent MIE (neck anastomosis 481; Ivor Lewis 580) between 1996 and 2011 [48]. Forty-five (4.5%) patients required conversion to open surgery; no intraoperative mortality occurred; overall 30-day mortality was 1.68%;

and vocal cord paresis/paralysis was significantly lower in the Ivor Lewis group (1%). Significant postoperative morbidity rate was 25% and included 5% anastomotic dehiscence rate requiring surgery. R0 resection was possible 98% with median lymph node harvest of 21. These results reinforced their faith in MIE.

A meta-analysis of ten studies (one trial and nine case-control studies) reported favorable short-term outcomes for MIE including lower complication rate, anastomotic leaks, blood loss, LOS, and mortality [49]. Several other groups have published similar good short-term results of MIE [50–54]. Studies also indicate favorable outcomes following MIE after neoadjuvant therapy in the era of multimodality treatment such as less intensive care unit (ICU) stay, early removal of nasogastric tube, and quicker initiation of oral diet as compared to open esophagectomy (OE) [55]. More importantly no significant difference has been found even in the oncologic outcomes between OE and MIE in terms of survival and recurrence rates across various studies and meta-analyses [56–58]. Robotic-assisted MIE is being successfully performed and results point to its feasibility and safety with perioperative outcomes similar to OE [59, 60]. In addition, in a retrospective study of 43 patients, robotic-assisted MIE was reported to have similar short-term outcomes (blood loss, lymph node yield, ICU stay, complications, operative time, LOS) compared with thoracoscopic MIE with no added advantages to the robotic group [61].

2.3.3 MIS in Head and Neck Cancer

MIS in head and neck cancer is evolving. Transoral Robotic Surgery (TORS) received approval by the Food and Drug Administration (FDA) in 2009 and has principally been used for early stage oropharyngeal and supraglottic cancers [62]. A multicenter study was conducted by Weinstein et al. [63] to assess the safety, feasibility, and the adequacy of surgical margins after TORS using pooled data from clinical trials in three different institutions. A total of 192 patients were initially screened, predominantly comprising 139 (78%) tumors arising in the oropharynx and 26 (15%) in the larynx. TORS was performed in 161 patients. TORS was deemed safe and feasible in the multidisciplinary management of head and neck cancer.

A retrospective multi-institutional study by De Almeida et al. [64] reported on the oncologic outcomes after TORS. Of 410 patients that underwent TORS between January 2007 and December 2012 across 11 institutions, 364 (88.8%) had oropharyngeal cancers. Eleven patients received radiation and/or chemotherapy before and 338 after TORS. They found favorable oncologic outcomes across institutions in a multidisciplinary network and supported the role of TORS in the treatment of selected oropharyngeal cancer, especially tonsillar neoplasms.

Transoral Laser Microsurgery (TLM) though initially used in early laryngeal cancer, has been applied in the treatment of oropharyngeal cancer with good survival, local control, and QOL [65]. A total of 204 patients with advanced tonsil and base of tongue (BOT) cancer across three centers treated with TLM were analyzed with a minimum follow-up of 2 years. There was good local control (97%) and 3 year OS was 86% with good swallowing function (87%) [66]. The use of TLM for oropharyngeal surgery remains limited to a few high-volume centers primarily as it often results in specimen disruption vis-à-vis an en bloc resection and there are concerns regarding resection margins.

2.3.3.1 MIS in Thyroid Cancer

Garner et al. [67] was the first person to report feasibility of endoscopic subtotal parathyroidectomy in 1995 done for primary hyperparathyroidism. This laid the path for minimal invasive thyroid surgery. In 2001, the same team published their study regarding endoscopic thyroidectomy for solitary thyroid nodule [68] in 18 patients and backed the approach with a better cosmesis and faster recovery compared to standard open thyroidectomy (OT).

Minimal invasive approach to thyroid is classified into three categories: (1) endoscopic approach with continuous gas insufflation access via neck or chest or axillary or breast, (2) gasless techniques with or without a wall lifter, (3) minimal invasive open surgery. Access to thyroid through the axilla was introduced by Ikeda et al. [69]. The MIVAT (Minimal Invasive Video-Assisted Thyroidectomy) technique was described by Miccoli in 1999 [70]. In 2015, Miccoli et al. [71] presented their landmark experience with MIVAT technique in a large group of 2412 patients. Of these, 800 patients had papillary thyroid carcinoma (PTC), 7 had medullary carcinoma, 15 patients were RET gene carriers, and 3 patients were affected by thyroglossal duct carcinoma carcinoma. The cure rate for MIVAT was 85% versus 80% in OT with a median follow-up of 7.5 years. Unilateral recurrent laryngeal nerve palsy was seen in 1.2% cases. The biggest advantage of MIS was that patients could be discharged a day after surgery and with a cosmetically better scar. Similarly, Del Rio et al. [72] reported insignificant difference in the cumulative Radioactive Iodine (RAI) dose and serum Thyroglobulin (Tg) level in a 5-year outcome study in patients with PTC treated with MIVAT versus conventional thyroidectomy and concluded MIVAT to be a safe procedure. The same authors [73] presented their 10 years' experience with MIVAT technique in various thyroid diseases including low to intermediate risk differentiated thyroid carcinoma reiterating its safety and minimal invasiveness to tissues. A prospective comparative study on video-assisted thyroidectomy and central compartment dissection versus conventional thyroidectomy in patients with PTC (52 patients in each group) by Lombardi et al. [74] in 2012 supported the use of video-assisted thyroidectomy in selected patients with similar short-term outcomes.

Wilhelm and Metzig in 2009 first published transoral thyroidectomy technique through the floor of the mouth in a 53-year-old patient after cadaveric and animal experiments in pigs [75]. Transoral Endoscopic Thyroidectomy Vestibular (premandibular) Approach (TOETVA) was described by Nakajo et al. in 2013, and Wang et al. reported the first randomized study in benign thyroid nodules with 12 patients in the vestibular (TOETVA) and 12 in the areola access endoscopic group with excellent results [76, 77]. In 2022, Sun H et al. published results of their retrospective study wherein they compared PTC patients who underwent total thyroidectomy and central compartment dissection in TOETVA ($n = 28$) versus conventional OT ($n = 56$). They reported comparable rates of central lymph node retrieval, transient hypothyroidism, rate of vocal cord paresis, and complications in both groups and rendered TOETVA as safe and feasible option in patients with PTC [78].

Robotic thyroidectomy (RoT) tends to overcome the shortcomings of endoscopic thyroidectomy enhancing the range of movement, minimizing surgeon hand tremor, excellent fine instruments, and 3D imaging. Furthermore, it is difficult to do cervical lymph node dissection through endoscopy, which limits its use to low-risk thyroid cancer and benign diseases. RoT also helps in cervical lymph node dissection. In a meta-analysis of 23 publications and 5200 cases of thyroid cancer, Pan et al. [79] in 2016 reported similar short-term outcomes for RoT but with significantly longer operative time, less lymph node yield, less blood loss, and higher postoperative Tg level versus OT and emphasized for more data and RCTs on the subject.

2.3.4 MIS in Lung Cancer

The first attempt to look into the pleural cavity was done by Francis Richard Cruise in 1865 [80, 81]. Forlanini et al. in 1882 observed that spontaneous pneumothorax or severe effusion led tubercular lung cavities to collapse. He pumped air through a needle placed in the anterior axillary line and created a pneumothorax artificially. This technique was highly successful in the era before streptomycin was discovered and was hence quickly adopted [80]. HC Jacobeus [82] in 1910 first reported the use of a cystoscope introduced through a trocar in examining the pleural and peritoneal cavities. Over the years thoracoscopy was evolved and utilized for multiple diagnostic and therapeutic interventions such as talc pleurodesis, sympathectomy, and with discovery of antibiotics and anesthesia in 1950 thoracoscopic-guided biopsies of lung lesions.

The first VATS (Video-Assisted Thoracoscopic Surgery) lobectomy was done in 1991 in Milan by Giancarlo Roviara [81]. Several studies subsequently refined the VATS trocar placement and dissection techniques and found favorable outcomes in both short-term and long-term of the procedure [82–86]. A systematic review consisting mainly of nonrandomized studies and only one RCT comparing lobectomy for early lung cancer between VATS and thoracotomy groups revealed faster recovery and better survival in the VATS group [87]. Similarly, another meta-analysis published in 2007 found reduced pain, quicker recovery, less perioperative morbidity, less delays in adjuvant therapy, and possibly better survival in the VATS group [87, 88].

A multi-port approach is commonly used for accessing the thoracic cavity for camera and other instruments. Further refinements in technique and technology led to introduction of two-port and one-port (uniportal) configurations among others and use of the robot in thoracic surgery [89, 90]. Uniportal VATS was the next milestone in minimal invasive thoracic approach and Geatano Rocco [91] first introduced the technique for wedge resections of peripheral lung nodules in his landmark publication in 2012. The Uniportal approach was rapidly and successfully adopted enabling not only lobectomies but also complex vascular, carinal, and bronchial sleeve resections and also enabled resections in non-intubated otherwise high-risk patients [92]. VATS has evolved as a standard of care now in early lung cancer and has come a long way ever since the first series of 45 patients with VATS lobectomy/pneumonectomy and mediastinal lymph node resection/sampling was reported in 1994 [93].

Initial reports with robotic thoracic lobectomy with mediastinal lymphadenectomy in lung cancer were encouraging, showing its utility, safety, and feasibility. With the first few robotic lobectomies published in and around 2003, ample data now exists on the feasibility and oncological safety of robotic lobectomy with results comparable to VATS and superior to traditional rib-splitting open thoracotomy with added ergonomic dexterity, superior optics, and magnification and maneuverability it offers to the surgeon [89, 90, 94, 95].

2.3.5 MIS in Gastric Cancer

2.3.5.1 MIS in Early Gastric Cancer (EGC)

Kitano et al. first described the technique of Bilroth I Laparoscopic-Assisted Distal Gastrectomy (LADG) for EGC in 1994 [96] by lifting the abdominal wall. This was followed by a series of retrospective studies from the eastern countries [97, 98]. The initial skepticism for the laparoscopic surgery in gastric cancer was dismissed by Kitano et al. in 2002 [99] who published the results of the first small RCT on the subject. Patients with EGC were randomized into LADG versus standard open distal gastrectomy (ODG) groups with 14 patients in each category. The laparoscopic group showed less pain, faster recovery, better pulmonary compliance, and equivalent histological parameters, thus oncological safety of the procedure. This was followed by reports of several laparoscopic procedures from Southeast Asian countries, namely, Japan, Korea, and China.

There were three important RCTs that were published in 2005. Lee et al. [100] randomized EGC patients to ODG ($n = 28$) or LADG ($n = 28$). It was noted that laparoscopic procedure resulted in significantly lower pulmonary complications and less LOS and analgesic requirement (though not significant). Blood loss and transfusion requirements were similar in both groups. Although lymph node yield was lower, though not significant, no recurrence was reported in 14 months of follow-up in either group. Another RCT by Hayashi et al. [101] with 14 EGC patients in each LADG and ODG groups, respectively, found that the LADG group required significantly fewer duration of postoperative epidural anesthesia and had lower levels of inflammatory markers (IL-6 and CRP), similar radicality with no major additional complications. Huscher et al. [102] published results in 2005 of their RCT with a 5-year follow-up on 30 patients who underwent laparoscopic radical subtotal gastrectomy versus

29 who underwent the same via open technique. The operative morbidity, mortality, number of resected lymph nodes, and 5-year OS and DFS were not significantly different among the groups. In addition, the laparoscopic arm had lower blood loss, early resumption of oral diet, and less LOS. A RCT by Kim et al. [103] in 2008 first revealed the comparative QOL data in 82 patients with $cT_1/N_{0,1}/M_0$ EGC who underwent LADG versus 82 in ODG group with a follow-up of 3 months. Besides confirming the shot-term surgery-related benefits of earlier studies, patients in LADG group scored significantly better in most QOL outcomes parameters. Similar results of significantly improved short-term postoperative outcomes and lower serum inflammatory markers (CRP, WBC) favoring the laparoscopic group were reported in a RCT by Sakuramoto et al. [104] in 2013, wherein all surgeries (ODG or LADG) were performed by highly experienced surgeons in 63 patients with EGC.

The Korean Laparoscopic Gastrointestinal Group (KLASS-01) was one of the largest multicenter, phase III, prospective RCT conducted across 13 major Korean hospitals by 15 surgeons to assess the outcomes of Stage I EGC after LADG or ODG [105]. The short-term outcomes reported in the interim analysis in 2010 found less blood loss, LOS, and postoperative complications in LADG group. The long-term results published showed similar 5-year OS and cancer-specific survival in both the groups confirming the oncological safety and non-inferiority of LADG over ODG in Stage I EGC.

2.3.5.2 MIS in Advanced Gastric Cancer (AGC)

Initial experience with Laparoscopic Total Gastrectomy (LTG) was described in 1999 by Azagra et al. [106]. The first successful totally LTG for cancer with distal pancreatosplenectomy and D2 lymphadenectomy was reported by Uyama et al. also in 1999 in two Advanced Gastric Cancer (AGC) patients [107]. Several retrospective studies also reported feasibility and safety of laparoscopic gastrectomy for AGC. In a retrospective analysis of 336 patients with AGC (cT2–T4) requiring D2 lymphadenectomy, Shinohara et al. [108] in 2013 reported that the laparoscopic group ($n = 186$) had lower blood loss and LOS, similar morbidity and mortality but longer operative time compared to the open group ($n = 150$). The 5-year DFS and OS and recurrence pattern were also similar. A large multicenter, retrospective study by Park et al. [109] involving 10 surgeons across 10 hospitals analyzed outcomes following 239 laparoscopy-assisted gastrectomies (193 subtotal/ 41 TG/ 5 proximal) for pathologically staged AGC. The long-term survival rates were similar to those reported for open gastrectomy previously and emphasized the need for RCT on the subject. Several reports such as by Lee et al. [110] started appearing confirming feasibility (acceptable morbidity) and oncological safety (good lymph node yield 60.5) of LTG with D2 lymphadenectomy with/without concomitant pancreatectomy/ splenectomy in 94 AGC patients but concerns regarding long-term results remained. A RCT conducted by Cai et al. [111] reported their results in 2011 wherein again LADG ($n = 61$) with D2 lymphadenectomy was proven to be a safe alternative to open gastrectomy ($n = 62$). A case-control study published by a major center in the West by Strong et al. [112] in 2009 compared 30 patients with AGC who underwent laparoscopic with 30 who underwent open subtotal gastrectomy and reported significantly longer operative time but less analgesic requirement, shorter LOS, and complications (both early and late) in the laparoscopic group with comparable oncological safety (margin status, lymph node harvest, and recurrence rates). A meta-analysis of 6 RCTs and 19 high-quality, nonrandomized studies comprising of 3055 patients was published by Vinuela et al. [113] comparing laparoscopic ($n = 1658$) and open ($n = 1397$) distal gastrectomy irrespective of pathological stage. The laparoscopic group had significantly favorable short-term outcomes (minor complications, medical complications, blood loss, and less LOS) but with longer operative time although major complications and mortality were similar. Total lymph node yield in the laparoscopic group was significantly less although the percentage with <15 lymph nodes harvested was similar between the groups and hence overall nodal staging remained unaffected.

2.3.5.3 Robotic Surgery in Gastric Cancer

Hashizume et al. [114] way back in 2022 had suggested that robotic platforms could enable a more precise MIS. The benefit of robotic gastrectomy over laparoscopic gastrectomy remains unclear due to lack of mature data on the subject. A decade ago in 2013, Hyun et al. [115] in 2013 carried out a meta-analyses of 9 nonrandomized observational studies comparing robotic versus laparoscopic versus open gastrectomy involving 7200 patients. While the robotic group fared better than the open group on most short-term parameters, its advantage over the laparoscopic group was not found. In fact, it was associated with longer operating time and higher costs. A recent meta-analysis [116] that analyzed data from 48 retrospective studies published between 2012 and 2022 comprising a total of 20,151 gastric cancer patients reported significantly lower blood loss, time for first feed, LOS but higher lymph node yield and operative time for the robotic (n = 6175) versus laparoscopic group (n = 13,976) while R0 resection rate, margin status, mortality, conversion rate, and 3-year OS were similar among both the groups.

2.3.6 MIS in Liver Cancer

Laparoscopic liver surgery also picked up closely following publication of reports on laparoscopy for colon resections with first laparoscopic liver resections (LLR) reported in 1992 for benign lesions. With improvement in skills and technology (LUS/liver resection tools and energy devices) the initial fear of blood loss, CO2 embolism, and recurrence was gradually overcome. Rao et al. in 2012 published the first meta-analysis of ten observational studies and reported significantly lower blood loss, positive margin status, complications, and LOS in the laparoscopic (n = 296) versus open (n = 404) hepatic resection groups for malignant lesions [117].

Ezaz et al. [118] from the Johns Hopkins University School of Medicine, Baltimore reported data of a national database analysis from 2000 to 2011. A large number of liver and pancreatic resections (n = 62,192; 95.6%) were still being performed by the open technique versus (n = 2841; 4.4%) by MIS approach. However, a gradual rise in the use of MIS was noted across the period from 2.3 to 7.5%. Although MIS was initially used for old patients with multiple comorbidities, the overall complication rate, in-hospital mortality, and LOS were significantly lower compared to the open group.

Robotic liver resection (RLR) soon followed with the first case reported in 2006 for focal nodular hyperplasia mass in segment 2/3. The first consensus meeting for LLR was held in 2008 laying down basic guidelines for the procedure and MIS liver surgery has come a long way since then and is widely being used for complex resections for both primary hepatocellular carcinoma (HCC) and secondary liver tumors such as colorectal liver metastases (CRLM) among others without adversely affecting the oncological outcomes in experienced high-volume centers in carefully selected group of patients [119].

MIS approach to intrahepatic cholangiocarcinoma (ICC) is discussed in the biliary section below.

2.3.7 MIS in Biliary Tract Cancer

2.3.7.1 MIS in Gallbladder Cancer (GBC)

Laparoscopic cholecystectomy was the first and most quickly adopted MIS. In contrast, laparoscopic Gallbladder Cancer (GBC) resection is still not widely practiced; the key concerns are tumor implantation during laparoscopic surgery, complexity of perihilar dissection, increased risk of iatrogenic gallbladder tumor perforation, and port site metastasis [120–122].

Cho et al. [123] in 2004 published their study on 36 patients with possible stage ≤T2 GBC with no evidence of liver invasion on radiological imaging. Thirty patients finally underwent laparoscopic radical cholecystectomy (LRC).

Eighteen of these 30 patients had GBC on frozen section biopsy and underwent laparoscopic lymphadenectomy along with LRC. All 18 patients survived disease free after 27 months of median follow-up.

Feasibility and short-term safety of LRC was reported by Gumbs et al. [124] on 15 GBC patients who underwent an LRC (10 suspected, 5 completion) with an average lymph node harvest of 4, all had R0 resection with no biliary leak, 1 conversion and 2 recurrences at 3 and 20 months of follow-up with no port-site recurrence. In a retrospective study, LRC ($n = 24$) was compared to open surgery ($n = 46$) in matched GBC patients by Aggarwal et al. [125] who found similar lymph node yield (median 10), morbidity, mortality, lower blood loss, and LOS but longer operating time in LRC group. Port site metastasis was not seen in any patient.

2.3.7.2 MIS in Cholangiocarcinoma (CC)

Considerable technical skills are needed to perform resection including lymph node dissection and complex reconstructions for cholangiocarcinoma (CC) unlike in HCC and hence MIS in the field is only slowly percolating across high-volume hospitals. The feasibility and utility of laparoscopic staging in Hilar CC was long proved by Barlow et al. [126] in their series of 100 patients with 45% overall yield. Russolillo et al. [127] reported that LUS complemented diagnostic laparoscopy in picking up unresectable cancer and thus obviating an unfruitful laparotomy in radiologically deemed resectable proximal biliary cancers (GBC, ICC but not in Hilar CC).

Two cases of totally laparoscopic left hepatectomy with caudate lobe resection for ICC were reported by Abu et al. in 2011 [128] stating its feasibility in selected patients when performed by experienced surgeons. Several studies have since then shown feasibility and oncological safety of LLR for ICC in terms of similar morbidity, mortality, resection margins, lymph node yield, recurrence free and OS with the advantages of less blood loss, short LOS, and early initiation of adjuvant therapy versus open surgery [129–132]. Favorable findings have also been reported by a recent large meta-analysis of 17 studies (3975 patients) showing better short-term outcomes including significantly better R0 resection and tumor recurrence rates with similar DFS and OS for LLR versus open surgery in ICC [133].

Most of the perihilar CC require extensive complex hepatectomies with periportal lymphadenectomy and bilio-enteric reconstruction and hence are less frequently approached with MIS. The first few reports on laparoscopic left hepatectomy with regional lymph node dissection appeared around 2011–2014 [134–136] with Yu et al. [136] cautioning against laparoscopic resection of type II perihilar CC owing to increased positive margins, bile leaks, and port-site metastases. A propensity score matched analysis published in 2022 also reported significantly inferior DFS and OS between 20 laparoscopic versus 47 open resections for perihilar CC [137]. A robot-assisted approach in perihilar CC (Bismuth-Corlette type II–IV) in 10 patients although was technically feasible faired significantly inferior to 32 patients in the open surgery group in terms of major complications, operative time, DFS, and with much higher costs [138].

Laparoscopic pancreaticoduodenectomy (LPD) was first reported in 1994 by Gagner and Pomp in a patient with chronic pancreatitis who had a prolonged postoperative stay due to complications though no Post-Operative Pancreatic Fistula (POPF) occurred [139]. Cases of totally LPD for CC lower 1/3rd bile duct started appearing from across the world confirming its feasibility and safety [140, 141]. There remained a general pessimism for LPD for quite some time owing to longer operating hours, complex anastomosis, and lack of evidence regarding its benefits.

2.3.8 MIS in Pancreatic Cancer

Surgery on the pancreas has always been challenging due to its location deep in the retroperitoneum, proximity to major vasculature where arterial aberrations are common, an active unpredictive and unpleasant gland, technically demanding anastomosis, and risk of life-threatening complications most importantly POPF and postpancreatectomy hemorrhage (PPH). It's even more challenging to do major pancreatic resections and reconstructions laparoscopically. Nevertheless, continuous perseverance has now resulted in an exponential rise of minimally invasive pancreatic surgery for both benign and malignant lesions with a curative intent.

2.3.8.1 Minimal Invasive Distal Pancreatectomy (MIDP)

Distal pancreatectomy (DP) is commonly performed laparoscopically especially for benign and low-grade malignant tumors and is considered safe and feasible [142]. Kooby et al. in 2012 published a multicenter comparative retrospective review of 23 of 212 patients who underwent laparoscopic distal pancreatectomy (LDP) with open DP (ODP) for pancreatic ductal adenocarcinoma (PDAC) and reported similar short-term and long-term outcomes with a significantly shorter LOS in LDP group [143]. Similar results were published by Hilal et al. in their study that included both benign and malignant pancreatic lesions, with significantly lower overall cost for LDP ($n = 35$) compared to ODP ($n = 16$) [144].

The LEOPARD Trial was a major patient-blinded RCT by the Dutch Pancreatic Cancer Group conducted across 14 high-volume centers and included benign, premalignant, and malignant pancreatic lesions confined to the distal pancreas and compared 51 minimally invasive DP (MIDP) with 57 open DP [145]. MIDP was significantly associated with faster functional recovery, less blood loss, less incidence of grade B/C DGE, and better QOL though with comparative longer operative time [145]. Results of another phase 3, patient-blinded RCT were published recently in 2023, the DIPLOMA trial, that was conducted across 35 high volume experienced centers world over and compared outcomes after 114 MIDP (laparoscopic or robotic) versus 110 OPD in patients with resectable pancreatic cancer of the body and tail. This trial proved non-inferiority of MIPD vis-à-vis OPD in pancreatic cancer with favorable R0 resection rate ($P_{non\text{-}inferiority} = 0.039$) and similar lymph node yield, functional recovery time, complications, intraperitoneal recurrence, and OS [146].

2.3.8.2 Minimal Invasive Pancreaticoduodenectomy (MIPD)

As discussed earlier in the preceding section, Gagner et al. was the first one to report feasibility of laparoscopic pancreaticoduodenectomy (LPD) in 1994 [139]. It is considered as one of the most complex procedures due to technical difficulty in manipulation during surgery and very laborious reconstruction. Many authors have compared their experience between open and LPD with all confirming its feasibility and have reported favorable outcomes for LPD on short-term operative and oncological parameters but with significantly longer operative time [147–149] with two studies stating no clear advantage of LPD over the open PD (OPD) [141, 150].

MIPD includes pure laparoscopic, robotic, and the hybrid approach (MIS for resection and open reconstruction/laparoscopic-robotic). Buchs et al. reported one of the first series of robotic PD ($n = 44$) versus OPD ($n = 39$) with significantly shorter operative time, lower blood loss, higher lymph node yield, and with similar overall complications mortality and LOS in the robotic group [151]. Although compared to OPD, MIDP demonstrated a longer operative time but with lower morbidity, blood loss, and shorter LOS [152, 153]. Zhang et al. [154] reported one of the earliest meta-analysis of open ($n = 203$) versus robotic ($n = 137$) pancreatectomies in 2012 wherein he included seven major studies (no RCT) on PD (5)/DP (1) central pancreatectomy (1). An absolute reduction of 12% in the overall complications, reduced margin positivity, and reoperation rates was found in patients undergoing robotic pancreatectomy with no significant difference in POPF and mortality.

LEOPARD-2 [155] trial by the Dutch Pancreatic Cancer Group was patient-blinded, multicenter, phase 2/3 RCT conducted across four high-volume centers in the Netherlands by experienced surgeons who had completed a dedicated training program and had performed at least 20 LPDs before trial. After analyzing the outcomes of the initial 40 patients enrolled in phase 2 part of the trial of which there were 3 mortalities in LPD (n = 20) versus 0 in OPD group, it was decided to proceed with phase 3. Overall, 99 of 105 patients underwent surgery in combined phase 2/3 with LPD (n = 50) versus OPD (n = 49). The trial had to be prematurely aborted due to more major complications (25/50 vs. 19/49) and related mortality (5/50 vs. 1/49) in the LPD versus OPD groups though the difference was not statistically significant (P = 0.20) as was the time to functional recovery 10 versus 8 days, respectively. This assumes significance in view of the fact that the procedures were carried out by highly trained surgeons in high-volume hospitals.

MIS has also been explored with success in various other pancreatic resections including total pancreatectomy (TP), pancreatic enucleation (PEN), and central pancreatectomy (CP) [156–164].

2.3.9 MIS in Gynecologic Cancers

Gynecologic malignancies are increasingly being managed with MIS. In an interesting survey of the members of Society of Gynecologic Oncology (SGO) published by Conrad et al. [165], it was observed that use of laparoscopic surgery was nearly static at 83% versus 84% in 2004 and 91% in 2007 whereas robotic surgery increased rapidly with 97% of respondents using the platform as compared to 27% in 2007. Robotic MIS was generally preferred for cervical cancer (75%) and overall management of uterine cancer remained the most commonly performed surgery with MIS technique (70%).

2.3.9.1 MIS in Endometrial Cancer

MIS for endometrial cancer became popular ever since the first few reports were published in around early 1990s on laparoscopic-assisted staging. A systematic review published in 2013 included data from 9 RCTs (3500 patients) comparing outcomes after open (n = 1361) versus laparoscopic (n = 2255) resection in endometrial cancer irrespective of stage. The laparoscopic approach had shorter LOS and fewer postoperative complications, although with longer operating room time and higher intraoperative complications but similar 3-year recurrence rates, OS, and pelvic lymph node yield [166]. Gallal et al. [167] carried out a review of 8 RCTs with overall 3644 women with early-stage endometrial cancer and reported similar OS, DFS, less morbidity, and LOS in the laparoscopic group versus open surgery group. The same authors updated their results in 2018 [168] with 9 RCTs including 4389 women re-enforcing their earlier findings favoring laparoscopy. Walker et al. [169] conducted a prospective RCT—LAP2 in which 2616 patients with stage I-IIA uterine cancer were randomized into laparoscopic (n = 1696) or open (n = 920) groups and underwent a variety of surgical staging procedures. Overall, the laparoscopic group had better short-term outcomes with early discharge and less postoperative complications without any added adverse intraoperative events. The update published in 2012 stated that though the trial failed to prove non-inferiority of laparoscopy over open surgery but 3-year recurrence rate was 11.4% versus 10.2%, respectively, and 5-year OS 89.8% in both the groups [170].

2.3.9.2 MIS in Cervical Cancer (CxC)

The first case of successful laparoscopic-assisted radical hysterectomy with para-aortic and pelvic lymph node dissection (PLND) in stage IA_2 cervical cancer (CxC) was reported by Nezhat and colleagues [171] in 1992 wherein the surgery was completed vaginally. Despite initial resistance, laparoscopic radical hysterectomy (LRH) continued to evolve with Spirtos and colleagues [172] in 2002, published outcomes following LRH in 78 patients with stage IA_2-1B CxC with a minimum of 3-year follow-up, and concluded it to be a safe procedure with acceptable morbidity. The use of LRH for CxC remained a hot subject for debate [173].

Meanwhile, in 2005 the FDA granted approval for use of the da Vinci robotic system in Gynecology and in 2006 the first case of robotic-assisted radical hysterectomy in a 43-year-old lady was reported by Sert et al. who found that robot enhanced surgical precision of dissection [174]. In 2008, the first series of 20 successful robotic radical hysterectomies with minimal complications and 2-year follow-up was published by Fanning and colleagues [175] for Stage IB-IIA CxC. With an increasing number of hospitals getting access to the robotic system, the SGO in 2011 came up with a consensus statement [176] stating the equivalence of robotic-assisted versus laparoscopic surgery in gynecological cancers though with added costs and emphasized on structured training programs.

While most data on MIS in early stage CxC was from retrospective studies, a landmark phase III multicenter trial across 33 centers worldwide, the LACC (Laparoscopic Approach to Cervical Cancer) trial, was initiated in 2008 to gather Level I evidence [177]. Patients enrolled had CxC stage IA_{1-2}/IB_1 and were randomized into MIS ($n = 319$) versus open ($n = 312$) radical hysterectomy groups. Not only was the recurrence rate higher (poorer DFS) but OS was also inferior in the MIS group and this led to premature suspension of the trial in November 2017 with 631 patients enrolled instead of the target of 740 eligible patients. Another observational retrospective study by Melamed and colleagues [178] in 2018 across certain accredited US hospitals and SEER database on women with early stage CxC (stage 1B/IIA) who underwent MIS versus open radical hysterectomy reported shorter OS in the MIS group. It further stated a continuous decline in the 4-year survival rate of these patients following introduction of the MIS at the rate of 0.8% per year since 2006. A large number of studies were subsequently published from across the world reporting inferior oncological results with MIS [179–184]. Thus the impact of publication of the LACC study and others had a profound effect and led to a tectonic shift in the surgical management of early-stage CxC with the rates of MIS radical hysterectomy dropping by half despite the prevailing controversies [185]. It was soon followed by modifications published by the NCCN [186], FIGO [187], the European Society of Gynaecological Oncology (ESGO) [188], and SGO [189] reiterating open surgery as the "gold-standard" approach for early-stage CxC.

2.3.9.3 MIS in Ovarian Cancer

Ovarian cancer is primarily treated with upfront optimal cytoreduction, followed by adjuvant chemotherapy in a large majority of cases [190]. Comprehensive surgical staging is traditionally carried out by open surgery. With advances in the field of MIS, attempts were made to use its benefits for ovarian cancer treatment as well. The first few reports in the early 1990s successfully explored and reported feasibility of the technique in staging, completion/interval cytoreduction/second look laparoscopy in selected patients, and the approach quickly evolved from a mere diagnostic to a therapeutic tool with all short-term benefits of MIS both for early and advanced ovarian cancer [191–193]. One of the earliest case series of 36 patients with a long follow-up of 55.9 months by Nezhat et al. [194] reported the feasibility and oncological safety of laparoscopic staging in early ovarian cancer.

Attempts were next made to explore the feasibility and safety of therapeutic laparoscopy in advanced ovarian/fallopian tube/primary peritoneal cancer and one such retrospective study was published in 2010 by Nezhat et al. [195]. Successful laparoscopic primary/interval cytoreduction was feasible with lower blood loss and shorter LOS in their series of 32 patients with longer time to recurrence in laparoscopy 31.7 versus 21.5 months in laparoscopy/laparotomy groups, respectively, though not statistically significant ($P = 0.3$). Similarly, Fanning et al. [196] in 2011 reported successful optimal laparoscopic cytoreduction in 23 of 25 stage III/IV ovarian cancer with no conversions and acceptable morbidity with a median OS of 3.5 years. Liang et al. in 2017 [197] published their data on 64 patients who underwent laparoscopic cytoreduction versus 68 matched controls in the laparotomy group with advanced epithelial ovarian cancer. No significant difference was observed among the groups with respect to lymph node retrieval, complications, progression-free survival, and OS with a median follow-up of 18 months. The conversion rate was 3.1% and shot-term outcomes favored the laparoscopic group. A large recent review based on retrospective studies also supports the use of MIS interval cytoreduction in highly selected group of patients with stage III/IV ovarian cancer following neoadjuvant chemotherapy with favorable outcomes [198]. Laparoscopic secondary/tertiary debulking for recurrent ovarian, fallopian tube, or primary peritoneal cancer has also been reported by a few studies [199, 200].

Robotic-assisted surgery for patients with ovarian cancer has been explored but remains controversial. Magrina et al. [201] reported the comparative results of their retrospective case-control study on ovarian cancer patients who had undergone robotic (n = 25) versus laparoscopic (n = 27) versus laparotomy (n = 119) primary surgery. The robotic group had significantly longer operative time but less blood loss and OS was similar among the groups (67.1% vs. 75.6% vs. 66%, respectively; $P = 0.11$). Open surgery was still recommended by the authors for patients requiring debulking with two or more major additional procedures. Feasibility of robotic interval cytoreduction has also been reported in selected patients with stage II/IV ovarian cancer [202].

Tumor rupture, access and maneuverability, port-site metastasis, and quality of debulking remain significant challenges in MIS approach for surgical treatment of ovarian cancer.

2.4 Conclusions

MIS in cancer has evolved from humble diagnostic experimental peritoneoscopies in the early 1900s to complex surgeries being performed today with a curative intent and greater precision resulting in better short-term and perhaps long-term outcomes compared to traditional open surgery. As more data accumulates in terms of Level-1 evidence, MIS will further find acceptance and may become a standard of care in the surgical management of certain cancers. Already, colon cancer, early gastric cancer, esophageal cancer, and prostate cancer are now preferentially resected with MIS techniques in experienced centers. There is a definite learning curve and slightly longer operative time, which is likely to improve with experience and as new technology and tools gets added to the MIS armamentarium.

References

1. Frampton S, Kneebone RL. John Wickham's new surgery: 'minimally invasive therapy', innovation, and approaches to medical practice in twentieth-century Britain. Soc Hist Med. 2017;30(3):544–66. Available at https://doi.org/10.1093/shm/hkw074. Accessed 1 May 2022
2. Lau WY, Leow CK, Li AK. History of endoscopic and laparoscopic surgery. World J Surg. 1997;21(4):444–53.
3. Chang J, Rattner DW. History of minimally invasive surgical oncology. Surg Oncol Clin. 2019;28(1):1–9.
4. Antoniou SA, Antoniou GA, Koutras C, Antoniou AI. Endoscopy and laparoscopy: a historical aspect of medical terminology. Surg Endosc. 2012;26(12):3650–4.
5. Litynski GS. Laparoscopy—the early attempts: spotlighting Georg Kelling and Hans Christian Jacobaeus. JSLS. 1997;1(1):83–5.
6. Kemp JA, Zuckerman RS, Finlayson SR. Trends in adoption of laparoscopic cholecystectomy in rural versus urban hospitals. J Am Coll Surg. 2008;206(1):28–32.
7. Pappas TN. Laparoscopic cholecystectomy: the standard of care for chronic and acute cholecystitis. Ann Med. 1991;23(3):231.
8. DeVita VT, Bagley CM, Goodell B, Kieffe DA, Trujillo NP. Peritoneoscopy in the staging of Hodgkin's disease. Cancer Res. 1971;31(11):1746–50.
9. Cuschieri A, Hall AW, Clark JO. Value of laparoscopy in the diagnosis and management of pancreatic carcinoma. Gut. 1978;19(7):672–7.
10. Easter DW, Cuschieri A, Nathanson LK, Lavelle-Jones M. The utility of diagnostic laparoscopy for abdominal disorders: audit of 120 patients. Arch Surg. 1992;127(4):379–83.
11. Cuschieri A. Role of video-laparoscopy in the staging of intra-abdominal lymphomas and gastrointestinal cancer. Semin Surg Oncol. 2001;20(2):167–72. New York: Wiley
12. Cuschieri A. Laparoscopic management of cancer patients. J R Coll Surg Edinb. 1995;40(1):1–9.
13. Gouma DJ, De Wit LT, Van Dijkum EN, Delden OV, Bemelman WA, Rauws EA, Van Lanschot JJ, Obertop H. Laparoscopic ultrasonography for staging of gastrointestinal malignancy. Scand J Gastroenterol. 1996;31(suppl 218):43–9.
14. Liu JB, Feld RI, Barbot DJ, Rosato FE, Goldberg BB. Laparoscopic ultrasound: its role in laparoscopic surgery. Semin Laparosc Surg. 1996;3(1):50–8.
15. Bemelman WA, de Wit LT, Van Delden OM, Smits NJ, Obertop H, Rauws EJ, Gouma DJ. Diagnostic laparoscopy combined with laparoscopic ultrasonography in staging of cancer of the pancreatic head region. Br J Surg. 1995;82(6):820–4.
16. Clinical Outcomes of Surgical Therapy Study Group. A comparison of laparoscopically assisted

and open colectomy for colon cancer. N Engl J Med. 2004;350(20):2050–9.
17. Robinson CN, Chen GJ, Balentine CJ, Sansgiry S, Marshall CL, Anaya DA, Artinyan A, Albo D, Berger DH. Minimally invasive surgery is underutilized for colon cancer. Ann Surg Oncol. 2011;18(5):1412–8.
18. Wittich P, Kazemier G, Schouten WR, Jeekel J, Lange JF, Bonjer HJ. The colon cancer laparoscopic or open resection (COLOR) trial. Ned Tijdschr Geneeskd. 1997;141(39):1870–1.
19. Jayne DG, Guillou PJ, Thorpe H, Quirke P, Copeland J, Smith AM, Heath RM, Brown JM. Randomized trial of laparoscopic-assisted resection of colorectal carcinoma: 3-year results of the UK MRC CLASICC Trial Group. J Clin Oncol. 2007;25(21):3061–8.
20. Abraham NS, Byrne CM, Young JM, Solomon MJ. Meta-analysis of non-randomized comparative studies of the short-term outcomes of laparoscopic resection for colorectal cancer. ANZ J Surg. 2007;77(7):508–16.
21. Franklin ME, Rosenthal D, Abrego-Medina D, Dorman JP, Glass JL, Norem R, Diaz A. Prospective comparison of open vs. laparoscopic colon surgery for carcinoma. Dis Colon Rectum. 1996;39(10):S35–46.
22. Lacy AM, Delgado S, Castells A, Prins HA, Arroyo V, Ibarzabal A, Pique JM. The long-term results of a randomized clinical trial of laparoscopy-assisted versus open surgery for colon cancer. Ann Surg. 2008;248(1):1–7.
23. Jeong SY, Park JW, Nam BH, Kim S, Kang SB, Lim SB, Choi HS, Kim DW, Chang HJ, Kim DY, Jung KH. Open versus laparoscopic surgery for mid-rectal or low-rectal cancer after neoadjuvant chemoradiotherapy (COREAN trial): survival outcomes of an open-label, non-inferiority, randomised controlled trial. Lancet Oncol. 2014;15(7):767–74.
24. Van der Pas MH, Haglind E, Cuesta MA, Fürst A, Lacy AM, Hop WC, Bonjer HJ, COlorectal cancer Laparoscopic or Open Resection II (COLOR II) Study Group. Laparoscopic versus open surgery for rectal cancer (COLOR II): short-term outcomes of a randomised, phase 3 trial. Lancet Oncol. 2013;14(3):210–8.
25. Cooper CR, Feingold DL. Laparoscopic colectomy for colonic malignancy: review of literature. Ann Laparosc Endosc Surg. 2019;4:3. Available at https://doi.org/10.21037/ales.2018.12.12. Accessed 1 May 2022
26. Arezzo A, Passera R, Scozzari G, Verra M, Morino M. Laparoscopy for extraperitoneal rectal cancer reduces short-term morbidity: Results of a systematic review and meta-analysis. UEG J. 2013;1(1):32–47.
27. Stevenson AR, Solomon MJ, Lumley JW, Hewett P, Clouston AD, Gebski VJ, Davies L, Wilson K, Hague W, Simes J, ALaCaRT Investigators. Effect of laparoscopic-assisted resection vs open resection on pathological outcomes in rectal cancer: the ALaCaRT randomized clinical trial. JAMA. 2015;314(13):1356–63.
28. Fleshman J, Branda M, Sargent DJ, Boller AM, George V, Abbas M, Peters WR, Maun D, Chang G, Herline A, Fichera A. Effect of laparoscopic-assisted resection vs open resection of stage II or III rectal cancer on pathologic outcomes: the ACOSOG Z6051 randomized clinical trial. JAMA. 2015;314(13):1346–55.
29. Creavin B, Kelly ME, Ryan E, Winter DC. Meta-analysis of the impact of surgical approach on the grade of mesorectal excision in rectal cancer. J Br Surg. 2017;104(12):1609–19.
30. Milone M, Manigrasso M, Burati M, Velotti N, Milone F, De Palma GD. Surgical resection for rectal cancer. Is laparoscopic surgery as successful as open approach? A systematic review with meta-analysis. PLoS One. 2018;13(10):e0204887. Available at https://doi.org/10.1371/journal.pone.0204887. Accessed 1 May 2022
31. Sara S, Poncet G, Voirin D, Laverriere MH, Anglade D, Faucheron JL. Can adequate lymphadenectomy be obtained by laparoscopic resection in rectal cancer? Results of a case–control study in 200 patients. J Gastrointest Surg. 2010;14(8):1244–7.
32. Boutros M, Hippalgaonkar N, Silva E, Allende D, Wexner SD, Berho M. Laparoscopic resection of rectal cancer results in higher lymph node yield and better short-term outcomes than open surgery: a large single-center comparative study. Dis Colon Rectum. 2013;56(6):679–88.
33. Penninckx F, Kartheuser A, Van De Stadt J, Pattyn P, Mansvelt B, Bertrand C, Van Eycken E, Jegou D, Fieuws S. Outcome following laparoscopic and open total mesorectal excision for rectal cancer. J Br Surg. 2013;100(10):1368–75.
34. Feliciotti F, Guerrieri MA, Paganini AM, De Sanctis A, Campagnacci R, Perretta S, D'Ambrosio G, Lezoche E. Long-term results of laparoscopic versus open resections for rectal cancer for 124 unselected patients. Surg Endosc Other Interv Tech. 2003;17(10):1530–5.
35. Bärlehner E, Benhidjeb T, Anders S, Schicke B. Laparoscopic resection for rectal cancer: outcomes in 194 patients and review of the literature. Surg Endosc Other Interv Tech. 2005;19(6):757–66.
36. Gao F, Cao YF, Chen LS. Meta-analysis of short-term outcomes after laparoscopic resection for rectal cancer. Int J Color Dis. 2006;21(7):652–6.
37. Aziz O, Constantinides V, Tekkis PP, Athanasiou T, Purkayastha S, Paraskeva P, Darzi AW, Heriot AG. Laparoscopic versus open surgery for rectal cancer: a meta-analysis. Ann Surg Oncol. 2006;13(3):413–24.
38. Pigazzi A, Ellenhorn JD, Ballantyne GH, Paz IB. Robotic-assisted laparoscopic low anterior resection with total mesorectal excision for rectal cancer. Surg Endosc. 2006;20:1521–5.
39. Baik SH, Kang CM, Lee WJ, Kim NK, Sohn SK, Chi HS, et al. Robotic total mesorectal excision for the treatment of rectal cancer. J Robot Surg. 2007;1:99–102.

40. Baik SH, Ko YT, Kang CM, Lee WJ, Kim NK, Sohn SK, et al. Robotic tumor-specific mesorectal excision of rectal cancer: short-term outcome of a pilot randomized trial. Surg Endosc. 2008;22:1601–8.
41. Jayne D, Pigazzi A, Marshall H, Croft J, Corrigan N, Copeland J, Quirke P, West N, Rautio T, Thomassen N, Tilney H. Effect of robotic-assisted vs conventional laparoscopic surgery on risk of conversion to open laparotomy among patients undergoing resection for rectal cancer: the ROLARR randomized clinical trial. JAMA. 2017;318(16):1569–80.
42. Atallah S, Albert M, Larach S. Transanal minimally invasive surgery: a giant leap forward. Surg Endosc. 2010;24(9):2200–5.
43. Atallah S, Martin-Perez B, Albert M, deBeche-Adams T, Nassif G, Hunter L, Larach S. Transanal minimally invasive surgery for total mesorectal excision (TAMIS–TME): results and experience with the first 20 patients undergoing curative-intent rectal cancer surgery at a single institution. Tech Coloproctol. 2014;18(5):473–80.
44. Luketich JD, Pennathur A, Awais O, Levy RM, Keeley S, Shende M, Christie NA, Weksler B, Landreneau RJ, Abbas G, Schuchert MJ. Outcomes after minimally invasive esophagectomy: review of over 1000 patients. Ann Surg. 2012;256(1):95.
45. DePaula AL, Hashiba K, Ferreira EA, de Paula RA, Grecco E. Laparoscopic transhiatal esophagectomy with esophagogastroplasty. Surg Laparosc Endosc. 1995;5(1):1–5.
46. Swanstrom LL, Hansen P. Laparoscopic total esophagectomy. Arch Surg. 1997;132(9):943–9.
47. Luketich JD, Nguyen NT, Weigel T, Ferson P, Keenan R, Schauer P. Minimally invasive approach to esophagectomy. JSLS. 1998;2(3):243.
48. Luketich JD, Pennathur A, Awais O, et al. Outcomes after minimally invasive esophagectomy. Ann Surg. 2012;256:95–103.
49. Biere SS, Cuesta MA, Van Der Peet DL. Minimally invasive versus open esophagectomy for cancer: a systematic review and meta-analysis. Minerva Chir. 2009;64(2):121–33.
50. Berger AC, Bloomenthal A, Weksler B, Evans N, Chojnacki KA, Yeo CJ, Rosato EL. Oncologic efficacy is not compromised, and may be improved with minimally invasive esophagectomy. J Am Coll Surg. 2011;212(4):560–6.
51. Parameswaran R, Veeramootoo D, Krishnadas R, Cooper M, Berrisford R, Wajed S. Comparative experience of open and minimally invasive esophagogastric resection. World J Surg. 2009;33(9):1868–75.
52. Smithers BM, Gotley DC, Martin I, Thomas JM. Comparison of the outcomes between open and minimally invasive esophagectomy. Ann Surg. 2007;245(2):232.
53. Zingg U, McQuinn A, DiValentino D, Esterman AJ, Bessell JR, Thompson SK, Jamieson GG, Watson DI. Minimally invasive versus open esophagectomy for patients with esophageal cancer. Ann Thorac Surg. 2009;87(3):911–9.
54. Sihag S, Kosinski AS, Gaissert HA, Wright CD, Schipper PH. Minimally invasive versus open esophagectomy for esophageal cancer: a comparison of early surgical outcomes from the Society of Thoracic Surgeons National Database. Ann Thorac Surg. 2016;101(4):1281–9.
55. Tapias LF, Mathisen DJ, Wright CD, Wain JC, Gaissert HA, Muniappan A, Lanuti M, Donahue DM, Morse CR. Outcomes with open and minimally invasive Ivor Lewis esophagectomy after neoadjuvant therapy. Ann Thorac Surg. 2016;101(3):1097–103.
56. Nagpal K, Ahmed K, Vats A, Yakoub D, James D, Ashrafian H, Darzi A, Moorthy K, Athanasiou T. Is minimally invasive surgery beneficial in the management of esophageal cancer? A meta-analysis. Surg Endosc. 2010;24(7):1621–9.
57. Sgourakis G, Gockel I, Radtke A, Musholt TJ, Timm S, Rink A, Tsiamis A, Karaliotas C, Lang H. Minimally invasive versus open esophagectomy: meta-analysis of outcomes. Dig Dis Sci. 2010;55(11):3031–40.
58. Sihag S, Wright CD, Wain JC, Gaissert HA, Lanuti M, Allan JS, Mathisen DJ, Morse CR. Comparison of perioperative outcomes following open versus minimally invasive Ivor Lewis oesophagectomy at a single, high-volume centre. Eur J Cardiothorac Surg. 2012;42(3):430–7.
59. Cerfolio RJ, Bryant AS, Hawn MT. Technical aspects and early results of robotic esophagectomy with chest anastomosis. J Thorac Cardiovasc Surg. 2013;145(1):90–6.
60. de la Fuente SG, Weber J, Hoffe SE, Shridhar R, Karl R, Meredith KL. Initial experience from a large referral center with robotic-assisted Ivor Lewis esophagogastrectomy for oncologic purposes. Surg Endosc. 2013;27(9):3339–47.
61. Weksler B, Sharma P, Moudgill N, Chojnacki KA, Rosato EL. Robot-assisted minimally invasive esophagectomy is equivalent to thoracoscopic minimally invasive esophagectomy. Dis Esophagus. 2012;25(5):403–9.
62. Byrd JK, Ferris RL. Is there a role for robotic surgery in the treatment of head and neck cancer? Curr Treat Options Oncol. 2016;17(6):1–2.
63. Weinstein GS, O'Malley BW Jr, Magnuson JS, Carroll WR, Olsen KD, Daio L, Moore EJ, Holsinger FC. Transoral robotic surgery: a multicenter study to assess feasibility, safety, and surgical margins. Laryngoscope. 2012;122(8):1701–7.
64. De Almeida JR, Li R, Magnuson JS, Smith RV, Moore E, Lawson G, Remacle M, Ganly I, Kraus DH, Teng MS, Miles BA. Oncologic outcomes after transoral robotic surgery: a multi-institutional study. JAMA Otolaryngol Head Neck Surg. 2015;141(12):1043–51.
65. Rich JT, Milov S, Lewis JS Jr, Thorstad WL, Adkins DR, Haughey BH. Transoral laser microsurgery (TLM) ± adjuvant therapy for advanced stage oro-

pharyngeal cancer: outcomes and prognostic factors. Laryngoscope. 2009;119(9):1709–19.
66. Haughey BH, Hinni ML, Salassa JR, Hayden RE, Grant DG, Rich JT, Milov S, Lewis JS Jr, Krishna M. Transoral laser microsurgery as primary treatment for advanced-stage oropharyngeal cancer: a United States multicenter study. Head Neck. 2011;33(12):1683–94.
67. Gagner M. Endoscopic subtotal parathyroidectomy in patients with primary hyperparathyroidism. J Br Surg. 1996;83(6):875.
68. Gagner M, Inabnet Iii WB. Endoscopic thyroidectomy for solitary thyroid nodules. Thyroid. 2001;11(2):161–3.
69. Ikeda Y, Takami H, Sasaki Y, Niimi M. Endoscopic neck surgery by the axillary approach. J Am Coll Surg. 2000;191:336–40.
70. Miccoli P, Berti P, Conte M, Bendinelli C, Marcocci C. Minimally invasive surgery for thyroid small nodules: preliminary report. J Endocrinol Invest. 1999;22(11):849–51.
71. Miccoli P, Biricotti M, Matteucci V, Ambrosini CE, Wu J, Materazzi G. Minimally invasive video-assisted thyroidectomy: reflections after more than 2400 cases performed. Surg Endosc. 2016;30(6):2489–95.
72. Del Rio P, Maestroni U, Sianesi M, Viani L, Vicente D, Stojadinovic A, Avital I. Minimally invasive video-assisted thyroidectomy for papillary thyroid cancer: a prospective 5-year follow-up study. Tumori J. 2015;101(2):144–7.
73. Del Rio P, Viani L, Montana CM, Cozzani F, Sianesi M. Minimally invasive thyroidectomy: a ten years experience. Gland Surg. 2016;5(3):295.
74. Lombardi CP, Raffaelli M, De Crea C, Sessa L, Rampulla V, Bellantone R. Video-assisted versus conventional total thyroidectomy and central compartment neck dissection for papillary thyroid carcinoma. World J Surg. 2012;36(6):1225–30.
75. Wilhelm T, Metzig A. Video. Endoscopic minimally invasive thyroidectomy: first clinical experience. Surg Endosc. 2010;24:1757–8. https://doi.org/10.1007/s00464-009-0820-9.
76. Nakajo A, Arima H, Hirata M, Mizoguchi T, Kijima Y, Mori S, et al. Trans-oral video-assisted neck surgery (TOVANS). a new transoral technique of endoscopic thyroidectomy with gasless premandible approach. Surg Endosc. 2013;27:1105–10. https://doi.org/10.1007/s00464-012-2588-6.
77. Wang C, Zhai H, Liu W, Li J, Yang J, Hu Y, et al. Thyroidectomy: a novel endoscopic oral vestibular approach. Surgery. 2014;155:33–8. https://doi.org/10.1016/j.surg.2013.06.010.
78. Sun H, Wang X, Zheng G, Wu G, Zeng Q, Zheng H. Comparison between transoral endoscopic thyroidectomy vestibular approach (TOETVA) and conventional open thyroidectomy for patients undergoing total thyroidectomy and central neck dissection: a propensity score-matching analysis. Front Oncol. 2022;12:856021. https://doi.org/10.3389/fonc.2022.856021.
79. Pan JH, Zhou H, Zhao XX, Ding H, Wei L, Qin L, Pan YL. Robotic thyroidectomy versus conventional open thyroidectomy for thyroid cancer: a systematic review and meta-analysis. Surg Endosc. 2017;31(10):3985–4001.
80. Braimbridge MV. The history of thoracoscopic surgery. Ann Thorac Surg. 1993;56(3):610–4.
81. Hytych V, Horazdovsky P, Pohnan R, Pracharova S, Taskova A, Konopa Z, Cernovska M, Demes R, Cermak J, Vasakova M, Benej R. VATS lobectomy, history, indication, contraindication and general techniques. Bratislavske Lekarske Listy. 2015;116(7):400–3.
82. Jacobaeus HV. On the possibility of using cystoscopy when examining serous cavities. (German) Munch Med Wschr. 1910;40:2090–2.
83. Landreneau RJ, Dowling RD, Castillo WM, Ferson PF. Thoracoscopic resection of an anterior mediastinal tumor. Ann Thorac Surg. 1992;54(1):142–4.
84. Landreneau RJ, Mack MJ, Hazelrigg SR, Dowling RD, Acuff TE, Magee MJ, Ferson PF. Video-assisted thoracic surgery: basic technical concepts and intercostal approach strategies. Ann Thorac Surg. 1992;54(4):800–7.
85. Park HS, Detterbeck FC, Boffa DJ, Kim AW. Impact of hospital volume of thoracoscopic lobectomy on primary lung cancer outcomes. Ann Thorac Surg. 2012;93(2):372–9.
86. Gopaldas RR, Bakaeen FG, Dao TK, Walsh GL, Swisher SG, Chu D. Video-assisted thoracoscopic versus open thoracotomy lobectomy in a cohort of 13,619 patients. Ann Thorac Surg. 2010;89(5):1563–70.
87. Whitson BA, Groth SS, Duval SJ, Swanson SJ, Maddaus MA. Surgery for early-stage non-small cell lung cancer: a systematic review of the video-assisted thoracoscopic surgery versus thoracotomy approaches to lobectomy. Ann Thorac Surg. 2008;86(6):2008–18.
88. Cheng D, Downey RJ, Kernstine K, Stanbridge R, Shennib H, Wolf R, Ohtsuka T, Schmid R, Waller D, Fernando H, Yim A. Video-assisted thoracic surgery in lung cancer resection: a meta-analysis and systematic review of controlled trials. Innovations. 2007;2(6):261–92.
89. Veronesi G, Galetta D, Maisonneuve P, Melfi F, Schmid RA, Borri A, Vannucci F, Spaggiari L. Four-arm robotic lobectomy for the treatment of early-stage lung cancer. J Thorac Cardiovasc Surg. 2010;140(1):19–25.
90. Ashton RC Jr, Connery CP, Swistel DG, et al. Robot-assisted lobectomy. J Thorac Cardiovasc Surg. 2003;126:292–3. https://doi.org/10.1016/S0022-5223(03)00201-0.
91. Rocco G. One-port (uniportal) video-assisted thoracic surgical resections—a clear advance. J Thorac Cardiovasc Surg. 2012;144(3):S27–31. Available

at https://doi.org/10.1016/j.jtcvs.2012.06.006 Accessed 1 May 2022
92. Gonzalez-Rivas D. Uniportal thoracoscopic surgery: from medical thoracoscopy to non-intubated uniportal video-assisted major pulmonary resections. Ann Cardiothorac Surg. 2016;5(2):85–91.
93. McKenna RJ Jr. Lobectomy by video-assisted thoracic surgery with mediastinal node sampling for lung cancer. J Thorac Cardiovasc Surg. 1994;107(3):879–82.
94. Giulianotti PC, Buchs NC, Caravaglios G, Bianco FM. Robot-assisted lung resection: outcomes and technical details. Interact Cardiovasc Thorac Surg. 2010;11(4):388–92.
95. Linsky P, Wei B. Robotic lobectomy. J Vis Surg. 2017;3:132. https://doi.org/10.21037/jovs.2017.08.12.
96. Kitano S, Iso Y, Moriyama M, Sugimachi K. Laparoscopy-assisted Billroth I gastrectomy. Surg Laparosc Endosc Percutan Tech. 1994;4(2):146–8.
97. Shimizu S, Uchiyama A, Mizumoto K, Morisaki T, Nakamura K, Shimura H, Tanaka M. Laparoscopically assisted distal gastrectomy for early gastric cancer. Surg Endosc. 2000;14(1):27–31.
98. Tanimura S, Higashino M, Fukunaga Y, Osugi H. Hand-assisted laparoscopic distal gastrectomy with regional lymph node dissection for gastric cancer. Surg Laparosc Endosc Percutan Tech. 2001;11(3):155–60.
99. Kitano S, Shiraishi N, Fujii K, Yasuda K, Inomata M, Adachi Y. A randomized controlled trial comparing open vs laparoscopy-assisted distal gastrectomy for the treatment of early gastric cancer: an interim report. Surgery. 2002;131(1 Suppl):S306–11.
100. Lee JH, Han HS. A prospective randomized study comparing open vs laparoscopy-assisted distal gastrectomy in early gastric cancer: early results. Surg Endosc Other Interv Tech. 2005;19(2):168–73.
101. Hayashi H, Ochiai T, Shimada H, Gunji Y. Prospective randomized study of open versus laparoscopy-assisted distal gastrectomy with extraperigastric lymph node dissection for early gastric cancer. Surg Endosc Other Interv Tech. 2005;19(9):1172–6.
102. Huscher CG, Mingoli A, Sgarzini G, Sansonetti A, Di Paola M, Recher A, Ponzano C. Laparoscopic versus open subtotal gastrectomy for distal gastric cancer: five-year results of a randomized prospective trial. Ann Surg. 2005;241(2):232.
103. Kim YW, Baik YH, Yun YH, Nam BH, Kim DH, Choi IJ, Bae JM. Improved quality of life outcomes after laparoscopy-assisted distal gastrectomy for early gastric cancer: results of a prospective randomized clinical trial. Ann Surg. 2008;248(5):721–7.
104. Sakuramoto S, Yamashita K, Kikuchi S, Futawatari N, Katada N, Watanabe M, Okutomi T, Wang G, Bax L. Laparoscopy versus open distal gastrectomy by expert surgeons for early gastric cancer in Japanese patients: short-term clinical outcomes of a randomized clinical trial. Surg Endosc. 2013;27(5):1695–705.
105. Kim HH, Han SU, Kim MC, Kim W, Lee HJ, Ryu SW, Cho GS, Kim CY, Yang HK, Park DJ, Song KY, Lee SI, Ryu SY, Lee JH, Hyung WJ, Korean Laparoendoscopic Gastrointestinal Surgery Study (KLASS) Group. Effect of laparoscopic distal gastrectomy vs open distal gastrectomy on long-term survival among patients with stage I gastric cancer: the KLASS-01 Randomized Clinical Trial. JAMA Oncol. 2019;5(4):506–13. https://doi.org/10.1001/jamaoncol.2018.6727.
106. Azagra JS, Goergen M, De Simone P, Ibanez-Aguirre J. Minimally invasive surgery for gastric cancer. Surg Endosc. 1999;13(4):351–7.
107. Uyama I, Sugioka A, Fujita J, Komori Y, Matsui H, Hasumi A. Laparoscopic total gastrectomy with distal pancreatosplenectomy and D2 lymphadenectomy for advanced gastric cancer. Gastric Cancer. 1999;2(4):230–4.
108. Shinohara T, Satoh S, Kanaya S, Ishida Y, Taniguchi K, Isogaki J, Inaba K, Yanaga K, Uyama I. Laparoscopic versus open D2 gastrectomy for advanced gastric cancer: a retrospective cohort study. Surg Endosc. 2013;27(1):286–94.
109. Park DJ, Han SU, Hyung WJ, Kim MC, Kim W, Ryu SY, Ryu SW, Song KY, Lee HJ, Cho GS, Kim HH. Long-term outcomes after laparoscopy-assisted gastrectomy for advanced gastric cancer: a large-scale multicenter retrospective study. Surg Endosc. 2012;26(6):1548–53.
110. Lee JH, Ahn SH, Park DJ, Kim HH, Lee HJ, Yang HK. Laparoscopic total gastrectomy with D2 lymphadenectomy for advanced gastric cancer. World J Surg. 2012;36(10):2394–9.
111. Cai J, Wei D, Gao CF, Zhang CS, Zhang H, Zhao T. A prospective randomized study comparing open versus laparoscopy-assisted D2 radical gastrectomy in advanced gastric cancer. Dig Surg. 2011;28(5–6):331–7.
112. Strong VE, Devaud N, Allen PJ, Gonen M, Brennan MF, Coit D. Laparoscopic versus open subtotal gastrectomy for adenocarcinoma: a case–control study. Ann Surg Oncol. 2009;16(6):1507–13.
113. Viñuela EF, Gonen M, Brennan MF, Coit DG, Strong VE. Laparoscopic versus open distal gastrectomy for gastric cancer: a meta-analysis of randomized controlled trials and high-quality nonrandomized studies. Ann Surg. 2012;255(3):446–56.
114. Hashizume M, Konishi K, Tsutsumi N, Yamaguchi S, Shimabukuro R. A new era of robotic surgery assisted by a computer-enhanced surgical system. Surgery. 2002;131(1):S330–3. Available at https://doi.org/10.1067/msy.2002.120119. Accessed 1 May 2022
115. Hyun MH, Lee CH, Kim HJ, Tong Y, Park SS. Systematic review and meta-analysis of robotic surgery compared with conventional laparoscopic and open resections for gastric carcinoma. J Br Surg. 2013;100(12):1566–78.

116. Baral S, Arawker MH, Sun Q, Jiang M, Wang L, Wang Y, Ali M, Wang D. Robotic versus laparoscopic gastrectomy for gastric cancer: a mega meta-analysis. Front Surg. 2022;9:895976.
117. Rao A, Rao G, Ahmed I. Laparoscopic vs. open liver resection for malignant liver disease. A systematic review. Surgeon. 2012;10:194–201.
118. Ejaz A, Sachs T, He J, Spolverato G, Hirose K, Ahuja N, Wolfgang CL, Makary MA, Weiss M, Pawlik TM. A comparison of open and minimally invasive surgery for hepatic and pancreatic resections using the Nationwide Inpatient Sample. Surgery. 2014;156(3):538–47.
119. Lo WM, Tohme ST, Geller DA. Recent advances in minimally invasive liver resection for colorectal cancer liver metastases—a review. Cancers (Basel). 2022;15(1):142. https://doi.org/10.3390/cancers15010142.
120. Z'graggen K, Birrer S, Maurer CA, Wehrli H, Klaiber C, Baer HU. Incidence of port site recurrence after laparoscopic cholecystectomy for preoperatively unsuspected gallbladder carcinoma. Surgery. 1998;124(5):831–8.
121. Gumbs AA, Milone L, Geha R, Delacroix J, Chabot JA. Laparoscopic radical cholecystectomy. Laparoendosc Adv Surg Tech A. 2009;19(4):519–20.
122. Agarwal AK, Kalayarasan R, Javed A, Gupta N, Nag HH. The role of staging laparoscopy in primary gall bladder cancer—an analysis of 409 patients: a prospective study to evaluate the role of staging laparoscopy in the management of gallbladder cancer. Ann Surg. 2013;258(2):318–23.
123. Cho JY, Han HS, Yoon YS, Ahn KS, Kim YH, Lee KH. Laparoscopic approach for suspected early-stage gallbladder carcinoma. Arch Surg. 2010;145(2):128–33.
124. Gumbs AA, Jarufe N, Gayet B. Minimally invasive approaches to extrapancreatic cholangiocarcinoma. Surg Endosc. 2013;27(2):406–14.
125. Agarwal AK, Javed A, Kalayarasan R, Sakhuja P. Minimally invasive versus the conventional open surgical approach of a radical cholecystectomy for gallbladder cancer: a retrospective comparative study. HPB. 2015;17(6):536–41.
126. Barlow AD, Garcea G, Berry DP, Rajesh A, Patel R, Metcalfe MS, Dennison AR. Staging laparoscopy for hilar cholangiocarcinoma in 100 patients. Langenbecks Arch Surg. 2013;398(7):983–8.
127. Russolillo N, D'Eletto M, Langella S, Perotti S, Lo Tesoriere R, Forchino F, Ferrero A. Role of laparoscopic ultrasound during diagnostic laparoscopy for proximal biliary cancers: a single series of 100 patients. Surg Endosc. 2016;30(3):1212–8.
128. Abu Hilal M, Badran A, Di Fabio F, Pearce NW. Pure laparoscopic en bloc left hemihepatectomy and caudate lobe resection in patients with intrahepatic cholangiocarcinoma. J Laparoendosc Adv Surg Tech. 2011;21(9):845–9.
129. Lee W, Park JH, Kim JY, Kwag SJ, Park T, Jeong SH, Ju YT, Jung EJ, Lee YJ, Hong SC, Choi SK. Comparison of perioperative and oncologic outcomes between open and laparoscopic liver resection for intrahepatic cholangiocarcinoma. Surg Endosc. 2016;30(11):4835–40.
130. Uy BJ, Han HS, Yoon YS, Cho JY. Laparoscopic liver resection for intrahepatic cholangiocarcinoma. J Laparoendosc Adv Surg Tech A. 2015;25(4):272–7.
131. Ratti F, Cipriani F, Ariotti R, Gagliano A, Paganelli M, Catena M, Aldrighetti L. Safety and feasibility of laparoscopic liver resection with associated lymphadenectomy for intrahepatic cholangiocarcinoma: a propensity score-based case-matched analysis from a single institution. Surg Endosc. 2016;30(5):1999–2010.
132. Takahashi M, Wakabayashi G, Nitta H, Takeda D, Hasegawa Y, Takahara T, Ito N. Pure laparoscopic right hepatectomy by anterior approach with hanging maneuver for large intrahepatic cholangiocarcinoma. Surg Endosc. 2013;27(12):4732–3.
133. Zhao X, Gao FW, Jiang KY, Yang J, Xie QY, Gong J, Yang MY, Mao TY, Lei ZH. Laparoscopic or open liver resection for intrahepatic cholangiocarcinoma: A meta-analysis and systematic review. Front Oncol. 2023;13:1096714.
134. Machado MA, Makdissi FF, Surjan RC, Mochizuki M. Laparoscopic resection of hilar cholangiocarcinoma. J Laparoendosc Adv Surg Tech. 2012;22(10):954–6.
135. Cho A, Yamamoto H, Kainuma O, Muto Y, Yanagibashi H, Tonooka T, Masuda T. Laparoscopy in the management of hilar cholangiocarcinoma. World J Gastroenterol. 2014;20(41):15153.
136. Yu H, Wu SD, Chen DX, Zhu G. Laparoscopic resection of Bismuth type I and II hilar cholangiocarcinoma: an audit of 14 cases from two institutions. Dig Surg. 2011;28(1):44–9.
137. Ma D, Wang W, Wang J, Zhang T, Jiang Z, Du G, Yang J, Zhang X, Qin G, Jin B. Laparoscopic versus open surgery for hilar cholangiocarcinoma: a retrospective cohort study on short-term and long-term outcomes. Surg Endosc. 2022;36(6):3721–31. https://doi.org/10.1007/s00464-021-08686-6.
138. Xu Y, Wang H, Ji W, Tang M, Li H, Leng J, Meng X, Dong J. Robotic radical resection for hilar cholangiocarcinoma: perioperative and long-term outcomes of an initial series. Surg Endosc. 2016;30(7):3060–70.
139. Gagner M, Pomp A. Laparoscopic pylorus-preserving pancreatoduodenectomy. Surg Endosc. 1994;8(5):408–10.
140. Menon KV, Hayden JD, Prasad KR, Verbeke CS. Total laparoscopic pancreaticoduodenectomy and reconstruction for a cholangiocarcinoma of the bile duct. J Laparoendosc Adv Surg Tech. 2007;17(6):775–80.
141. Kendrick ML, Cusati D. Total laparoscopic pancreaticoduodenectomy: feasibility and outcome in an early experience. Arch Surg. 2010;145(1):19–23.
142. DiNorcia J, Schrope BA, Lee MK, Reavey PL, Rosen SJ, Lee JA, Chabot JA, Allendorf JD. Laparoscopic distal pancreatectomy offers shorter hospital stays

with fewer complications. J Gastrointest Surg. 2010;14:1804–12.
143. Kooby DA, Hawkins WG, Schmidt CM, Weber SM, Bentrem DJ, Gillespie TW, Sellers JB, Merchant NB, Scoggins CR, Martin RC III, Kim HJ. A multicenter analysis of distal pancreatectomy for adenocarcinoma: is laparoscopic resection appropriate? J Am Coll Surg. 2010;210(5):779–85.
144. Abu Hilal M, Hamdan M, Di Fabio F, Pearce NW, Johnson CD. Laparoscopic versus open distal pancreatectomy: a clinical and cost-effectiveness study. Surg Endosc. 2012;26:1670–4.
145. De Rooij T, van Hilst J, van Santvoort H, Boerma D, van den Boezem P, Daams F, van Dam R, Dejong C, van Duyn E, Dijkgraaf M, van Eijck C, Festen S, Gerhards M, Groot Koerkamp B, de Hingh I, Kazemier G, Klaase J, de Kleine R, van Laarhoven C, Luyer M, Patijn G, Steenvoorde P, Suker M, Abu Hilal M, Busch O, Besselink M, Dutch Pancreatic Cancer Group. Minimally invasive versus open distal pancreatectomy (LEOPARD): a multicenter patient-blinded randomized controlled trial. Ann Surg. 2019;269(1):2–9.
146. Korrel M, Jones LR, van Hilst J, Balzano G, Björnsson B, Boggi U, Bratlie SO, Busch OR, Butturini G, Capretti G, Casadei R. Minimally invasive versus open distal pancreatectomy for resectable pancreatic cancer (DIPLOMA): an international randomised non-inferiority trial. Lancet Reg Health Eur. 2023;31:100673.
147. Asbun HJ, Stauffer JA. Laparoscopic vs open pancreaticoduodenectomy: overall outcomes and severity of complications using the Accordion Severity Grading System. J Am Coll Surg. 2012;215:810–9.
148. Kuroki T, Adachi T, Okamoto T, Kanematsu T. A non-randomized comparative study of laparoscopy-assisted pancreaticoduodenectomy and open pancreaticoduodenectomy. Hepato-Gastroenterology. 2012;59:570–3.
149. Zureikat AH, Breaux JA, Steel JL, Hughes SJ. Can laparoscopic pancreaticoduodenectomy be safely implemented? J Gastrointest Surg. 2011;15:1151–7.
150. Cho A, Yamamoto H, Nagata M, Takiguchi N, Shimada H, Kainuma O, Souda H, Gunji H, Miyazaki A, Ikeda A, Tohma T. Comparison of laparoscopy-assisted and open pylorus-preserving pancreaticoduodenectomy for periampullary disease. Am J Surg. 2009;198(3):445–9.
151. Buchs NC, Addeo P, Bianco FM, Ayloo S, Benedetti E, Giulianotti PC. Robotic versus open pancreaticoduodenectomy: a comparative study at a single institution. World J Surg. 2011;35:2739–46.
152. Chalikonda S, Aguilar-Saavedra JR, Walsh RM. Laparoscopic robotic-assisted pancreaticoduodenectomy: a case-matched comparison with open resection. Surg Endosc. 2012;26:2397–402.
153. Zhou NX, Chen JZ, Liu Q, Zhang X, Wang Z, Ren S, Chen XF. Outcomes of pancreatoduodenectomy with robotic surgery versus open surgery. Int J Med Robot Comput Assist Surg. 2011;7(2):131–7.
154. Zhang J, Wu WM, You L, Zhao YP. Robotic versus open pancreatectomy: a systematic review and meta-analysis. Ann Surg Oncol. 2013;20:1774–80.
155. Van Hilst J, de Rooij T, Bosscha K, Brinkman DJ, van Dieren S, Dijkgraaf MG, Gerhards MF, de Hingh IH, Karsten TM, Lips DJ, Luyer MD. Laparoscopic versus open pancreatoduodenectomy for pancreatic or periampullary tumours (LEOPARD-2): a multicentre, patient-blinded, randomised controlled phase 2/3 trial. Lancet Gastroenterol Hepatol. 2019;4(3):199–207.
156. Dallemagne B, de Oliveira AT, Lacerda CF, D'Agostino J, Mercoli H, Marescaux J. Full laparoscopic total pancreatectomy with and without spleen and pylorus preservation: a feasibility report. J Hepatobiliary Pancreat Sci. 2013;20:647–53.
157. Boggi U, Palladino S, Massimetti G, Vistoli F, Caniglia F, De Lio N, Perrone V, Barbarello L, Belluomini M, Signori S, Amorese G. Laparoscopic robot-assisted versus open total pancreatectomy: a case-matched study. Surg Endosc. 2015;29:1425–32.
158. Kuroki T, Eguchi S. Laparoscopic parenchyma-sparing pancreatectomy. J Hepatobiliary Pancreat Sci. 2014;21(5):323–7.
159. Dalla Valle R, Cremaschi E, Lamecchi L, Guerini F, Rosso E, Iaria M. Open and minimally invasive pancreatic neoplasms enucleation: a systematic review. Surg Endosc. 2019;33(10):3192–9.
160. Crippa S, Bassi C, Warshaw AL, Falconi M, Partelli S, Thayer SP, Pederzoli P, Fernández-del CC. Middle pancreatectomy: indications, short-and long-term operative outcomes. Ann Surg. 2007;246(1):69.
161. Machado MA, Epstein MG, Makdissi FF. Laparoscopic central pancreatectomy: a review of 51 cases. Surg Laparosc Endosc Percutan Tech. 2013;23(6):486–90.
162. Kang CM, Kim DH, Lee WJ, Chi HS. Initial experiences using robot-assisted central pancreatectomy with pancreaticogastrostomy: a potential way to advanced laparoscopic pancreatectomy. Surg Endosc. 2011;25:1101–6.
163. Rompianesi G, Montalti R, Giglio MC, Caruso E, Ceresa CD, Troisi RI. Robotic central pancreatectomy: a systematic review and meta-analysis. HPB (Oxford). 2022;24(2):143–51.
164. Zureikat AH, Moser AJ, Boone BA, Bartlett DL, Zenati M, Zeh HJ III. 250 robotic pancreatic resections: safety and feasibility. Ann Surg. 2013;258(4):554.
165. Conrad LB, Ramirez PT, Burke W, Naumann RW, Ring KL, Munsell MF, Frumovitz M. Role of minimally invasive surgery in gynecologic oncology: an updated survey of members of the Society of Gynecologic Oncology. Int J Gynecol Cancer. 2015;25(6):1121–7.
166. He H, Zeng D, Ou H, Tang Y, Li J, Zhong H. Laparoscopic treatment of endometrial cancer: systematic review. J Minim Invasive Gynecol. 2013;20(4):413–23.

167. Galaal K, Bryant A, Fisher AD, Al-Khaduri M, Kew F, Lopes AD. Laparoscopy versus laparotomy for the management of early stage endometrial cancer. Cochrane Database Syst Rev. 2012;9:CD006655. Available at https://doi.org/10.1002/14651858.CD006655.pub2. Accessed 1 May 2022
168. Galaal K, Donkers H, Bryant A, Lopes AD. Laparoscopy versus laparotomy for the management of early stage endometrial cancer. Cochrane Database Syst Rev. 2018;10:CD006655. https://doi.org/10.1002/14651858.CD006655.pub3. Accessed 27 Apr 2022
169. Walker JL, Piedmonte MR, Spirtos NM, Eisenkop SM, Schlaerth JB, Mannel RS, Spiegel G, Barakat R, Pearl ML, Sharma SK. Laparoscopy compared with laparotomy for comprehensive surgical staging of uterine cancer: Gynecologic Oncology Group Study LAP2. J Clin Oncol. 2009;27(32):5331–6.
170. Walker JL, Piedmonte MR, Spirtos NM, Eisenkop SM, Schlaerth JB, Mannel RS, et al. Recurrence and survival after random assignment to laparoscopy versus laparotomy for comprehensive surgical staging of uterine cancer: Gynecologic Oncology Group LAP2 Study. J Clin Oncol. 2012;30(7):695–700. https://doi.org/10.1200/JCO.2011.38.8645. Epub 30 Jan 2012. Erratum in: J Clin Oncol. 2012;30(13):1570
171. Nezhat CR, Burrell MO, Nezhat FR, Benigno BB, Welander CE. Laparoscopic radical hysterectomy with paraaortic and pelvic node dissection. Am J Obstet Gynecol. 1992;166(3):864–5.
172. Spirtos NM, Eisenkop SM, Schlaerth JB, Ballon SC. Laparoscopic radical hysterectomy (type III) with aortic and pelvic lymphadenectomy in patients with stage I cervical cancer: surgical morbidity and intermediate follow-up. Am J Obstet Gynecol. 2002;187(2):340–8.
173. Dargent DF. Laparoscopic surgery in gynecologic oncology—some disputable applications and one fruitful indication. Gynecol Oncol. 2005;97(3):725–6.
174. Sert BM, Abeler VM. Robotic-assisted laparoscopic radical hysterectomy (Piver type III) with pelvic node dissection-case report. Eur J Gynaecol Oncol. 2006;27(5):531–3.
175. Fanning J, Fenton B, Purohit M. Robotic radical hysterectomy. Am J Obstet Gynecol. 2008;198(6):649.e1–4. Available at https://doi.org/10.1016/j.ajog.2007.11.002. Accessed 1 May 2022
176. Ramirez PT, Adams S, Boggess JF, Burke WM, Frumovitz MM, Gardner GJ, Havrilesky LJ, Holloway R, Lowe MP, Magrina JF, Moore DH. Robotic-assisted surgery in gynecologic oncology: a Society of Gynecologic Oncology consensus statement: the Society of Gynecologic Oncology's clinical practice robotics task force. Gynecol Oncol. 2012;124(2):180–4.
177. Ramirez PT, Frumovitz M, Pareja R, Lopez A, Vieira M, Ribeiro R, Buda A, Yan X, Shuzhong Y, Chetty N, Isla D. Minimally invasive versus abdominal radical hysterectomy for cervical cancer. N Engl J Med. 2018;379(20):1895–904.
178. Melamed A, Margul DJ, Chen L, Keating NL, Del Carmen MG, Yang J, Seagle BL, Alexander A, Barber EL, Rice LW, Wright JD. Survival after minimally invasive radical hysterectomy for early-stage cervical cancer. N Engl J Med. 2018;379(20):1905–14.
179. Uppal S, Gehrig PA, Peng K, Bixel KL, Matsuo K, Vetter MH, Davidson BA, Cisa MP, Lees BF, Brunette LL, Tucker K. Recurrence rates in patients with cervical cancer treated with abdominal versus minimally invasive radical hysterectomy: a multi-institutional retrospective review study. J Clin Oncol. 2020;38(10):1030–40.
180. Cusimano MC, Baxter NN, Gien LT, Moineddin R, Liu N, Dossa F, Willows K, Ferguson SE. Impact of surgical approach on oncologic outcomes in women undergoing radical hysterectomy for cervical cancer. Am J Obstet Gynecol. 2019;221(6):619-e1–24.
181. Paik ES, Lim MC, Kim MH, Kim YH, Song ES, Seong SJ, Suh DH, Lee JM, Lee C, Choi CH. Comparison of laparoscopic and abdominal radical hysterectomy in early stage cervical cancer patients without adjuvant treatment: ancillary analysis of a Korean Gynecologic Oncology Group study (KGOG 1028). Gynecol Oncol. 2019;154(3):547–53.
182. Kim SI, Lee M, Lee S, Suh DH, Kim HS, Kim K, Chung HH, No JH, Kim JW, Park NH, Song YS. Impact of laparoscopic radical hysterectomy on survival outcome in patients with FIGO stage IB cervical cancer: a matching study of two institutional hospitals in Korea. Gynecol Oncol. 2019;155(1):75–82.
183. Chen X, Zhao N, Ye P, Chen J, Nan X, Zhao H, Zhou K, Zhang Y, Xue J, Zhou H, Shang H. Comparison of laparoscopic and open radical hysterectomy in cervical cancer patients with tumor size ≤ 2 cm. Int J Gynecol Cancer. 2020;30(5):564–71.
184. Pedone Anchora L, Turco LC, Bizzarri N, Capozzi VA, Lombisani A, Chiantera V, De Felice F, Gallotta V, Cosentino F, Fagotti A, Ferrandina G. How to select early-stage cervical cancer patients still suitable for laparoscopic radical hysterectomy: a propensity-matched study. Ann Surg Oncol. 2020;27(6):1947–55.
185. Charo LM, Vaida F, Eskander RN, Binder P, Saenz C, McHale M, Plaxe S. Rapid dissemination of practice-changing information: a longitudinal analysis of real-world rates of minimally invasive radical hysterectomy before and after presentation of the LACC trial. Gynecol Oncol. 2020;157(2):494–9.
186. Koh WJ, Abu-Rustum NR, Bean S, Bradley K, Campos SM, Cho KR, Chon HS, Chu C, Clark R, Cohn D, Crispens MA. Cervical cancer, version 3.2019, NCCN clinical practice guidelines in oncology. J Natl Compr Cancer Netw. 2019;17(1):64–84.
187. FIGO Gynecologic Oncology Committee. FIGO statement on minimally invasive surgery in cervical cancer. Int J Gynaecol Obstet. 2020;149(3):264.

Available at https://doi.org/10.1002/ijgo.13141. Accessed 1 May 2022
188. Querleu D, Cibula D, Concin N, Fagotti A, Ferrero A, Fotopoulou C, Knapp P, Kurdiani D, Ledermann JA, Mirza MR, Morice P. Laparoscopic radical hysterectomy: a European Society of Gynaecological Oncology (ESGO) statement. Int J Gynecol Cancer. 2020;30(1):15.
189. The Society of Gynaecologic Oncology. SGO member update: emerging data on the surgical approach for radical hysterectomy in the treatment of women with cervical cancer. Available at https://www.sgo.org/clinical-practice/guidelines/sgo-member-update-emerging-data-on-the-surgical-approach-for-radical-hysterectomy-in-the-treatment-of-women-with-cervical-cancer/. Accessed 8 Oct 2023
190. Matulonis UA, Sood AK, Fallowfield L, Howitt BE, Sehouli J, Karlan BY. Ovarian cancer. Nat Rev Dis Primers. 2016;2(1):1–22.
191. Querleu D, Leblanc E. Laparoscopic infrarenal paraaortic lymph node dissection for restaging of carcinoma of the ovary or fallopian tube. Cancer. 1994;73(5):1467–71.
192. Amara DP, Nezhat C, Teng NN, Nezhat F, Rosati M. Operative laparoscopy in the management of ovarian cancer. Surg Laparosc Endosc. 1996;6(1):38–45.
193. Liu CS, Nagarsheth NP, Nezhat FR. Laparoscopy and ovarian cancer: a paradigm change in the management of ovarian cancer? J Minim Invasive Gynecol. 2009;16(3):250–62.
194. Nezhat FR, Ezzati M, Chuang L, Shamshirsaz AA, Rahaman J, Gretz H. Laparoscopic management of early ovarian and fallopian tube cancers: surgical and survival outcome. Am J Obstet Gynecol. 2009;200(1):83-e1–6.
195. Nezhat FR, DeNoble SM, Liu CS, Cho JE, Brown DN, Chuang L, Gretz H, Saharia P. The safety and efficacy of laparoscopic surgical staging and debulking of apparent advanced stage ovarian, fallopian tube, and primary peritoneal cancers. JSLS. 2010;14(2):155–68.
196. Fanning J, Yacoub E, Hojat R. Laparoscopic-assisted cytoreduction for primary advanced ovarian cancer: success, morbidity and survival. Gynecol Oncol. 2011;123(1):47–9.
197. Liang H, Guo H, Zhang C, Zhu F, Wu Y, Zhang K, Li H, Han J. Feasibility and outcome of primary laparoscopic cytoreductive surgery for advanced epithelial ovarian cancer: a comparison to laparotomic surgery in retrospective cohorts. Oncotarget. 2017;8:113239–47. Retrieved from https://www.oncotarget.com/article/22573/text/
198. Yang H, Wei Y, Deng P, Ou H, Nie H, Zhuang Y. Feasibility and safety of minimally invasive technology for interval cytoreductive surgery during advanced ovarian cancer after neoadjuvant chemotherapy. Eur J Gynaecol Oncol. 2022;43(6):4–12.
199. Trinh H, Ott C, Fanning J. Feasibility of laparoscopic debulking with electrosurgical loop excision procedure and argon beam coagulator at recurrence in patients with previous laparotomy debulking. Am J Obstet Gynecol. 2004;190(5):1394–7.
200. Nezhat FR, Denoble SM, Cho JE, Brown DN, Soto E, Chuang L, Gretz H, Saharia P. Safety and efficacy of video laparoscopic surgical debulking of recurrent ovarian, fallopian tube, and primary peritoneal cancers. JSLS. 2012;16(4):511–8.
201. Magrina JF, Zanagnolo V, Noble BN, Kho RM, Magtibay P. Robotic approach for ovarian cancer: perioperative and survival results and comparison with laparoscopy and laparotomy. Gynecol Oncol. 2011;121(1):100–5.
202. Abitbol J, Gotlieb W, Zeng Z, Ramanakumar A, Kessous R, Kogan L, Pare-Miron V, Rombaldi M, Salvador S, Kucukyazici B, Brin S. Incorporating robotic surgery into the management of ovarian cancer after neoadjuvant chemotherapy. Int J Gynecol Cancer. 2019;29(9)

3 Minimally Invasive Esophagectomy

Koji Otsuka, Satoru Goto, Tomotake Ariyoshi, Takeshi Yamashita, Yoshihito Sato, Akira Saito, Masahiro Kohmoto, Kentaro Motegi, Rei Kato, Koichiro Fujimasa, Tetsuo Sawatani, and Masahiko Murakami

Abstract

Esophagectomy with total mediastinal lymph node dissection is performed as the standard procedure to control lymph node metastasis. However, esophagectomy by the thoracotomy is invasive and can result in a high incidence of complications, particularly pulmonary complications [Watson. World J Surg. 1994;18(3):361–6]. We introduce a novel operative technique to dissect lymph nodes adjacent to the recurrent laryngeal nerve and can prevent recurrent laryngeal nerve palsy by minimally invasive procedure, which we called the *native tissue preservation* technique. In this technique, there was no damage to the recurrent laryngeal nerve, which was kept in its anatomical position. Although a small incision is important, we believe that preventing complications is a more important issue, and this is a minimally invasive esophagectomy. In this chapter, we explain minimally invasive esophagectomy with total mediastinal lymph node dissection.

Keywords

Esophagectomy · Radical lymphadenectomy · Nerve paralysis · Prevent complications · Native tissue preservation technique · Microanatomical layer

3.1 Introduction

Esophageal cancer has a poor prognosis and high mortality rate, and squamous cell carcinoma relative lesions account for more than 95% of esophageal cancer cases in Japan. Esophagectomy with total mediastinal lymph node dissection is performed as the standard procedure to control lymph node metastasis. However, esophagectomy by thoracotomy is invasive and make a high incidence of complications, particularly pulmonary complications [1]. Cuschieri et al. initially reported performing thoracoscopic operation of esophageal cancer in 1992 [2]. Palanivelu et al. first described thoracoscopic esophagectomy in the prone position in 2006 [3], and many esophageal surgeons in Japan performed this position [4, 5]. Palanivelu et al. suggested that fewer respiratory complications occurred and securing ample working space was relatively easy, resulting in the shortening of the operative time

Supplementary Information The online version contains supplementary material available at https://doi.org/10.1007/978-981-97-7059-5_3.

K. Otsuka (✉) · S. Goto · T. Ariyoshi · T. Yamashita · Y. Sato · A. Saito · M. Kohmoto · K. Motegi · R. Kato · K. Fujimasa · T. Sawatani · M. Murakami
Showa University Esophageal Cancer Center, Shinagawa-ku, Tokyo, Japan
e-mail: kojiotsuka@med.showa-u.ac.jp

M. Tewari (ed.), *Minimally Invasive Surgery in Cancer*,
https://doi.org/10.1007/978-981-97-7059-5_3

in prone position [3]. However, this method has some difficulty for performing in the upper mediastinal lymph node dissection. Because when we dissected in the upper mediastinal lymph node dissection, we need crossing over the trachea. This problem can result in thermal injury to the trachea by the coagulation device and pulling up the left recurrent laryngeal nerve when we dissect the left recurrent laryngeal nerve lymph nodes. Depending on this difficulty, we can find the lymph node dissection except for the left recurrent laryngeal nerve lymph node dissection in the international conferences and manuscripts. In contrast, the visual field on the ventral side of the left recurrent laryngeal nerve can be easily exposed by only a slight deviation of the trachea in the left lateral decubitus position. We have been performing minimally invasive esophagectomy with artificial pneumothorax in the left lateral decubitus position since 1996 [6], with over 1700 cases up till now. Minimally invasive esophagectomy is particularly beneficial in reducing the incidence of postoperative respiratory complications rather than the thoracotomy, but it may be associated with a higher incidence of left recurrent laryngeal nerve palsy according to a large Japanese study [7]. Although it depends on the extent of lymph node dissection, the reported incidence of recurrent laryngeal nerve paralysis (RLNP) after esophagectomy varies from 8.3 to 40.9% [8–10]. Neural injury during surgery is caused by thermal damage, stretching, and vascular compromise of the nerve. These injuries are more frequent in the left recurrent laryngeal nerve than in the right recurrent laryngeal nerve because of its anatomical position, longer course, and vulnerability within the mediastinum. Although minimally invasive esophagectomy is particularly beneficial in reducing the incidence of postoperative respiratory complications, it may be associated with a higher incidence of left recurrent nerve palsy. However, we previously introduced the lymph node dissection technique, to avoid recurrent laryngeal nerve injury (native tissue preservation techniques) [11]. In this chapter, we explain minimally invasive esophagectomy with total mediastinal lymph node dissection.

3.2 Indication

The inclusion criteria were without serious cardiac or respiratory disease that would perform safety operation under general anesthesia. Moreover, clinical stage is without metastases to other organs such as the lung or liver, and lower than cT4b stage. We do not have age limitation; the oldest patient at our institute was 96 years of age.

3.3 Surgical Procedure

3.3.1 Anesthesia, Patients' Position, and Port Arrangement

Surgery was performed after the induction of general anesthesia. In general, one-lung pulmonary ventilation with an 8-Fr spiral tube and inserted blocker balloon in the right bronchus was used during the thoracoscopic procedure. The thoracic procedure was performed in the left lateral decubitus position with a 15° head elevation and the video monitor was placed on the patient's head side. The surgeon stood on the dorsal side of the patient, and the assistant operator and camera operator stood on the patient's ventral side. The first camera port (12 mm) was placed in the fifth intercostal space in the anterior axillary line. Carbon dioxide pneumothorax was injected at a pressure of 8–10 mmHg, and the right lung was decompressed. Two ports (5 mm) for the operator into the fifth and eighth intercostal spaces at the posterior axillary line. A 5-mm port for the thoracoscope was inserted into the eighth intercostal space at the midaxillary line, and 12-mm ports for the assistant were inserted in the third intercostal space at the anterior axillary line (Fig. 3.1).

3.3.2 Total Mediastinal Lymph Node Dissection

The thoracic procedure is performed as follows:

1. *Dissection of the lymph nodes around the right recurrent laryngeal nerve*
2. *Transection of the esophagus*

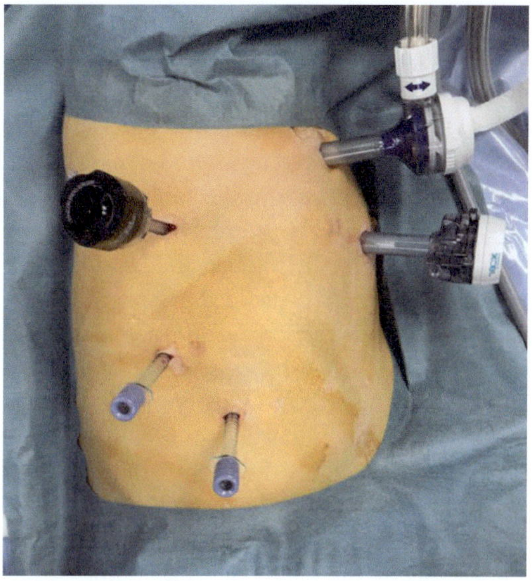

Fig. 3.1 A 5-mm port for the thoracoscope was inserted into the eighth intercostal region at the midaxillary line, and 12-mm ports for the assistant were inserted in a slightly ventral position in the third intercostal space at the anterior axillary line

3. *Dissection of the lymph nodes around the left recurrent laryngeal nerve*
4. *Dissection of the lower mediastinal lymph nodes including the supradiaphragmatic lymph nodes and anterior thoracic para-aortic lymph nodes*
5. *Dissection of the tracheal bifurcation area lymph nodes*
6. *Dissection of the middle mediastinal lymph nodes including the pulmonary ligament lymph node around the left inferior pulmonary vein*
7. *Drainage tube insertion*

3.3.2.1 Dissection of the Lymph Nodes Around the Right Recurrent Laryngeal Nerve

The right recurrent laryngeal nerve lymph nodes were resected. Three to four narrow branches ran from the right recurrent laryngeal nerve toward the esophagus, we cut these branches with an ultrasonic device carefully. We usually use HARMONIC® HD 1100 (Johnson and Johnson, New Brunswick, NJ, USA). This ultrasonic device is useful for dividing the microanatomical layer and can be used as a dissection device. We preserved the thin connective tissue around the right recurrent laryngeal nerve with careful attention to the risk of thermal damage. It will be avoiding traction on the nerve when dissecting the right recurrent laryngeal nerve lymph node (Fig. 3.2). This preservation of thin native tissue overlying the right recurrent laryngeal nerve can avoid the recurrent laryngeal nerve palsy.

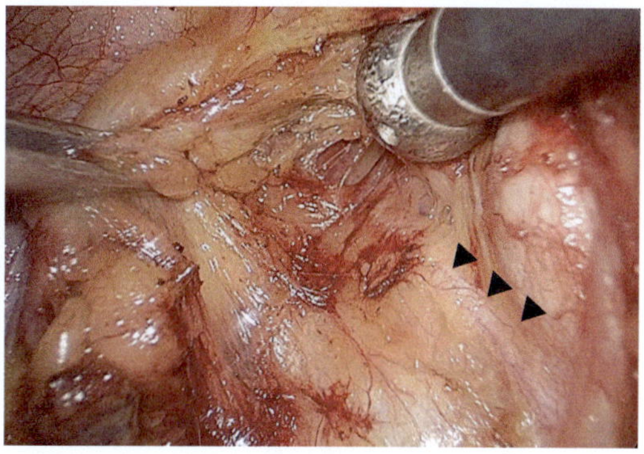

Fig. 3.2 We preserved the thin layer of connective tissue around the right recurrent laryngeal nerve. Black triangle shows the right recurrent laryngeal nerve

3.3.2.2 Transection of the Esophagus

We dissected the line between the trachea and esophagus using an ultrasonic device. First, we dissected the dorsal side of trachea. After dissected this line, the left recurrent laryngeal nerve and lymph nodes were separated with the esophagus from trachea. We should dissect this procedure until we could confirm the overlying shiny thin layer of connective tissues. This shiny thin layer is on the cardiac branch of the sympathetic nerve and preserving this layer can avoid cardiac arrhythmias (Fig. 3.3). After dissection of the cervicothoracic junction to the inferior of the aortic arch around the thoracic esophagus, we cut the thoracic esophagus using an automatic suture device (Echelon Gold 60 mm, Johnson and Johnson, New Brunswick, NJ, USA). Both sides of the transected esophagus were ligated by strings, and the cranial side of the esophagus was pulled up to the cranial side, while the caudal side of the esophagus was pulled down to the caudal side. We could then see this area with a good view without the esophagus.

3.3.2.3 Dissection of the Lymph Nodes Around the Left Recurrent Laryngeal Nerve

We can obtain a good view of the fatty tissue, including the left recurrent laryngeal nerve and lymph nodes, without the esophagus.

3.3.3 Native Tissue Preservation Technique of the Recurrent Laryngeal Nerve

We developed this technique to prevent recurrent laryngeal nerve palsy. The aim of this technique was the opinion that if the recurrent laryngeal nerve stays on the normal anatomical position, without touching the nerve, traction and injury to the recurrent laryngeal nerve will be limited. We rotated the lymph nodes and fatty tissue counterclockwise from the ventral side to the dorsal side about the axis of the left recurrent laryngeal nerve (Fig. 3.4). By preserving the thin native tissue layer around the left recurrent laryngeal nerve, injury of the nerve by traction and bending were avoided. We carefully avoided grasping the fatty tissue, avoiding traction on the nerve and not touching the nerve when dissecting around the left recurrent laryngeal nerve lymph nodes. We mainly used the ultrasonic dissector to avoid thermal damage while dissecting around the left recurrent laryngeal nerve. We used a short pitch dissection technique, which prevents thermal damage due to the longer dissection time. A few transverse vessels around the left recurrent laryngeal nerve were dissected by ultrasonic dissection. We confirmed the location of the left recurrent laryngeal nerve under the thin layer of connective tissue, after the fatty tissue and lymph nodes were rotated dorsally to the left recurrent laryngeal nerve. These lymph nodes were dissected from caudal to cranial because of small branches of the left recurrent laryngeal nerve passing from caudal to cranial, and these branches should be divided in the same direction to avoid injury to the main nerve. We could dissect the left recurrent laryngeal nerve lymph nodes with an adequate margin from the nerve after lymph nodes were already rotated toward the dorsal side of the left recurrent laryngeal nerve (Fig. 3.5).

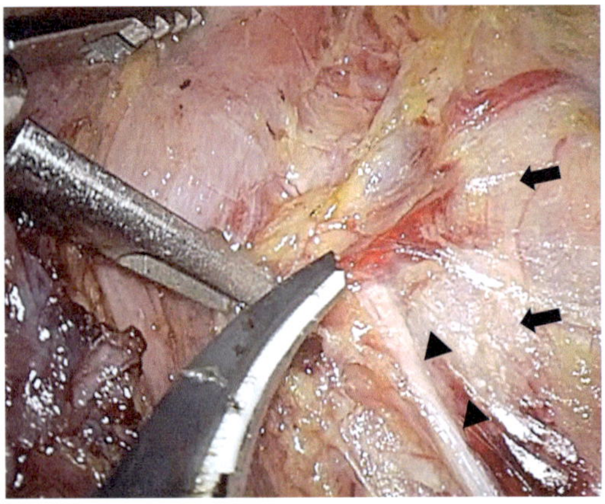

Fig. 3.3 The shiny thin layer is on the cardiac branch of the sympathetic nerve and is preserved to avoid cardiac arrhythmias. Black triangle shows the left recurrent laryngeal nerve. Black arrow shows the sympathetic nerve

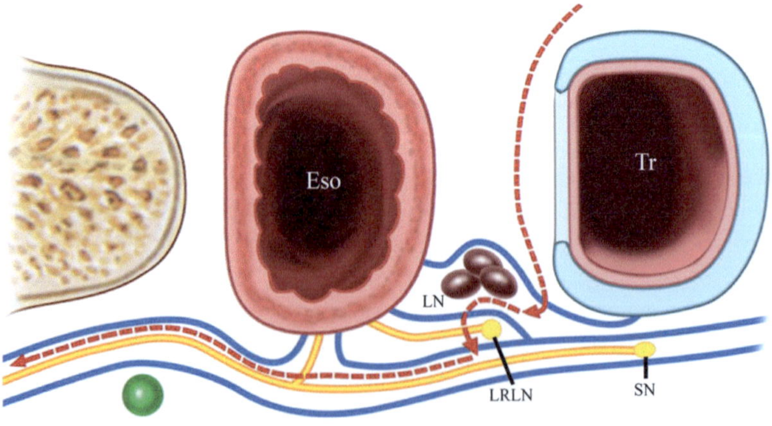

Fig. 3.4 Illustration of the anatomical layer. *Eso* esophagus, *Tr* trachea, *LN* lymph node, *LRLN* left recurrent laryngeal nerve, *SN* sympathetic nerve

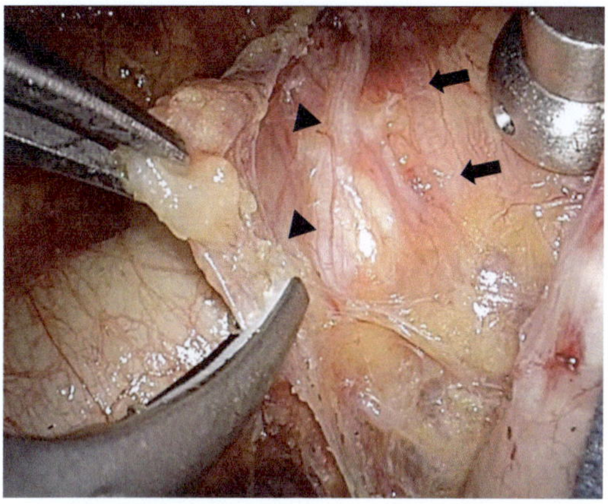

Fig. 3.5 We could then see this area with a good view without the esophagus. Black triangle shows the left recurrent laryngeal nerve. Black arrow shows the sympathetic nerve

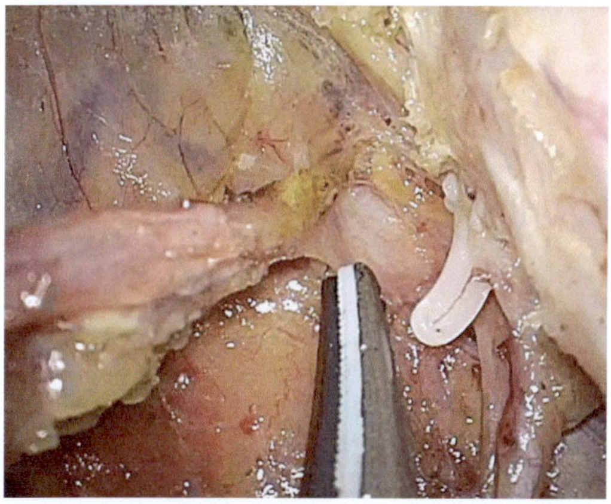

Fig. 3.6 The cranial landmark was marked with a clip to facilitate confirmation of the location during the cervical procedure

The intrathoracic cranial landmark clip placed on the left recurrent laryngeal nerve lymph node could help confirm the location of the lymph node. This clip provides the information on the extent to which the lymph node can be dissected during the cervical procedure (Figs. 3.6 and 3.7). The left recurrent laryngeal nerve lymph nodes were removed while maintaining the normal anatomical position without touching or stretching the nerve.

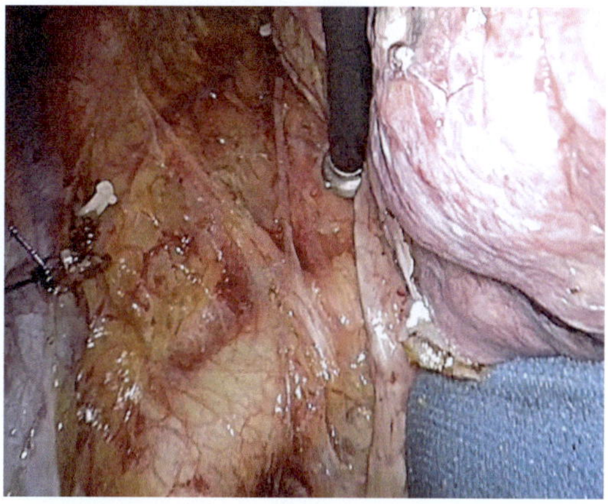

Fig. 3.7 After dissection view

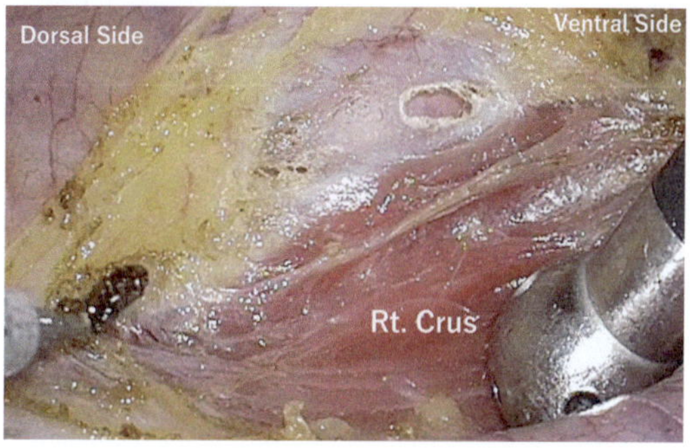

Fig. 3.8 We dissected the mediastinal pleura on the dorsal and ventral sides above the crus of the diaphragm *Rt. Crus* right crus of the diaphragm

3.3.3.1 Dissection of the Lower Mediastinal Lymph Nodes, Including the Supradiaphragmatic Lymph Nodes and Anterior Thoracic Para-Aortic Lymph Nodes

First, we dissected the right pulmonary ligament and pulmonary ligament lymph nodes. Lung injury should be considered when dissecting the ligament. Next, we dissected the mediastinal pleura on the dorsal and ventral sides above the crus of the diaphragm (Fig. 3.8). The ventral side of the esophagus was the supradiaphragmatic lymph nodes, and we dissected the mediastinal pleura from here to the right main bronchus

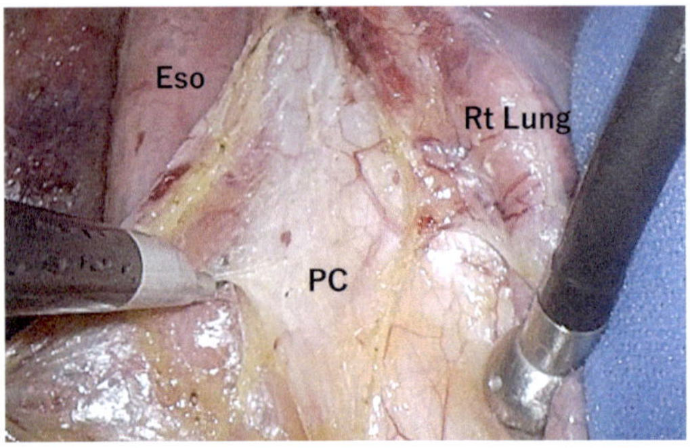

Fig. 3.9 We dissected the mediastinal pleura from the ventral side of the esophagus to the right main bronchus. *Eso* esophagus, *PC* pericardium, *Rt Lung* right lung

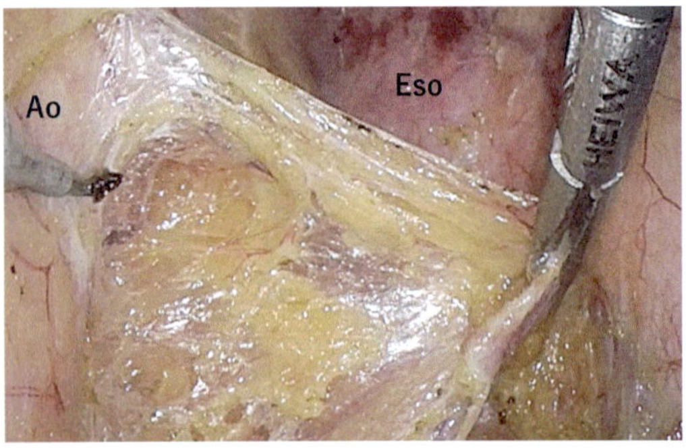

Fig. 3.10 We dissected the anterior thoracic mediastinal pleura from the diaphragm to the azygos vein. *Eso* esophagus, *Ao* descending aorta

(Fig. 3.9). We also dissected the connecting tissue on the dorsal side of the pericardium. This lymph node is a paraesophageal lymph node from the middle to the lower esophagus. Next, we dissected the anterior thoracic mediastinal pleura from the diaphragm to the azygos vein (Fig. 3.10). When we dissect this fat and connecting tissue including the anterior thoracic para-aortic lymph nodes, we should ligate by clip or cut the proper esophageal artery using an energy device (Fig. 3.11). We should dissect this fat and connect the tissue around the left side of the mediastinum from the dorsal side to the ventral side (Fig. 3.12). We usually use electric cautery and ultrasonic devices when dissecting this area (Fig. 3.13).

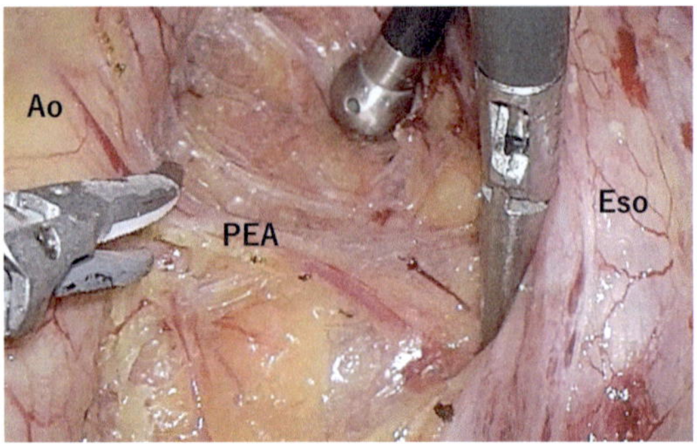

Fig. 3.11 We should ligate by clip or cut the proper esophageal artery using an energy device. *Eso* esophagus, *Ao* descending aorta, *PEA* proper esophageal artery

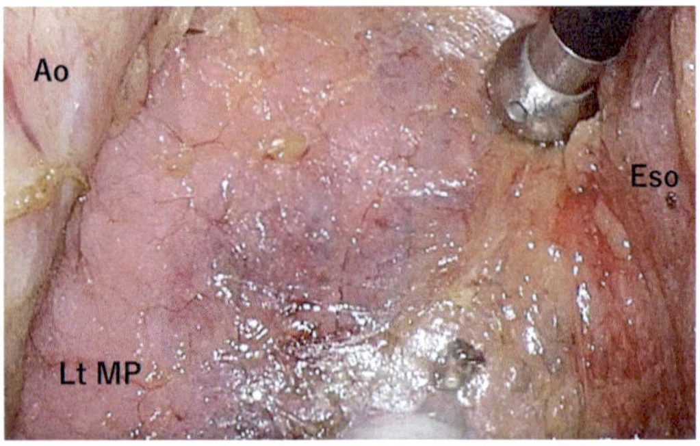

Fig. 3.12 We should dissect paraesophageal lymph node from the middle to the lower esophagus until we can see the left side of the mediastinum from the dorsal side to the ventral side. *Eso* esophagus, *Ao* descending aorta, *Lt MP* left mediastinal pleura

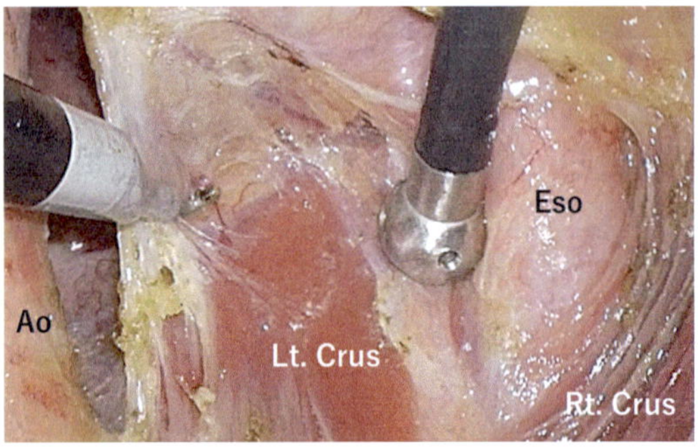

Fig. 3.13 After finishing the dissection of the lower mediastinal lymph nodes, including the supradiaphragmatic lymph nodes and anterior thoracic para-aortic lymph nodes. *Eso* esophagus, *Ao* descending aorta, *Rt. Crus* right crus of the diaphragm, *Lt. Crus* left crus of the diaphragm

3.3.3.2 Dissection of the Tracheal Bifurcation Area Lymph Nodes

First, we dissected the mediastinal pleura under the right main bronchus from the periphery to the bifurcation (Fig. 3.14). We could see the periphery of the right bronchial artery and one of the lung branches from the right vagus nerve under the right main bronchus, and we cut it to perform radical dissection of these lymph nodes. Next, we dissected the mediastinal pleura under the left main bronchus from the periphery to the bifurcation (Fig. 3.15). In this area, we could see a few left vagus nerves and cut them under the left main bronchus. We believe that we can clearly observe the peripheral lymph nodes under the left main bronchus after cutting the left vagus nerves. Bleeding occurs at the top of the bifurcation lymph node when it is dissected because it is usually connected to the paratracheal lymph nodes (Fig. 3.16).

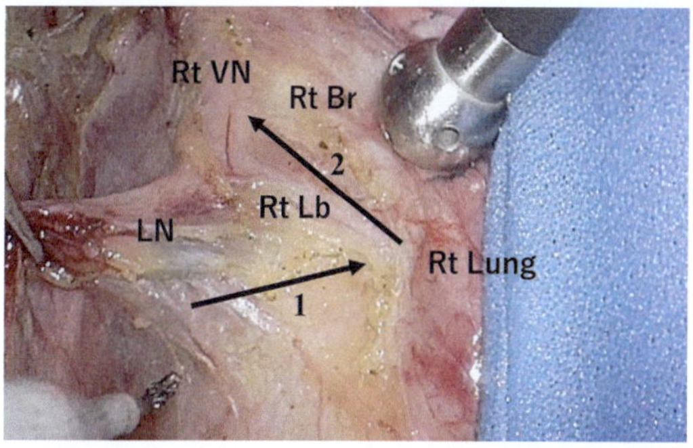

Fig. 3.14 We dissected the mediastinal pleura under the right main bronchus from the periphery to the bifurcation. *LN* Tracheal bifurcation area lymph nodes, *Rt Lung* right lung, *Rt Br* right bronchus, *Rt VN* right vagus nerve, *Rt Lb* the lung branches from the right vagus nerve

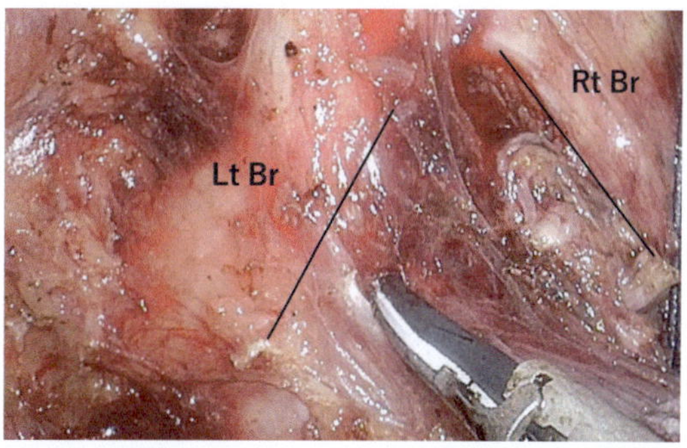

Fig. 3.15 We dissected the mediastinal pleura under the left main bronchus from the periphery to the bifurcation. *Rt Br* right bronchus, *Lt Br* left bronchus

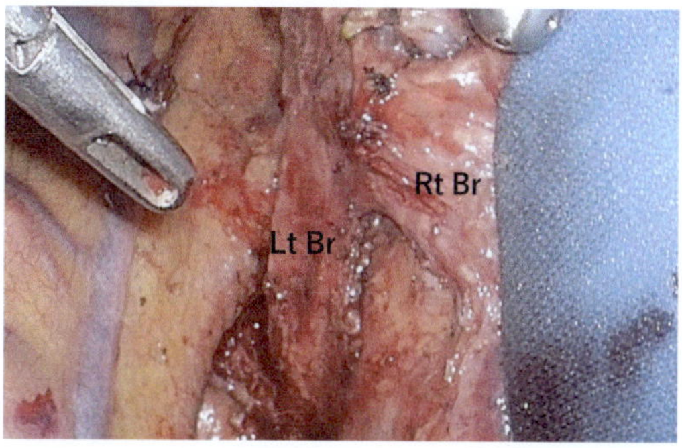

Fig. 3.16 After dissection view of the tracheal bifurcation area lymph nodes. *Rt Br* right bronchus, *Lt Br* left bronchus

3.3.3.3 Dissection of the Middle Mediastinal Lymph Nodes Including the Pulmonary Ligament Lymph Node Around the Left Inferior Pulmonary Vein

Dissection of a large proportion of the middle to lower mediastinal lymph nodes was completed after performing *(4) dissection of the lower mediastinal lymph nodes including the supradiaphragmatic lymph nodes and anterior thoracic para-aortic lymph nodes*. However, we noticed the existence of a lymph node above and below the left inferior pulmonary vein (Fig. 3.17). It should be dissected until we can confirm the left mediastinal pleura. Traction of the caudal side by the ligated esophagus provides a clear view in this area.

3.3.3.4 Drainage Tube Insertion

After total mediastinal lymph node dissection was completed, the drainage tube was inserted from the 5-mm port of the operator (Fig. 3.18). We usually use a 10-Fr brake drain (J-VAC drain, Johnson and Johnson, New Brunswick, NJ, USA). This drainage tube was removed after checking for no air leakage and less than 200 mL/day. We believe that such a narrow drainage tube helps control pain in patients.

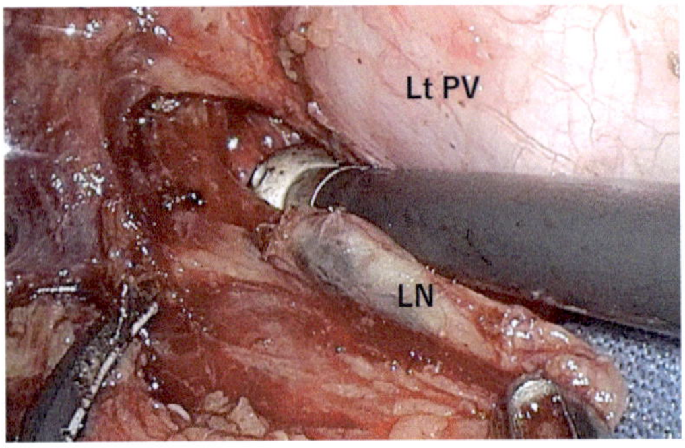

Fig. 3.17 We noticed the existence of a lymph node above and below the left inferior pulmonary vein. It should be dissected until we can confirm the left mediastinal pleura. *LN* lymph node below the left inferior pulmonary vein, *Lt PV* left inferior pulmonary vein

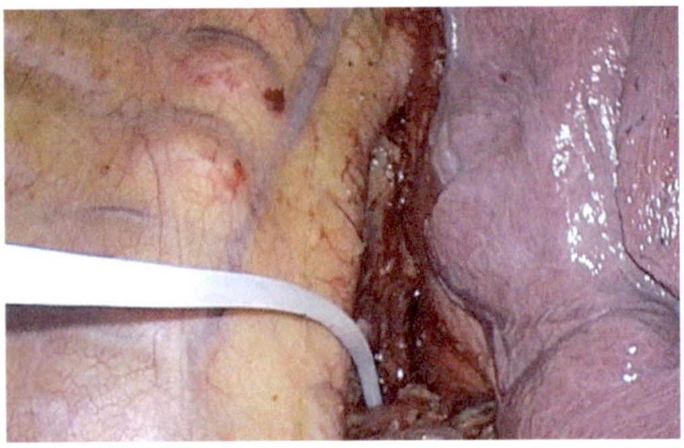

Fig. 3.18 10-Fr brake drain was inserted from the 5-mm port of the operator

3.4 Evaluation for RLNP

The presence of RLNP was assessed by an anesthesiologist at extubation. An otolaryngologist using a flexible laryngoscope (postoperative day 7) evaluates the presence or absence of hoarseness or paralysis. We and nurses also evaluated hoarseness until discharge. The RLNP grade was classified according to the Clavien-Dindo classification [12] and supplementary criteria advocated by the Japan Clinical Oncology Group [13]. If a patient was found to have RLNP, they were continuously followed up regarding hoarseness of their voice once every month in the first 6 months and every 3 months thereafter at the outpatient clinic.

3.5 Postoperative Management

The tracheal tube was removed immediately after surgery. Patients were treated in the intensive care unit on the day after surgery and transferred to a high care unit, started walking and drinking water on postoperative day 1. Patients returned to the general surgical ward, started drinking liquid nutrition on postoperative day 3, started eating food on day 5, and were discharged on day 9 or later.

3.6 Outcome

Although our recent results show that the overall complication rate was 16%, including anastomotic leak in 3.6% and postoperative bleeding in 3.6% of cases [11], there were no instances of grade II or higher postoperative RLNP (Clavien-Dindo classification). However, temporary hoarseness (Clavien-Dindo grade I) was observed in one patient who recovered without specific therapy within 2 months. Arrhythmias, pulmonary thrombosis, atelectasis, and pneumonia were observed in 7.2%, 1.8%, 1.8%, and 3.6%, respectively. Reoperation within 30 days was necessary in 3.6% of patients due to postoperative bleeding of cervical area. No mortality occurred within 30 days.

3.7 Conclusion

We introduced a minimally invasive esophagectomy in the left lateral decubitus position. Our technique, the *native tissue preservation technique*, prevents recurrent laryngeal nerve palsy during lymph node dissection. Many surgeons perform minimally invasive esophagectomy in the prone position worldwide, but the left lateral decubitus position is beneficial for upper mediastinal lymph node dissection. Both techniques should allow for the esophageal operation, but total mediastinal lymph node dissection without complications is an important technique for minimally invasive esophagectomy. Although a small incision is significant, we believe that preventing complications is a more important issue, and this is a minimally invasive esophagectomy.

Disclosures The authors declare no conflicts of interest.

References

1. Watson A. Operable esophageal cancer: current results from the West. World J Surg. 1994;18(3):361–6.
2. Cuschieri A, Shimi S, Banting S. Endoscopic oesophagectomy through a right thoracoscopic approach. J R Coll Surg Edinb. 1992;37(1):7–11.
3. Palanivelu C, Prakash A, Senthilkumar R, Senthilnathan P, Parthasarathi R, Rajan PS, et al. Minimally invasive esophagectomy: thoracoscopic mobilization of the esophagus and mediastinal lymphadenectomy in prone position—experience of 130 patients. J Am Coll Surg. 2006;203(1):7–16.
4. Noshiro H, Iwasaki H, Kobayashi K, Uchiyama A, Miyasaka Y, Masatsugu T, et al. Lymphadenectomy along the left recurrent laryngeal nerve by a minimally invasive esophagectomy in the prone position for thoracic esophageal cancer. Surg Endosc. 2010;24(12):2965–73.
5. Daiko H, Nishimura M. A pilot study of the technical and oncologic feasibility of thoracoscopic esophagectomy with extended lymph node dissection in the prone position for clinical stage I thoracic esophageal carcinoma. Surg Endosc. 2012;26(3):673–80.
6. Murakami M, Otsuka K, Goto S, Ariyoshi T, Yamashita T, Aoki T. Thoracoscopic and hand assisted laparoscopic esophagectomy with radical lymph node dissection for esophageal squamous cell carcinoma in the left lateral decubitus position: a single center retrospective analysis of 654 patients. BMC Cancer. 2017;17(1):748.
7. Takeuchi H, Miyata H, Ozawa S, Udagawa H, Osugi H, Matsubara H, et al. Comparison of short-term outcomes between open and minimally invasive esophagectomy for esophageal cancer using a nationwide database in Japan. Ann Surg Oncol. 2017;24(7):1821–7.
8. Booka E, Takeuchi H, Nishi T, Matsuda S, Kaburagi T, Fukuda K, et al. The impact of postoperative complications on survivals after esophagectomy for esophageal cancer. Medicine (Baltimore). 2015;94(33):e1369.
9. Ninomiya I, Osugi H, Fujimura T, Fushida S, Okamoto K, Maruzen S, et al. Thoracoscopic esophagectomy with extended lymph node dissection in the left lateral position: technical feasibility and oncologic outcomes. Dis Esophagus. 2014;27(2):159–67.
10. Takemura M, Hori T, Fujiwara Y. Clinical outcomes and prognosis after thoracoscopic esophagectomy with two-field lymph node dissection for lower thoracic esophageal cancer. Anticancer Res. 2013;33(2):601–8.
11. Otsuka K, Murakami M, Goto S, Ariyoshi T, Yamashita T, Saito A, et al. Minimally invasive esophagectomy and radical lymph node dissection without recurrent laryngeal nerve paralysis. Surg Endosc. 2020;34(6):2749–57.
12. Clavien PA, Strasberg SM. Severity grading of surgical complications. Ann Surg. 2009;250(2):197–8.
13. Katayama H, Kurokawa Y, Nakamura K, Ito H, Kanemitsu Y, Masuda N, et al. Extended Clavien-Dindo classification of surgical complications: Japan Clinical Oncology Group postoperative complications criteria. Surg Today. 2016;46(6):668–85.

Minimally Invasive Gastrectomy

4

Original and Practical Reconstruction Methods in Minimally Invasive Surgery for Gastric Cancer

Suguru Yamauchi, Seira Honjo, Hajime Orita, Jun Chen, Hiroyuki Egawa, Yutaro Yoshimoto, Akira Kubota, Osamu Itose, Yukinori Yube, Sanae Kaji, and Tetsu Fukunaga

Abstract

Minimally invasive surgical techniques for gastric cancer have progressed rapidly over the past decade. In our institution, laparoscopic or robot-assisted surgery is the first choice in the surgical treatment of gastric cancer. For laparoscopic or robot-assisted gastrectomies for gastric cancer, the reconstruction method is critical for a better outcome. However, the optimal reconstruction technique remains controversial. In this chapter, we reported the augmented rectangle technique as a reconstruction option for totally laparoscopic Billroth-I reconstructions after distal gastrectomy and hemi-double stapling technique performed with an EEA™OrVil™ circular stapler for totally laparoscopic esophagojejunostomy after total gastrectomy and its innovations and tips.

Keywords

Laparoscopic · Distal gastrectomy · Total gastrectomy · Reconstruction · Billroth-I · Augmented rectangle technique · Esophagojejunostomy · OrVil · EEA

4.1 Introduction

Currently, reconstruction after gastrectomy using totally laparoscopic surgery is widely performed, but various complications and difficulties in the procedure were reported [1]. Based on our experiences, we introduce a new reconstruction method for stable results [2–7]. In this chapter, we describe the technical details of the totally laparoscopic anastomotic method after gastrectomy for gastric cancer, Billroth-I (B-I) reconstruction after distal gas-

Supplementary Information The online version contains supplementary material available at https://doi.org/10.1007/978-981-97-7059-5_4.

S. Yamauchi (✉)
Department of Upper Gastroenterological Surgery, Juntendo University Faculty of Medicine, Tokyo, Japan

Department of Surgery, Johns Hopkins University School of Medicine, Baltimore, MD, USA
e-mail: s.yamauchi.gk@juntendo.ac.jp

S. Honjo · H. Orita · J. Chen · H. Egawa
Y. Yoshimoto · A. Kubota · O. Itose · Y. Yube · S. Kaji
T. Fukunaga
Department of Upper Gastroenterological Surgery, Juntendo University Faculty of Medicine, Tokyo, Japan

M. Tewari (ed.), *Minimally Invasive Surgery in Cancer*,
https://doi.org/10.1007/978-981-97-7059-5_4

trectomy using augmented rectangle technique (ART), and hemi-double stapling technique (HDST) performed with an EEA™OrVil™ circular stapler (CS), in which anvil can be inserted orally for esophagojejunostomy after total gastrectomy.

4.2 Patient Positioning and Operating Room Setup

Patients are placed in the lithotomy position under general anesthesia. The 4K monitors are placed near the patient's head and faced the operator, assistant, and scopist to view the same screen (Fig. 4.1). At the start of the surgery, the surgeon stands on the left side of the patient with the assistant standing on the patient's right. The surgeon and assistant change positions according to the progress of the surgery.

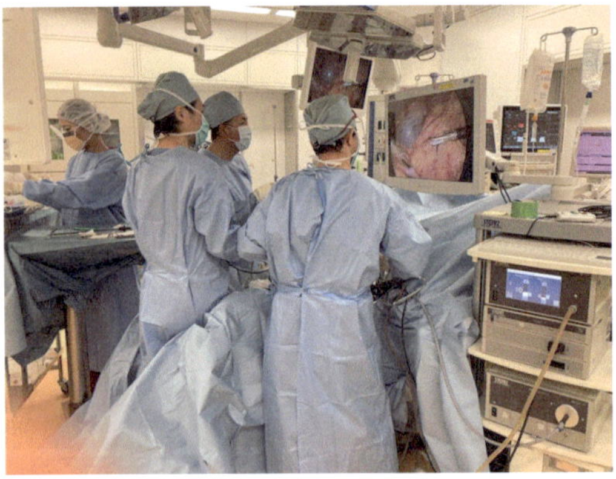

Fig. 4.1 Operating room setup. Patients are placed in the lithotomy position under general anesthesia. The 4K monitors are placed near the patient's head and faced the operator, assistant, and scopist to view the same screen

4.3 List of Specific Instruments/Gadgets Used

4K Camara System (IMAGE1 S™; Karl Storz), Ultrasonically activated devices (SonoSurg®; OLYMPUS, Sonicision®; Medtronic, HARMONIC®; ETHICON), Vessel sealing system (LigaSure™ Blunt Tip Jaw; Medtronic), Endoscopic linear staplers (Signia™; Medtronic), Endoscopic CS (DST Series™ EEA™ & DST Series™ EEA™ OrVil™ Device; Medtronic), Internal Organ Retractor™ (Aesculap)

4.4 Port Setting

The ports were positioned in a reverse trapezoid shape as usual. The size of the port below the right hypochondrium is 5 mm, and that of the umbilical port and the other three ports are 12 mm (Fig. 4.2). The development of the left hepatic lobe is important in the intraoperative field of view for laparoscopic gastrectomy. Especially, during reconstruction in total gastrectomy, adequate liver traction to establish a clear surgical field is one of the factors for smooth and appropriate reconstruction. We used an internal organ retractor to expand the surgical field in the left hepatic lobe. We also used a 30° rigid video laparoscope.

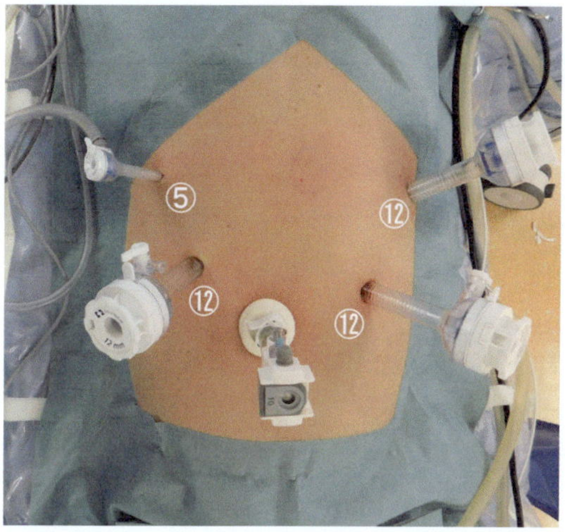

Fig. 4.2 Port setting. The ports were positioned in a reverse trapezoid shape as usual. The size of the port below the right hypochondrium is 5 mm, and that of the umbilical port and the other three ports are 12 mm

4.5 The Operative Technique in a Detailed Stepwise Manner

We are applying totally laparoscopic gastrectomy for advanced gastric cancer. Recently, it has been expanded to apply in cStage IIIB, including cN (+) cases. Lymph node dissection was decided according to the Japanese Classification of Gastric Carcinoma by the Japanese Gastric Cancer Association. Recently, a new "Outside-In approach" was developed for lymph node dissection. The typical surgical procedures for D2 lymph node dissection for totally laparoscopic distal gastrectomy are described as follows. The gastrocolic ligament, along with lymph node station 4d, was separated using ultrasonically activated instruments (USADs). While continuing to dissect the gastrocolic ligament toward the right side, sufficient space between the front layer of the transverse mesocolon and the second portion of the duodenum was created before proceeding with the lymph node dissection at station 6. After the division of the origin of the right gastroepiploic vein, the right gastroepiploic artery was confirmed to branched gastroduodenal artery and was separated, utilizing a clip and USADs at station 6. Subsequently, the gastrocolic ligament, encompassing lymph node station 4sb, was incised 4 cm below the epiploic arcade, and the origin of the left gastroepiploic vein and artery were severed using a combination of a clip and USADs. Following the confirmation of the upper boundary of lymph node dissection at station 12a, the point where the right and left hepatic arteries bifurcate was exposed. Next, the right gastric artery and vein were severed at their origins using a combination of a clip and USADs, allowing for the comprehensive dissection of lymph nodes at stations 12a and 5, after which the dissection of suprapancreatic lymph nodes at stations 11p, 9, 7, and 8a was performed. The "Outside-In approach" is particularly effective in the dissection of the suprapancreatic lymph node dissection. The dissection of the pancreatic capsule was carried out with the assistance of USADs, extending from the suprapancreatic border to the pancreatic tail, all the way to the root of the posterior gastric artery. The dissection involved lymph nodes positioned between the splenic artery and vein at station 11p. Exposing and dividing the left gastric artery and vein was done using a clip and USADs. The common hepatic artery was then uncovered and skeletonized, followed by the dissection of lymph node station 8a in a cephalic direction to expose the right crus of the diaphragm. Subsequently, removal of the cardiac lymph nodes at station 1 and the lymph nodes along the lesser curvature of the stomach at station 3 was performed. After lymph node dissection, the stomach was resected and removed, and reconstruction was performed.

4.5.1 ART for Laparoscopic Billroth-I Reconstruction

ART is a Billroth-I reconstruction method after totally laparoscopic distal gastrectomy using Linear Stapler (LS). The advantages of ART are (1) a large rectangle of the anastomosis can be secured, (2) true end-to-end anastomosis, (3) no ischemic area remains, and (4) no need for supporting suture, and the procedure is simple.

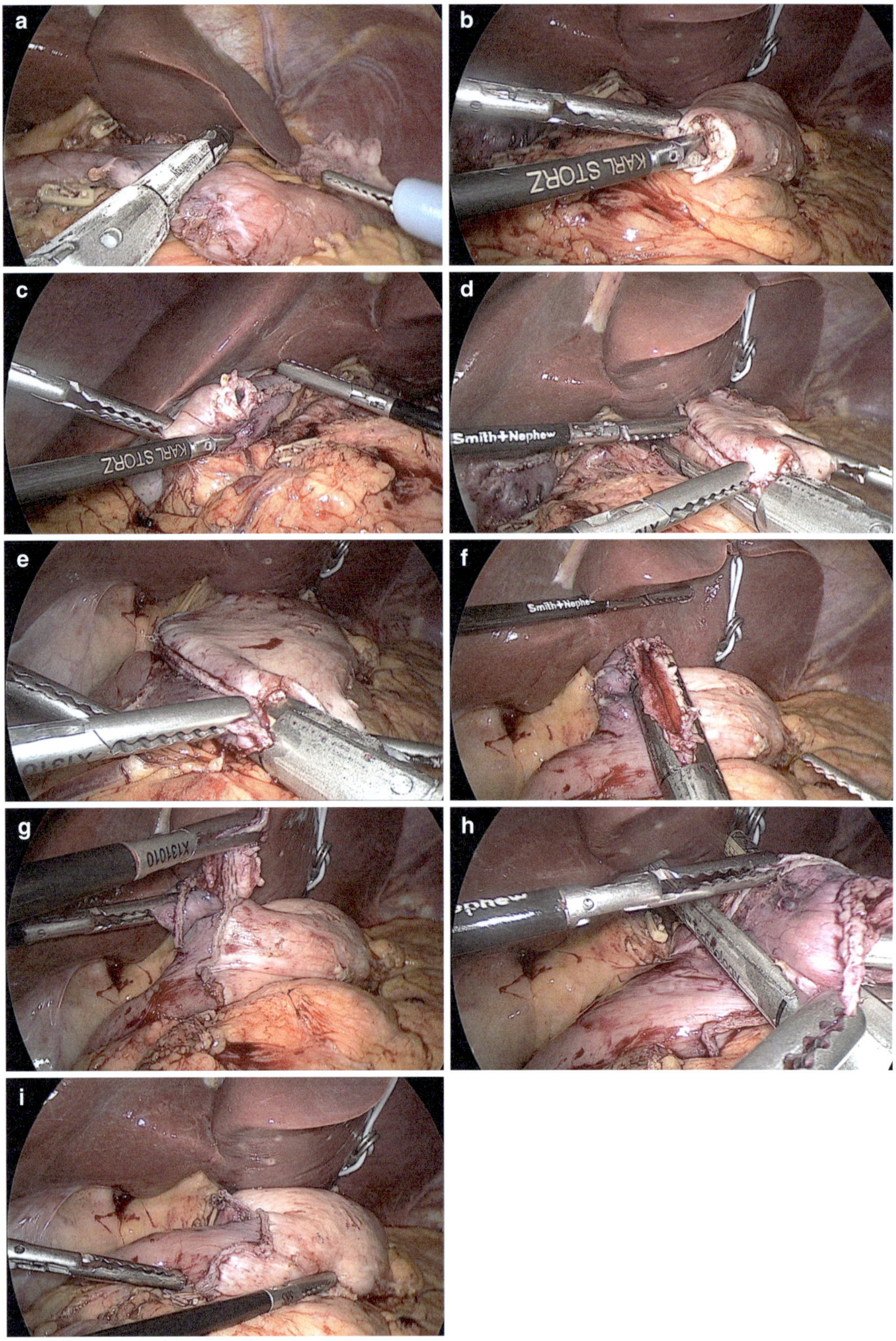
a
b
KARL STORZ
c
KARL STORZ
d
Smith+Nephew
e
f
Smith+Nephew
g
X13010
h
i

Fig. 4.3 (**a**) Duodenal dissection. A 60-mm LS was used to transect the duodenum and the stomach, from the greater curvature to the lesser curvature. (**b**) Creating a gastric stump insertion hole. The resection margin at the greater curvature of the gastric stump was left open to create an insertion hole for the LS. (**c**) Creating a duodenal stump insertion hole. The resection margin at the greater curvature of the duodenal stump was left open to create an insertion hole for the LS. (**d**) Insertion of LS into the stomach. The thicker jaw of the first 60-mm LS was inserted into the stomach via the lower left port. (**e**) First suture (creation of posterior and cranial wall). The posterior wall of the stomach and the posterior duodenum should not be shifted. While grasping the stomach and duodenum, the LS was fired. (**f**) Second suture (creation of tail side wall). Using a 30-mm LS, we closed the duodenal wall and the gastric wall near the greater curvature to close the previous insertion hole. This suture should be stopped just before the duodenal dissection line. (**g**) Third suture preparation and line setting. A 60-mm LS was used to create the anterior sidewall of the rectangle while the entire stapled duodenal stump was being removed. (**h**) Third suture (creation of anterior side wall). Meanwhile, the assistant adjusted the position of the LS to ensure overlap between the two suture lines, the first being along the second staple line, and the second being along with the gastric stump. (**i**) Completion of ART. The end-to-end anastomosis with an augmented rectangular gastroduodenal anastomotic stoma was completed

4.5.1.1 Duodenal and Gastric Dissection

A 60-mm LS was used to transect the duodenum and the stomach, from the greater curvature to the lesser curvature. It does not need to twist from the posterior wall to the anterior wall, but it should be cut as close to the pyloric ring as possible to insert the 60-mm LS into the duodenum (Fig. 4.3). The superior duodenal vessels along the lesser curvature were transected to mobilize the duodenum.

4.5.1.2 Creating an Insertion Hole

An insertion hole was deliberately left in the resection margin along the greater curvature of both the gastric and duodenal stump, with the purpose of creating an access point for the LS (Fig. 4.3b, c). By separating from the staple line side, the displacement between the mucous membrane and the muscular layer was reduced, and an accurate diameter could be created.

4.5.1.3 Insertion of LS into the Stomach and Movement to the Duodenum Side

The thicker jaw of the initial 60-mm LS device found its way into the stomach through the lower left port. Subsequently, with precision, the LS tip was firmly applied against the posterior gastric wall, consistently keeping it 2 cm apart from the gastric resection margin. This strategic placement allowed us to skillfully secure the tissue near the suture line in close proximity to the insertion hole using the LS (Fig. 4.3d). The LS that grips the stomach toward the duodenal transection margin should be handled carefully.

4.5.1.4 Induction of the Duodenum

The LS was opened, and the duodenum was slowly inserted into the LS so that the surgeon covered the thinner jaw. At this time as well, the assistant could grasp the duodenal dissection staple line and guide it to cover this jaw to avoid duodenal injury. The duodenal dissection staple line should be placed closer to the gastric dissection staple line near the insertion hole. The margin of resection at the lesser curvature end of the duodenum was rotated externally by 90°.

4.5.1.5 First Suture (Creation of Posterior and Cranial Wall)

The posterior wall of the stomach and the posterior duodenum should not be shifted. While grasping the stomach and duodenum, the LS was fired (Fig. 4.3e). This first firing to open the separation line created two sides, which become the rectangular posterior and cranial wall. Then, we removed the LS jaw while closing it and observed the anastomotic site through the lumen to confirm that the traction was appropriate without bleeding.

4.5.1.6 Second Suture (Creation of Tail Side Wall)

Next, the valgus suture of the anterior wall and the tail side wall was systematically performed twice. Using a 30-mm LS, we closed the duodenal wall and the gastric wall near the greater curvature to close the previous insertion hole. This suture should be stopped just before the duodenal dissection line (Fig. 4.3f). The surgeon should grasp the cranial and caudal ends of a V-shaped suture line created with the first LS to ensure that the gastric and duodenal resection margins remain closed together. This created the tail sidewall of a rectangle.

4.5.1.7 Third Suture (Creation of Anterior Side Wall)

Following this step, a 60-mm LS was employed to shape the anterior sidewall of the rectangle while simultaneously removing the entire stapled duodenal stump. The surgeon applied caudolateral tension to manipulate the duodenal stump (Fig. 4.3g). Meanwhile, the assistant made adjustments to the LS's position to ensure that the two suture lines overlapped correctly. The first suture line followed the second staple line, while the second suture line ran alongside the gastric stump (Fig. 4.3h). This suturing technique concluded the end-to-end anastomosis, resulting in the creation of an augmented rectangular gastroduodenal anastomotic stoma (Fig. 4.3i).

4.5.2 HDST Using EEA™OrVil™ for Esophagojejunostomy in Laparoscopic Total Gastrectomy

We perform an HDST in esophagojejunostomy with EEA™OrVil™ in which HDST at the left end of the esophagus (greater curvature end) was selected to guide the tube and to bury the suture easily at the intersection of the LS and CS. The advantages of esophagojejunostomy using EEA™OrVil™ are (1) it can be reconstructed by the same procedure as open surgery, (2) the anastomosis can be placed without opening the digestive tract, (3) the anastomosis can be induced despite the patient's body shape, (4) minimal esophageal detachment can be anastomosed, and (5) higher anastomosis and additional excision are also possible.

4.5.2.1 Esophageal Dissection

After lymph node dissection, we inserted a 60-mm LS from the lower right abdominal port and dissected the esophagus. It is important to dissect the esophagus slightly diagonally from the lesser curvature side to the greater curvature side with respect to the long axis direction (Fig. 4.4).

4.5.2.2 Preparation of Elevated Jejunum and Y Limb (Added Aboral Pouch)

Laparoscopically, the jejunum was marked 30 cm from the Treitz ligament and pulled out of the abdominal cavity through a small incision in the umbilical region.

Then, the jejunum was dissected at the marked site using a 60-mm LS. The distance from the esophagojejunostomy to the Y limb was approximately 40 cm. We added an aboral pouch to the Y limb to reduce postoperative weight loss and improve quality of life (Fig. 4.4b).

Fig. 4.4 (**a**) Esophageal dissection. We inserted a 60-mm LS from the lower right abdominal port and dissect the esophagus. (**b**) Preparation of elevated jejunum and Y limb (added aboral pouch). The distance from the esophagojejunostomy to the Y limb was approximately 40 cm. We added an aboral pouch to the Y limb. (**c**) Circular stapler insertion. An incision was made at the blind end of the elevated jejunum, and the EEA™CS (25XL) was inserted into the Roux limb end. (**d**) Intraperitoneal insertion of CS with surgical gloves. The CS was guided into the abdominal cavity through a small umbilical incision using surgical gloves. (**e**) The OrVil™ tube transorally insertion. After confirming that the tip of the tube (valve tip) has reached the esophageal stump, it was pressed lightly against the left end (greater curvature end) of the esophageal stump to make a small hole. (**f**) Join the anvil. With the use of left-hand forceps, the anvil's plastic collar is held, and the CS is operated on with the surgeon's right hand to join the anvil. (**g**) Esophagojejunostomy. The anvil is adjusted with the surgeon's left-hand so that the axis and angle match, and confirm that firmly joined to the orange mark on the CS. (**h**) Reinforcement of the anastomotic site. The intersection of the LS and the CS is buried with a serosal muscular layer suture. (**i**) Duodenal stump burial and elevated jejunum fixation. The duodenal stump is buried with non-absorbable 3-0-VLoc™ followed by fixation of the elevated jejunum to the duodenal stump

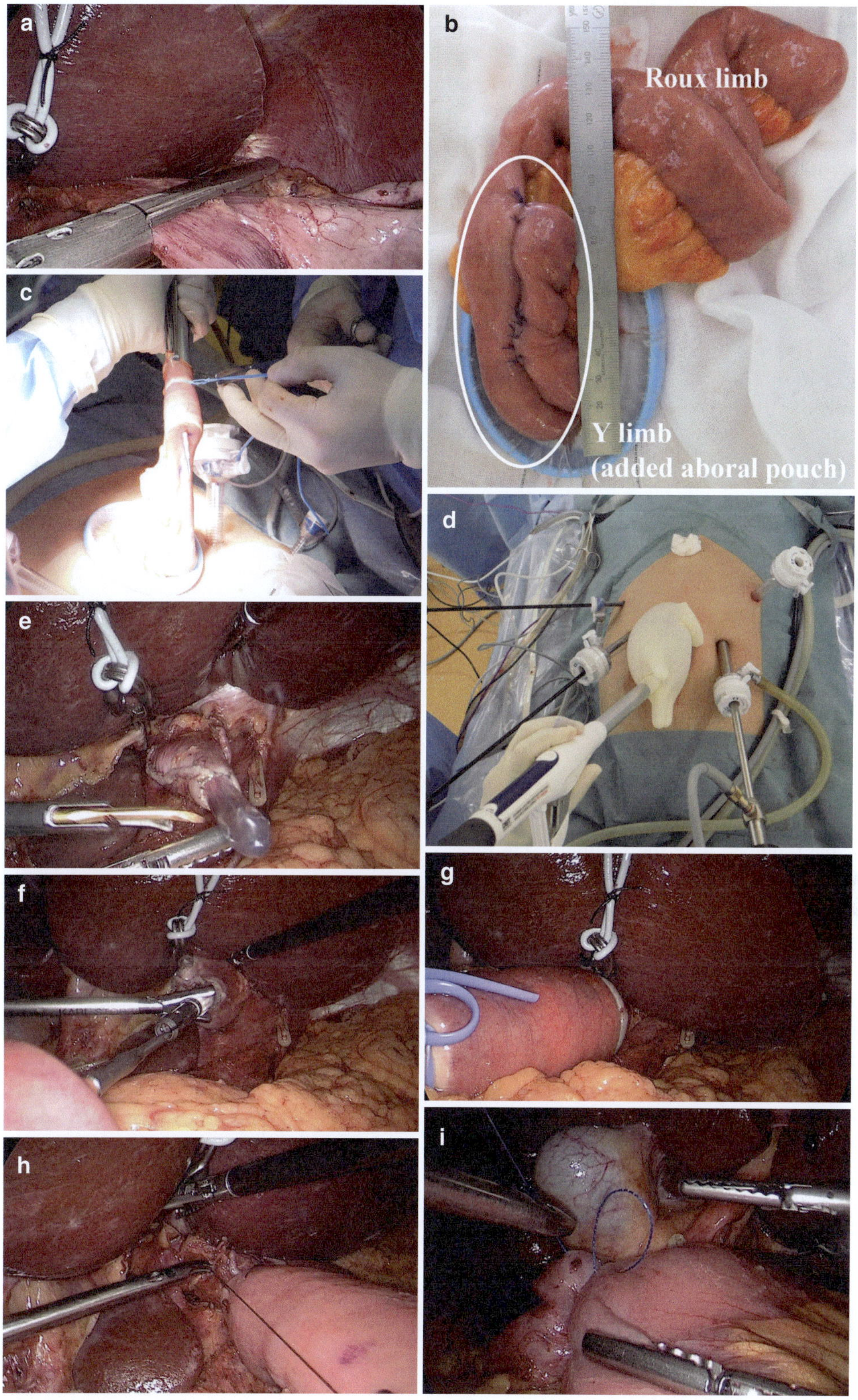
a
b
Roux limb
Y limb
(added aboral pouch)
c
d
e
f
g
h
i

4.5.2.3 CS Insertion

An incision was made at the blind end of the elevated jejunum, and the EEA™CS (25XL) was inserted into the Roux limb end. The insertion length of the CS into the Roux limb end was approximately 10 cm, and it was fixed with a vessel loop, and the center rod of the CS was pulled out from the center of the jejunum (Fig. 4.4c). The CS was guided into the abdominal cavity through a small umbilical incision using surgical gloves (Fig. 4.4d).

4.5.2.4 The OrVil™ Tube Transoral Insertion

We usually used a 25 mm OrVil™ to insert through the oral cavity while expanding the larynx. When inserting the tube, the anvil head should pass horizontally through the pharynx and slowly guide it until it disappeared from the oral cavity. Upon verifying that the tube's tip (valve tip) had reached the esophageal stump, it was gently applied to the left extremity (greater curvature end) of the esophageal stump to create a small triangular hole, approximately 5 mm in size (Fig. 4.4e) with caution not to make them too large holes. Then, the guide tube was readied and carefully drawn out through the small hole, leading it into the abdominal cavity until the anvil reached the esophageal stump. While the tube was slowly guided with the feeling of the resistance of the tube with the operator's forceps, the assistant pulled it out of the abdominal cavity from the upper left abdominal trocar. Before passing through the physiological stricture of the esophagus (corresponding to the area marked approximately 25–30 cm on the tube in OrVil™), the assistant removed the patient's pillow, extended the neck, and raised the lower jaw. This treatment avoids esophageal damage and enables smooth insertion. When the plastic collar of the center rod comes out, grasp it with forceps. Following that, one end of the thread securing the anvil was severed, and the tube connected to the anvil was extricated from the extraperitoneal space. As a result, the anvil is fixed to the left end (greater curvature end) of the esophageal stump.

4.5.2.5 Esophagojejunostomy

With the use of left-hand forceps, the anvil's plastic collar is held, and the CS is operated on with the surgeon's right hand to join the anvil (Fig. 4.4f). At this time, the anvil is adjusted with the surgeon's left hand so that the axis and angle match, and confirm that it is firmly joined to the orange mark on the CS. It is important to grasp the elevated jejunum using left-hand forceps and deploy it to the head side and ensure that there is no twist or entanglement (Fig. 4.4g). The insertion position of the camera is changed as appropriate to confirm the anastomosis status from various directions. Then, the CS is closed, and the tightening index is checked and fired. At the time of anastomosis, one should be careful to push the CS instead of pulling the anvil. Then, the vessel loop is cut, the CS is removed, and the blind end of the elevated jejunum is closed with a 60-mm LS to complete the esophagojejunostomy. The intersection of the LS and the CS is buried with a serosal muscular layer suture (Fig. 4.4h).

4.5.2.6 Duodenal Stump Burial and Elevated Jejunum Fixation

The duodenal stump is buried with nonabsorbable 3-0-VLoc™ followed by fixation of the elevated jejunum to the duodenal stump to prevent internal hernia, twisting of the elevated jejunum to reduce anastomotic tension (Fig. 4.4i). Petersen's defect is closed with sutures.

4.6 Postoperative Management

Drinking water was resumed on the 1st day after the operation, and liquid diet was started on the 3rd or 4th day after the operation and gradually returned to the normal diet. Postoperative fluoroscopy was not routine. Normally, a closed drain was placed on the pancreas until after resuming meals with no problems. Doctors, nurses, and dietitians continued to provide dietary and nutritional guidance.

4.7 Complications

Table 4.1 shows the operative results of our institution. Anastomosis-related complications are very low. Recently, good results on long-term postgastrectomy syndrome and quality of life were reported [8].

Table 4.1 Operative results

July 2016 to March 2020		
	TLDG ART (*n* = 137)	TLTG HDST OrVil (*n* = 52)
Operative time (median) (min)	276	340
Bleeding (median) (mL)	33	15
Postoperative complication CD3≦	10 (7.3%)	3 (5.7%)
Anastomotic-related complication		
Anastomotic leakage	2 (1.4%)	1 (1.9%)
Anastomotic bleeding	1 (0.7%)	0 (0%)
Anastomotic stenosis	0 (0%)	0 (0%)

TLDG totally laparoscopic distal gastrectomy, *ART* augmented rectangle technique. *TLTG* totally laparoscopic total gastrectomy, *HDST* hemi-double stapling technique, *CD* Clavien-Dindo

4.8 Personal Experience

We have innovatively developed and delineated a minimally invasive reconstruction technique following totally laparoscopic gastrectomy. This approach stands out for its simplicity, safety, and exceptionally low postoperative complication rates, rendering it an invaluable method. We obtained the necessary permissions to utilize the figures and tables featured in this chapter.

Acknowledgments All authors acknowledge no forms of financial support, including technical assistance and advice. We would like to thank Enago (www.enago.jp) for the English language review.

Funding No funding was received for this report.

Conflicts of Interest Statement The authors declare that they have no conflicts of interests.

References

1. Shen J, Ma X, Yang J, et al. Digestive tract reconstruction options after laparoscopic gastrectomy for gastric cancer. World J Gastrointest Oncol. 2020;12(1):21–36.
2. Fukunaga T, Hiki N, Tokunaga M, et al. Left-sided approach for suprapancreatic lymph node dissection in laparoscopy-assisted distal gastrectomy without duodenal transection. Gastric Cancer. 2009;12(2):106–12.
3. Fukunaga T, Hiki N, Kubota T, et al. Oncologic outcomes of laparoscopy-assisted distal gastrectomy for gastric cancer. Ann Surg Oncol. 2013;20(8):2676–82.
4. Fukunaga T, Ishibashi Y, Oka S, et al. Augmented rectangle technique for Billroth I anastomosis in totally laparoscopic distal gastrectomy for gastric cancer. Surg Endosc. 2018;32(9):4011–6.
5. Wu JZ, Fukunaga T, Oka S, et al. Comparative study of outcomes of Roux-en-Y reconstruction and Billroth I reconstruction performed after radical distal gastrectomy. Asian J Surg. 2019;42(1):379–85.
6. Wu JZ, Orita H, Zhang S, et al. Easy fixation effects the prevention of Peterson's hernia and Roux stasis syndrome. World J Gastrointest Surg. 2020;12(8):346–54.
7. Ishibashi Y, Oka S, Kanda S, et al. Hemi-double stapling technique performed with a transorally inserted anvil for esophagojejunostomy in the surgical treatment of gastric cancer. Asian J Endosc Surg. 2020;13(2):168–74.
8. Yamauchi S, Orita H, Chen J, et al. Long-term outcomes of postgastrectomy syndrome after total laparoscopic distal gastrectomy using the augmented rectangle technique. World J Gastrointest Surg. 2022;14(2):120–31.

Minimally Invasive Anatomic Liver Resection

5

Yusuke Ome and Goro Honda

Abstract

In laparoscopic anatomic liver resection (LALR), correct dissection of the Glissonean pedicles and careful exposure of the hepatic veins are essential. Therefore, LALR requires not only basic knowledge and procedures but also advanced techniques.

In laparoscopic liver resection (LLR), it is essential to control bleeding. The Pringle maneuver, which suppresses bleeding from both the inflow and outflow systems, should be usually prepared before initiating liver parenchymal dissection. To prevent venous bleeding, we have to understand the relationship among the central venous pressure, airway pressure, and pneumoperitoneal pressure, and adjust those pressures appropriately. The direction of approach to the hepatic veins is also important to avoid a split injury, which may cause critical bleeding. The hepatic veins should be approached from the central to the peripheral side.

The secondary or tertiary branches of the Glissonean pedicles are dissected in LALR. In open liver resection (OLR), the secondary branches are comparatively easy to dissect extrahepatically from the hepatic hilum. However, the correct dissection of these branches by laparoscopic surgery is sometimes difficult owing to restrictions in the manipulation of laparoscopic instruments. As for the tertiary branches, it is more difficult to dissect correctly even in OLR because the tertiary branches often ramify in the deep portions inside the liver. We have developed various approaches to isolate secondary and tertiary branches safely, taking advantage of laparoscopic surgery. The Arantius-first approach in left hemihepatectomy, caudate lobe-first approach in right hemihepatectomy or right posterior sectionectomy, and intrahepatic Glissonean approach to G7 or G8 are useful procedures, and described here in detail.

Keywords

Laparoscopic liver resection · Anatomic liver resection · Glissonean approach · Pringle maneuver · Hemihepatectomy · Sectionectomy · Segmentectomy

Supplementary Information The online version contains supplementary material available at https://doi.org/10.1007/978-981-97-7059-5_5.

Y. Ome · G. Honda (✉)
Department of Surgery, Institute of Gastroenterology, Tokyo Women's Medical University, Shinjuku-ku, Tokyo, Japan
e-mail: honda.goro@twmu.ac.jp

M. Tewari (ed.), *Minimally Invasive Surgery in Cancer*,
https://doi.org/10.1007/978-981-97-7059-5_5

5.1 Introduction

Laparoscopic liver resection (LLR) has been rapidly developed recently, and its feasibility and efficacy have been reported in various studies [1–4]. In anatomic liver resection, correct dissection of the Glissonean pedicles and careful exposure of the hepatic veins are essential. Therefore, laparoscopic anatomic liver resection (LALR) requires not only basic knowledge and procedures but also advanced techniques. The Second International Consensus Conference on LLR held in Morioka in 2014 concluded that major LLR, defined as trisectionectomy, bisectionectomy, hemihepatectomy, and resection of the posterosuperior segments comprising segment (S)1, S7, and S8 remains an innovative procedure and is still in the exploratory learning phase [5].

LLR has many advantages over open liver resection (OLR). A magnified caudodorsal view of the laparoscope enables meticulous procedures and unique laparoscopic approaches different from OLR [6–13]. Additionally, pneumoperitoneal pressure (PPP) in laparoscopic surgery potentially reduces blood loss from the hepatic veins during liver parenchymal dissection. On the contrary, LLR has some disadvantages, such as lack of tactile sense, instrument movement restriction, and direction misidentification. We have devised and standardized various procedures in LALR with the benefits of laparoscopic surgery, overcoming its disadvantages. In this section, we describe the basic procedures and unique laparoscopic approaches of LALR, focusing on how to dissect the Glissonean pedicles and expose the hepatic veins.

5.2 Indications for LALR

The indications for LLR have gradually expanded. Currently, almost all types of procedures, including major hepatectomy but excluding extrahepatic bile duct resection, can be successfully performed in experienced institutes. We have performed approximately 1000 LLR, and all types of LALR have been already standardized. Rehepatectomy is also aggressively performed laparoscopically. In fact, conversions to open surgery and blood transfusions are extremely rare in our institute. However, there are several limitations to LLR in terms of technical aspects, tumor characteristics, and the patients' condition, among others, owing to prolonged operation time, decreased curability, and increased risks of bleeding and severe complications. The true goal of LLR is to be minimally invasive for the patient. Therefore, the indication criteria for LALR should be rigorously determined with an understanding of the limitations of laparoscopic surgery [14].

5.3 Preoperative Management

Blood tests including hepatitis B virus antigen, hepatitis C virus antibody, hepatobiliary enzymes, tumor markers, and indocyanine green (ICG) retention test are performed to evaluate liver function and operative tolerance. Dynamic contrast-enhanced computed tomography (DCE-CT) and gadolinium-ethoxybenzyl-diethylenetriamine pentaacetic acid magnetic resonance imaging (EOB-MRI) are used to diagnose the tumor and to understand the intrahepatic vascular anatomy. If possible, preoperative simulation is helpful using 3D image construction to recognize the location of the tumor and vascular structures from a laparoscopic view. The resected and residual liver volume are measured, and the appropriate surgical procedure is determined in consideration of liver function [15].

5.4 Basic Knowledge and Procedures for LALR

5.4.1 Pringle Maneuver (Video 5.1)

During hepatectomy, bleeding control is the most important. The Pringle maneuver, which is an intermittent vascular occlusion technique implemented by clamping the hepatoduodenal ligament, is widely used for reducing blood loss in both OLR and LLR. The Pringle maneuver not only suppresses bleeding from the inflow systems, including the hepatic artery and portal vein, but also decreases venous bleeding due to a reduction in blood flowing into the liver. We previously reported a convenient laparoscopic method for the Pringle maneuver, using an extracorporeal tourniquet system [16]. The Pringle maneuver is usually performed before initiating liver parenchymal transection.

First, a 5 mm trocar is inserted where you plan to place the tourniquet for the Pringle maneuver. The foramen of Winslow should be carefully observed and checked for adhesions. The forceps are then inserted via the rightmost lateral trocar and advanced through the foramen of Winslow toward the lesser omentum (Fig. 5.1a). After a small incision is made in the lesser omentum, the tip of the forceps is exposed. The hepatoduodenal ligament is taped by pulling the tape out with forceps. Both ends of the tape with the 5 mm trocar are pulled outside the body. The tape is passed through a 22 Fr catheter with a length of 20 cm, and the catheter is inserted into the abdominal cavity through the 5 mm trocar hole. A 22 Fr catheter fits perfectly into a 5 mm trocar and prevents air leaks. When the tourniquet is closed, the inflow is transiently blocked (Fig. 5.1b). The tourniquet system can be freely and easily opened and closed from outside the body. The Pringle maneuver is initiated only when the operative field cannot be kept dry due to bleeding.

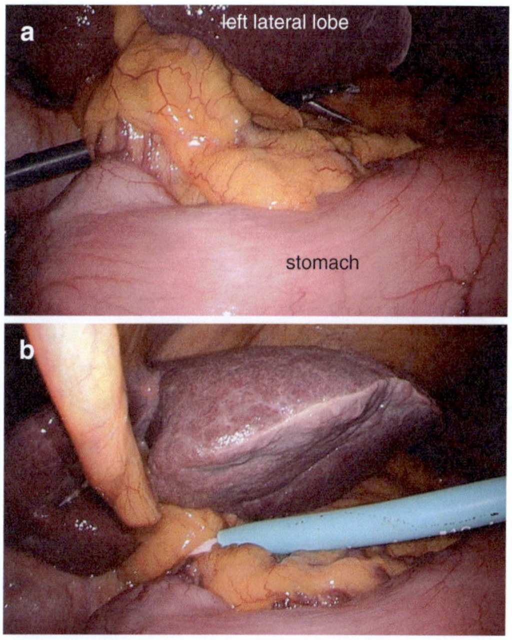

Fig. 5.1 Pringle maneuver. (**a**) Isolation of the hepatoduodenal ligament, (**b**) extracorporeal tourniquet system

5.4.2 Pressure Control Associated with LLR

To prevent venous bleeding in LLR, it is particularly important to correctly understand the relationship among three pressures and to adjust them appropriately: the central venous pressure (CVP), airway pressure (AWP), and PPP [17].

It is widely acknowledged that CVP must be kept low to reduce bleeding from the hepatic veins. In close cooperation with anesthesiologists, the amount of fluid infusion should be reduced as much as possible until the liver parenchymal division is completed. Additionally, Yoneda et al. [18] reported that CVP can be lowered by setting the body to the reverse Trendelenberg position. In LLR, the patient is usually tilted to the head-up position, or the reverse Trendelenberg position, in order to pull out the liver existing in the diaphragmatic fossa and move it to a position where it is easy to operate. Raising the hepatic dissection site higher than the inferior vena cava (IVC) also reduces the hepatic vein pressure and bleeding.

PPP is beneficial to reduce bleeding from the hepatic veins. To reduce bleeding, some surgeons may elevate the PPP. However, PPP elevation is associated with the risk of pulmonary gas embolism [19]. The following should be well understood. As previously reported, there are positive correlations between AWP and CVP, and between PPP and CVP. Under high AWP, CVP is persistently higher than PPP, even when PPP is increased. That is, bleeding from the hepatic veins cannot be reduced through PPP elevation under high AWP. Under low AWP, CVP does not increase relative to PPP and often decreases when PPP is increased. Therefore, PPP may become much higher than CVP under low AWP, and the risk of pulmonary gas embolism increases. Reducing AWP lowers CVP, and is effective for controlling bleeding from the hepatic veins and is safer than increasing PPP. It is recommended that PPP is never elevated for bleeding reduction; instead, the AWP is reduced and sometimes ventilation is stopped for hemostasis. In LALR, the liver parenchyma is divided along the hepatic veins; therefore, appropriate pressure control of CVP, AWP, and PPP is especially important. We always maintain PPP at 10 mmHg and keep CVP as low as possible in cooperation with the anesthesiologist. AWP is not lowered under normal circumstances, but is lowered only in the event of massive bleeding.

5.4.3 Approach to Hepatic Veins (Video 5.2)

During liver parenchymal dissection, hepatic veins appear in the cutting plane. In LALR, a thicker hepatic vein, usually one of the major hepatic veins or their thick branches, is exposed in the cutting plane, and thinner hepatic vein branches into the thicker vein have to be divided at the confluence. Dissection of the hepatic branches from the peripheral side sometimes causes a split injury, which extends to the thicker side of the thicker hepatic vein, and may cause severe and critical bleeding. This type of injury can be prevented by exposing the hepatic vein trunk from the thicker (root) side toward the thinner (peripheral) side [20] (Fig. 5.2). We mainly used CUSA® EXcel (Integra LifeSciences Corporation, Plainsboro, NJ, USA) and always tried to approach the major hepatic veins and all hepatic vein branches moving the tip of the CUSA® from the thicker (root) side toward the thinner (peripheral) side. The CUSA® also performs sucking and stanching as well as fracturing of the liver parenchyma as a single device, by applying electrocautery at soft coagulation mode. The device does not need to be changed frequently, and the liver parenchyma can be dissected while keeping a dry surgical field. We usually do not use other suction or hemostatic devices.

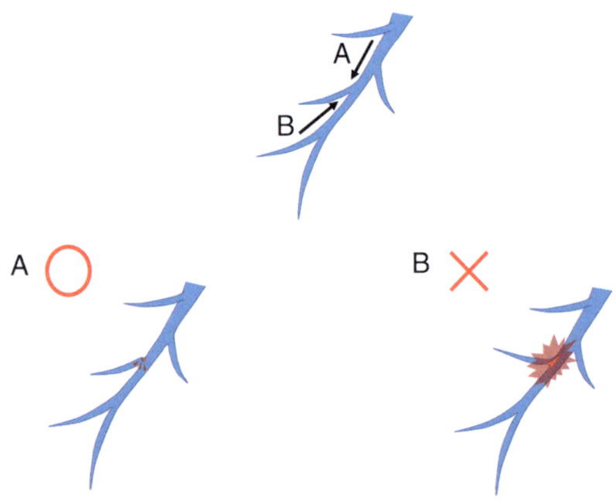

Fig. 5.2 Proper approach to hepatic veins

5.4.4 Glissonean Approach

In major anatomic liver resection such as hemihepatectomy and sectionectomy, there are two methods for dividing the inflow systems: one is the individual dissection of the hepatic artery, portal vein, and bile duct, and the other is the Glissonean approach. The Glissonean approach is a safe and useful method and is preferred except in cases where tumor invades the vicinity of the hepatic hilum. The Glissonean pedicle is composed of the hepatic artery, portal vein, and bile duct, all wrapped with connective tissue. In this approach, the pedicle is divided all at once, and the territory fed by the Glissonean pedicle is confirmed as the ischemic area and is removed [21]. The Glissonean approach is standard for anatomic resections smaller than a sectionectomy. Here, we describe the Glissonean approach.

The Glissonean pedicles are approached extrahepatically or intrahepatically. In the extrahepatic Glissonean approach, the Glissonean pedicle is dissected from the liver parenchyma at the hepatic hilum. The secondary branches of the Glissonean pedicles are located outside the liver, and more peripheral branches run inside the liver. Therefore, the secondary branches can be relatively easily dissected and encircled extrahepatically during OLR. However, the correct dissection of these branches by laparoscopic surgery is sometimes difficult owing to restrictions in the manipulation of laparoscopic instruments. Therefore, we devised procedures for easy and safe dissection of the secondary Glissonean branches [9, 10, 13].

Tertiary branches can be dissected by further dissection along the secondary branches toward the periphery when the pedicles ramify close to the hepatic hilum. However, that procedure is technically difficult, depending on the branching patterns. The tertiary branches in the left lobe are comparatively easy to dissect because these branches originate from the umbilical portion. On the other hand, the branches in the right lobe, especially the branches feeding S7 and S8, ramify in the deep portions inside the liver, and are difficult to approach from the hepatic hilum. In such cases, the intrahepatic Glissonean approach is useful. Tertiary and more peripheral branches can be approached intrahepatically after initially dissecting the liver parenchyma [21, 22]. The initial cutting line is determined by clamping the secondary pedicle or by referring to the hepatic vein that runs on the intersegmental plane because the thick hepatic veins, including the major hepatic vein trunks such as the left, middle, and right hepatic veins, usually run on the boundary between the segments or sections.

The intrahepatic Glissonean approach has several advantages. In the extrahepatic approach to the Glissonean branch of S7 (G7) and of S8 (G8), the secondary branches and other Glissonean pedicles that must be preserved have to be exposed, and small branches from the hepatic hilum or the secondary branches may be injured. These factors can increase the risk of postoperative biliary leakage and delayed biliary strictures. Furthermore, it is beneficial for the next hepatectomy, which is often required for hepatocellular carcinoma and colorectal liver metastases, to keep the hepatic hilum intact as much as possible. Therefore, we adopted the intrahepatic Glissonean approach for the anatomic resection of S7 and S8 [8, 11, 12].

5.5 Laparoscopic Unique Approach Utilizing a Laparoscopic Caudodorsal View (Videos 5.3 and 5.4)

OLR is usually performed in a ventral view, in which the Glissonean pedicles and hepatic veins cross each other (Fig. 5.3a). By contrast, a caudodorsal view is typical because a laparoscope is inserted from around the umbilicus or the caudal side of the liver (Fig. 5.3b). In a caudodorsal view, the origins of the Glissonean branches and hepatic veins are located on the dorsal center side of the liver, and they run radially and branch similar to a tree [23]. Therefore, we can easily predict and recognize the direction in which the vessels run. The major hepatic vein trunk runs in the intersegmental plane, which is the border between the segments and sectors. Theoretically, no Glissonean branch runs in this plane. During sectionectomy or hemihepatectomy, we can easily identify and dissect along the correct intersegmental plane by initiating parenchymal transection at the root of the Glissonean tree (i.e., the hepatic hilum) and continuing it toward the periphery, exposing the major hepatic vein trunk (Fig. 5.3c). Moreover, dissection along the hepatic vein from the root side toward the periphery can prevent a split injury. The caudodorsal approach is thus suitable and advantageous for laparoscopic surgery, and LLR can be performed using a different procedure from the open one. However, since the laparoscopic magnified operative view is significantly different from the open view, it is important to recognize landmarks to avoid disorientation. We present our standardized unique laparoscopic approach with exposed landmarks.

5.5.1 The Arantius-First Approach in Left Hemihepatectomy [7, 13]

In left hemihepatectomy, the left Glissonean pedicle (Glt) should be correctly divided, and the middle hepatic vein (MHV) is exposed on the cutting plane. The Arantius' duct is an important landmark to divide the Glt safely and identify an appropriate cutting plane. The Arantius' duct connects the root of the umbilical portion of the left portal branch and the root of the left hepatic vein (LHV) or the common trunk of the LHV and MHV, and is the border between the left and the Spiegel lobe. A bile duct from the right lobe (e.g., the right posterior branch) sometimes joins the

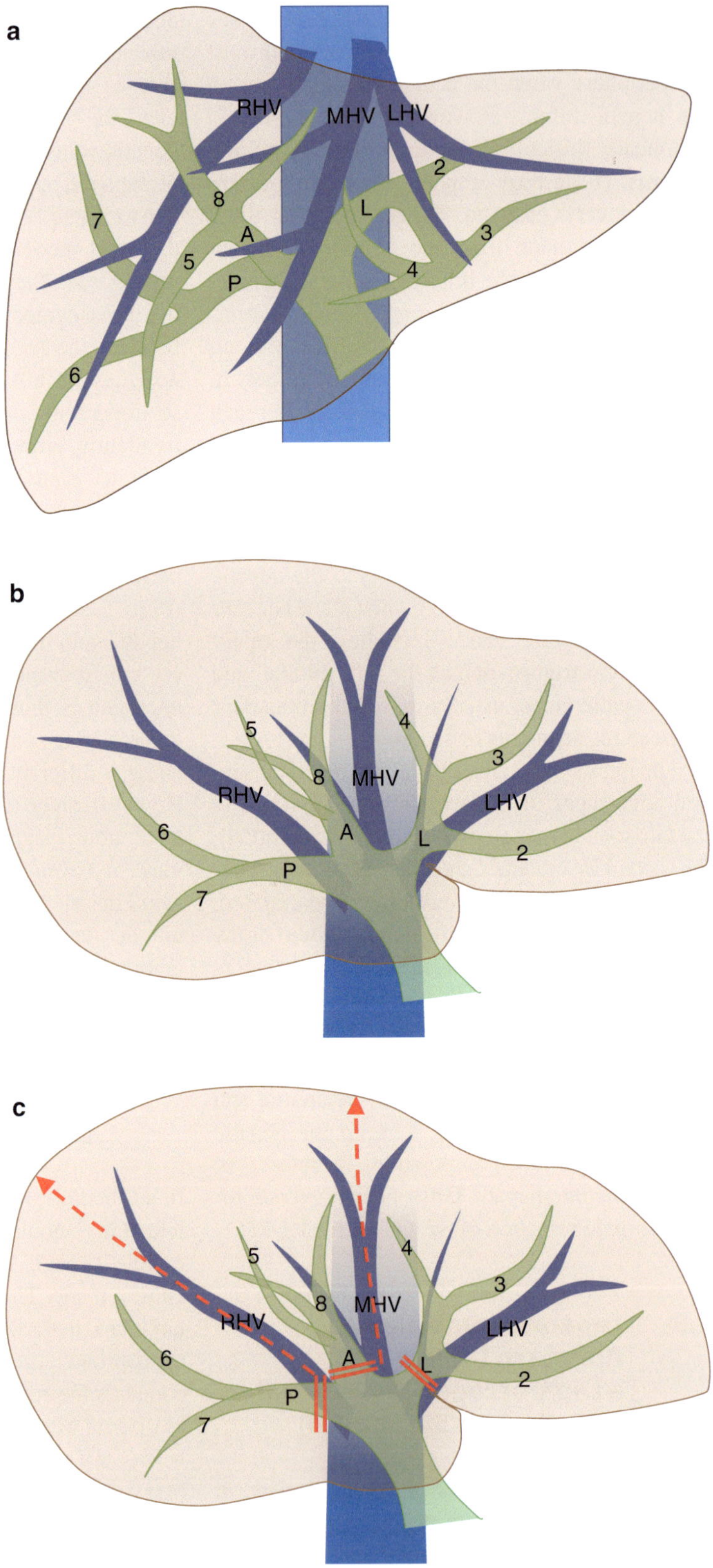

Fig. 5.3 The differences of the operative view between OLR and LLR. (**a**) Ventral view of the liver (typical view in OLR), (**b**) Caudodorsal view of the liver (typical view in LLR), (**c**) caudodorsal approach in LLR

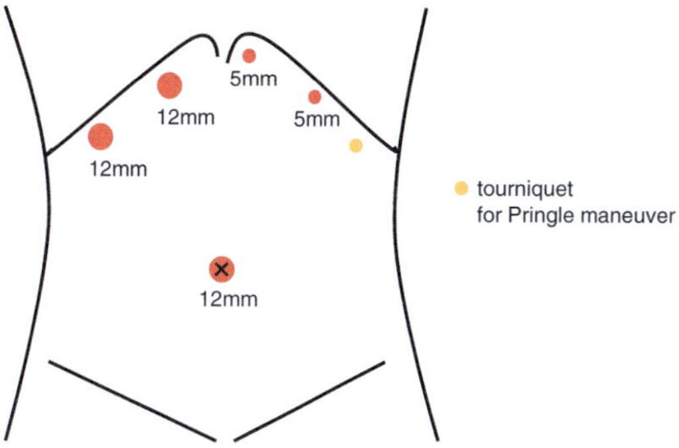

Fig. 5.4 The trocar placement in laparoscopic left hemihepatectomy

left hepatic duct below the bifurcation of the Arantius' duct. The Glt can be divided safely just above the bifurcation of the Arantius' duct without injury to the bile duct from the right lobe.

The patient is placed in a supine position. The trocar placement is illustrated in Fig. 5.4. Following mobilization of the left lateral section and exposure of the roots of the LHV and MHV, the Arantius' duct is identified between the left lateral section and the Spiegel's lobe, upturning the left lateral section (Fig. 5.5a). Liver parenchyma just above the Arantius' duct is dissected

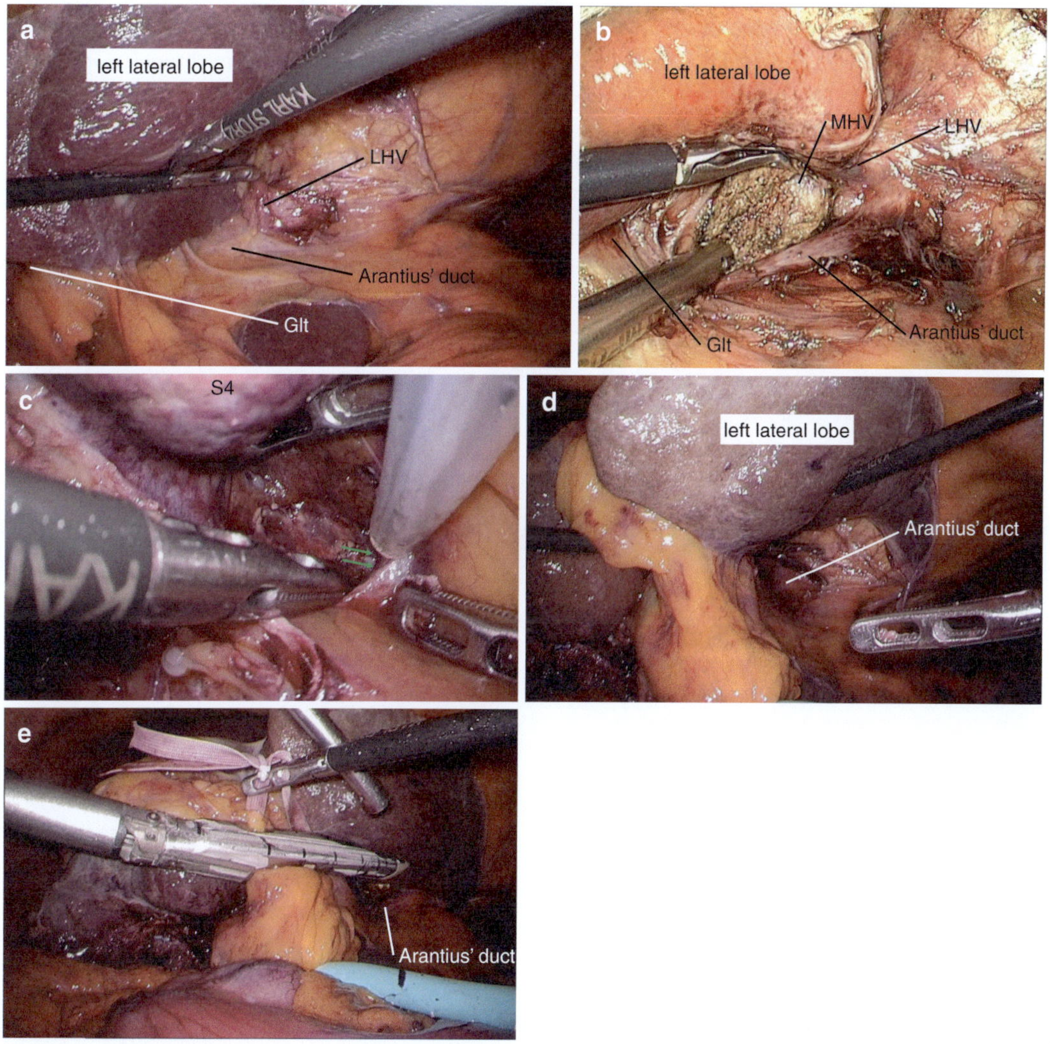

Fig. 5.5 Arantius-first approach. (**a**) Identification of Arantius' duct, (**b**) exposure of the posterior aspect of Gleft and the MHV, (**c**) dissection of the right aspect of Gleft, arrow: the right aspect of Gleft, (**d**) dissection of Gleft, (**e**) division of Gleft

and opened widely between the root of the LHV and the Glt. The left posterior aspect of the Glt is exposed, and some space is reserved behind the Glt. In the same operative view, the root of the MHV can be identified at a deeper portion of the root of the LHV (Fig. 5.5b). Then, the left medial section (S4) is separated from the hilar plate and the right aspect of the Glt (Fig. 5.5c). Because some space has already been reserved behind the Glt, Glt can be easily and safely encircled (Fig. 5.5d) and divided using a linear stapler inserted via the 12 mm trocar at the right most lateral below the right costal arch (Fig. 5.5e). After the division of the Glt, the parenchyma is dissected from the caudal edge of the liver along the demarcation line. The MHV is approached from its dorsal side by holding up the left lobe and continuously exposed from the root side toward the periphery (Fig. 5.6a). After the main trunk of the MHV is exposed, the liver parenchyma between the MHV and the demarcation line on the liver surface is divided cranially by moving the tip of the CUSA® from the MHV side toward the demarcation line, i.e., from the dorsal to the ventral side (Fig. 5.6b). Finally, the LHV is divided at its origin, and left hemihepatectomy is completed (Fig. 5.6c).

5.5.2 The Caudate Lobe-First Approach in Right Hemihepatectomy or Right Posterior Sectionectomy [9, 10]

The caudate lobe-first approach is useful for easy and safe dissection of the right Glissonean pedicle (Grt) or the right posterior branch (Gpost), as well as early exposure of the IVC, which is an important landmark for advancing the division of the liver parenchyma along the correct intersegmental plane.

The patient is placed in a modified left semidecubitus position in which only the upper body

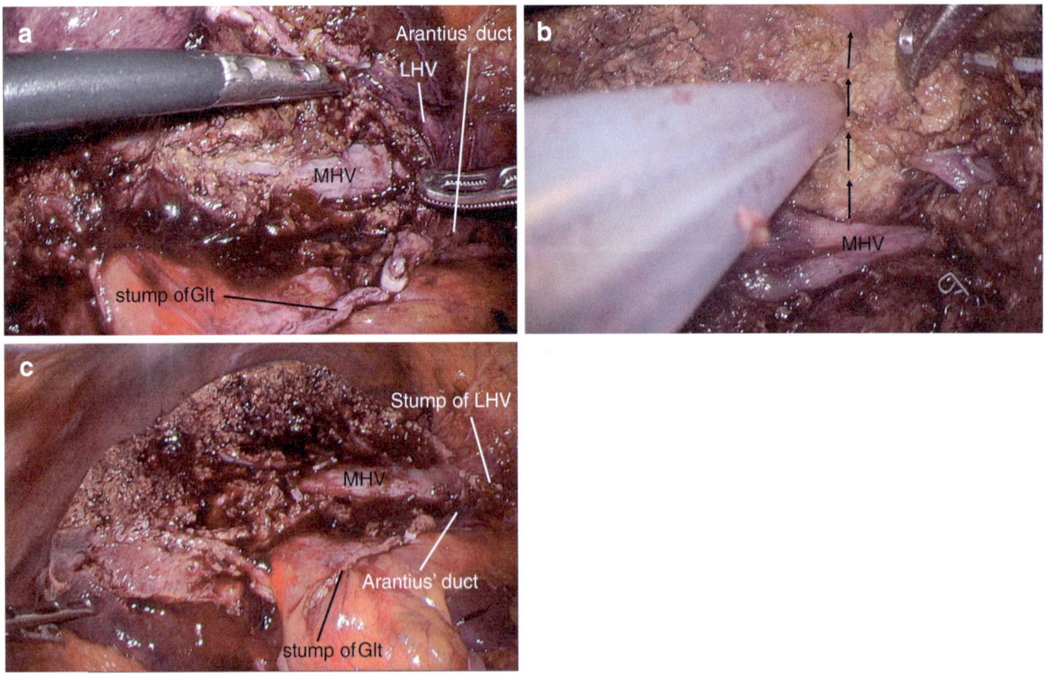

Fig. 5.6 Liver parenchymal transection. (**a**) Dissection along the MHV from the dorsal side, (**b**) the liver parenchymal transection between the MHV and the demarcation line, arrow: the direction of moving the tip of CUSA®, (**c**) the completion of the left hemihepatectomy

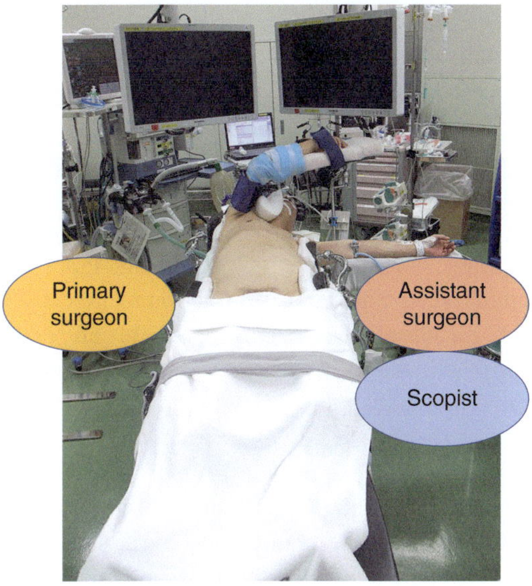

Fig. 5.7 Modified left semi-decubitus position

is twisted to the left while the pelvis and legs are kept in the supine position (Fig. 5.7). In this position, the right subphrenic cavity moves closer to the umbilicus, and approaching the posterosuperior area becomes easy from the caudal side.

The trocar placement is illustrated in Fig. 5.8. The right lobe is completely mobilized, and the roots of the MHV and the right hepatic vein (RHV) are exposed before liver parenchymal transection. Following dissection of the caudate lobe from the IVC, dividing the short hepatic veins, the caudate lobe transection is initiated from the caudal edge above the midline or the right border of the IVC (Fig. 5.9a). The initial cutting line depends on the type of procedure, i.e., right hemihepatectomy or right posterior sectionectomy, and the location of the tumor. The caudate lobe is divided as far as possible to

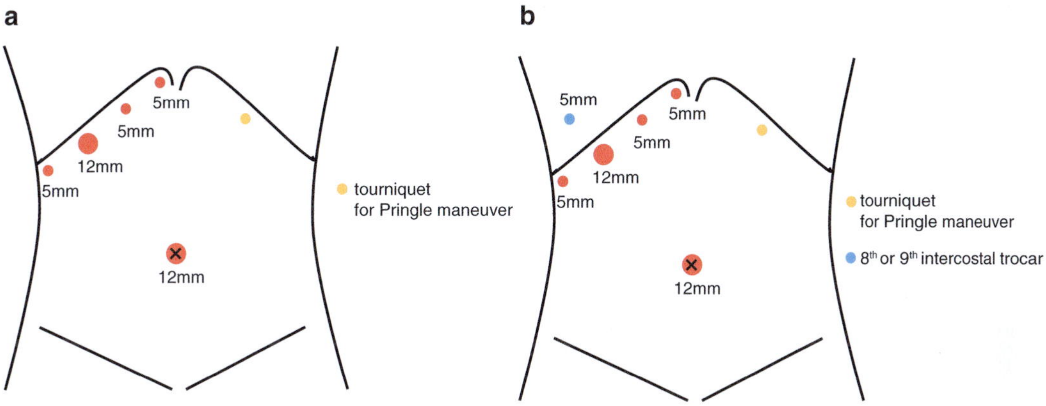

Fig. 5.8 Trocar placement. (**a**) In right hemihepatectomy, (**b**) in right posterior sectionectomy. The eighth or ninth intercostal trocar is sometimes added when the manipulation of the instrument for the primary surgeon's left hand is difficult via the trocar below the costal arch

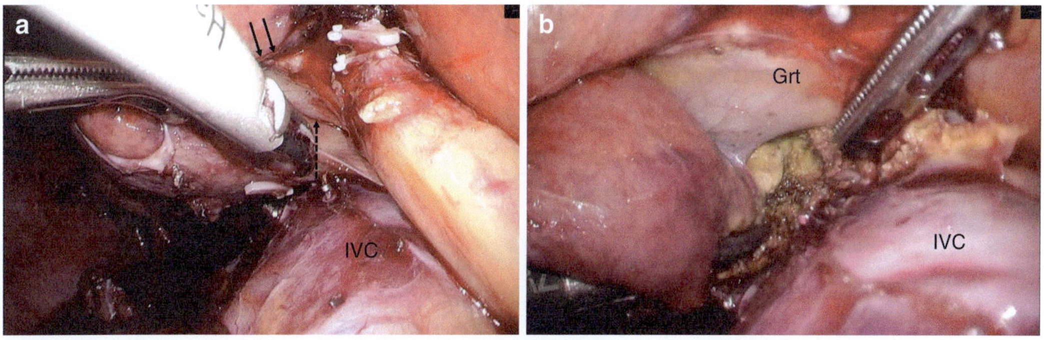

Fig. 5.9 Caudate lobe-first approach. (**a**) Initiation of the caudate lobe transection, arrow: Rouvière sulcus, dashed arrow: initial cutting line of the caudate lobe, (**b**) exposure of the posterior aspect of Grt

the cranial side beyond the hilar plate, and the posterior aspect of the Grt or Gpost is exposed (Fig. 5.9b). In right hemihepatectomy, the ventral aspect of Grt is dissected from the liver after whole-layer cholecystectomy (Fig. 5.10). The dissection of the gallbladder with a cystic plate naturally continues to the ventral aspect of the right anterior Glissonean branch (Gant). Grt can be easily isolated because its dorsal side has already been opened (Fig. 5.11). Gpost is also easily isolated using the caudate lobe-first approach after dissection of the ventral aspect without cholecystectomy (Fig. 5.12). After liver parenchymal dissection along the major hepatic fissure and creating a wide space around the hepatic hilum, Gant and Gpost are separately divided using linear staplers inserted directly from the ventral side to the posterior side. Grt should not be divided all at once because the procedure may cause injury or stenosis of the left portal vein and left hepatic duct. A linear stapler can be inserted safely because a large space has been prepared behind the Grt by the caudate lobe-first approach. This approach has another advantage in right posterior sectionectomy. The extrahepatic Glissonean approach to Gpost sometimes misses G7 because G7 often ramifies close to the root of Gpost. Gpost is often isolated using the subtraction method after the isolation of Grt and Gant in an open approach, and this method is somewhat complicated and takes longer time in laparoscopic surgery. However, in the caudate lobe-first approach, the posterior aspect of G7 and the Glissonean branch of S6 (G6) is also dissected sufficiently to the cranial side by dividing the caudate lobe above the IVC. G6 and G7 can be certainly isolated.

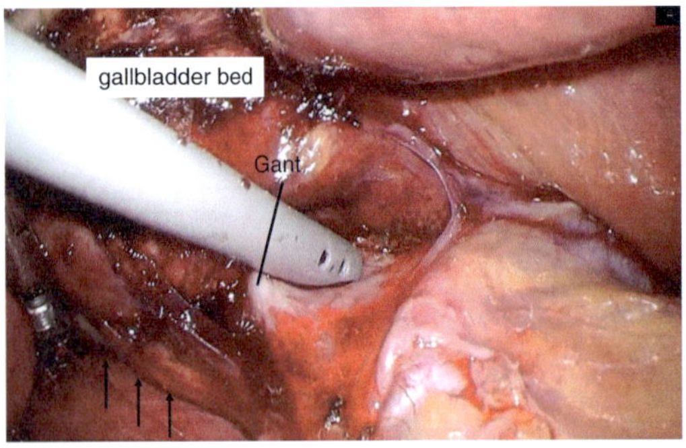

Fig. 5.10 Dissection of the ventral aspect of Grt. Arrow: Rouvière sulcus

After the division of the Glissonean pedicles, the demarcation line and IVC are landmarks to dissect the liver on the correct intersegmental plane (Fig. 5.13). The liver parenchyma is dissected from caudal to cranial by moving the tip of the CUSA® from the IVC side (dorsal side) to the demarcation line on the liver surface (ventral side). The posterior and right aspects of the MHV or the RHV are first exposed, and the vein is continuously exposed toward the IVC on the remnant liver cutting plane (Fig. 5.14). After the hepatic vein trunk is exposed, the division of the liver parenchyma between the hepatic vein trunk and the demarcation line is advanced by moving the tip of the CUSA® from the hepatic vein trunk to the demarcation line (Fig. 5.15).

Fig. 5.11 Isolation of Grt

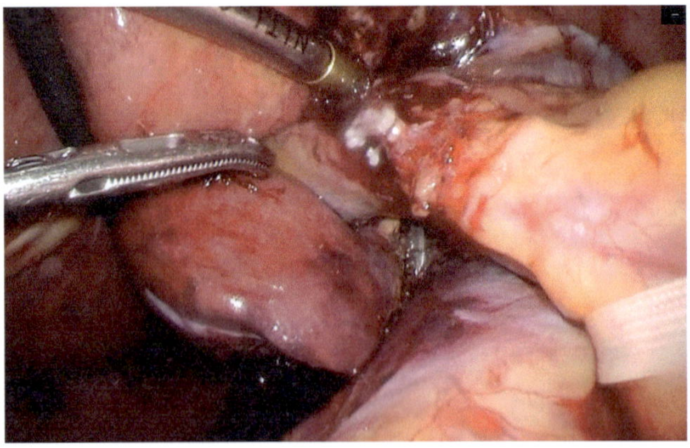

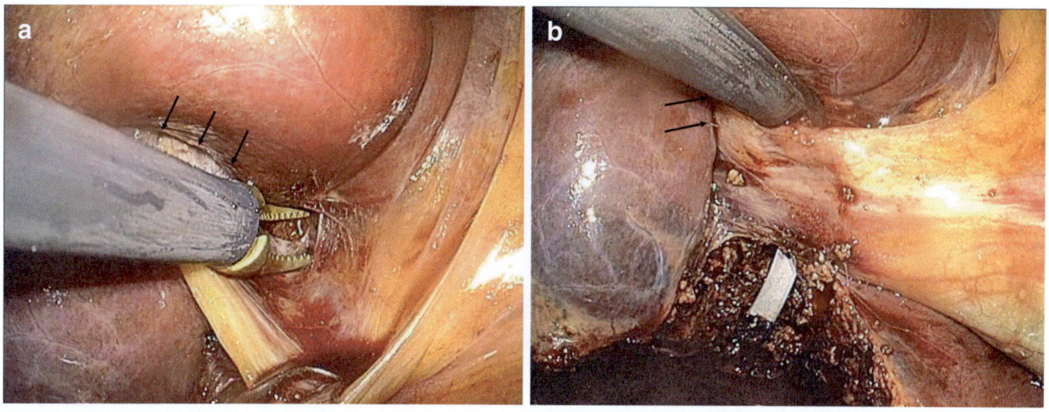

Fig. 5.12 Isolation of Gpost. (**a**) Dissection of the ventral aspect of Gpost, (**b**) isolation of Gpost. Arrow: Rouvière sulcus

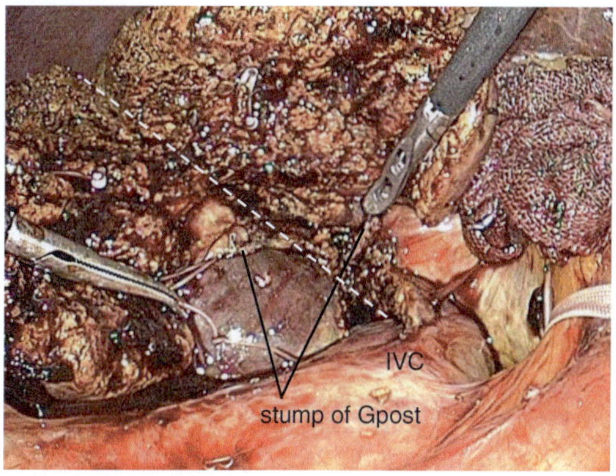

Fig. 5.13 The dissection line referring to IVC and the demarcation line in right posterior sectionectomy. Dashed line: line connecting the IVC and the demarcation line on the liver surface

5.5.3 Intrahepatic Glissonean Approach to G7 in LALR of S7 [8, 11]

Anatomic live resection of S7 is considered technically difficult even in OLR because of its position, which is located deep in the subphrenic cavity, and difficulty in approaching G7 and the RHV. However, these factors are dispelled when using a laparoscopic caudodorsal view.

The patient is placed in a modified left semidecubitus position (Fig. 5.8). The trocar placement is illustrated in Fig. 5.16. There are two methods for the intrahepatic approach to G7, depending on the branching portion of G7 from Gpost. When G7 ramifies slightly farther from the hepatic hilum, G7 usually passes through the dorsal side of the RHV, close to the posterior liver surface. G7 can be easily approached from the dorsal side of the liver, taking advantage of laparoscopic view. After mobilizing the right lobe completely, G7 is found by ultrasonography from the dorsal side, and the branching point of G7 is marked. Liver parenchymal dissection is initiated above the right border of the IVC from the root of the RHV toward the marked branching point of G7 (Fig. 5.17a). G7 can be identified, isolated, and divided in the shallow portion from the dorsal side (Fig. 5.17b).

On the other hand, when G7 ramifies close to the hepatic hilum, G7 runs deeper from the posterior liver surface. In that case, the approach described above is not suitable, but an approach similar to the caudate lobe-first approach is useful. After the caudate lobe is divided cranially from the caudal edge just above the IVC, the posterior aspect of the Gpost is exposed (Fig. 5.18a). The posterior

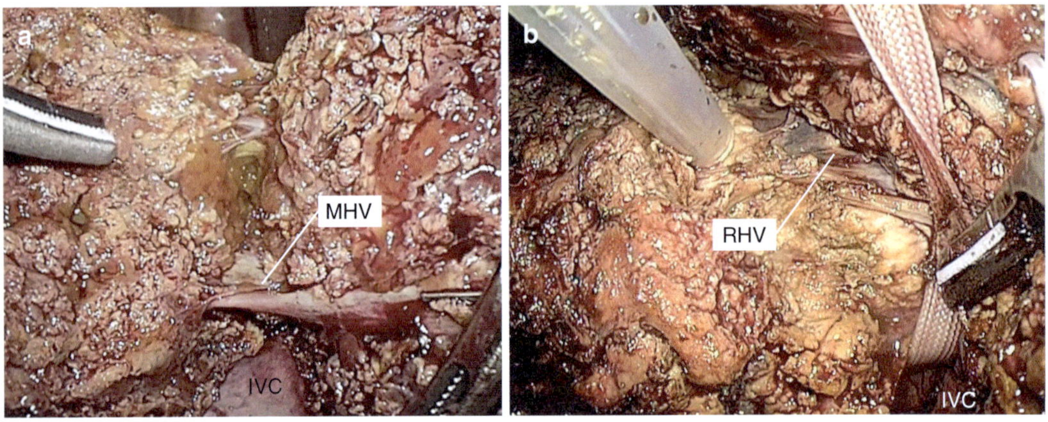

Fig. 5.14 Liver parenchymal dissection exposing the major hepatic vein. (**a**) Exposure of the MHV in right hemihepatectomy, (**b**) exposure of the RHV in right posterior sectionectomy

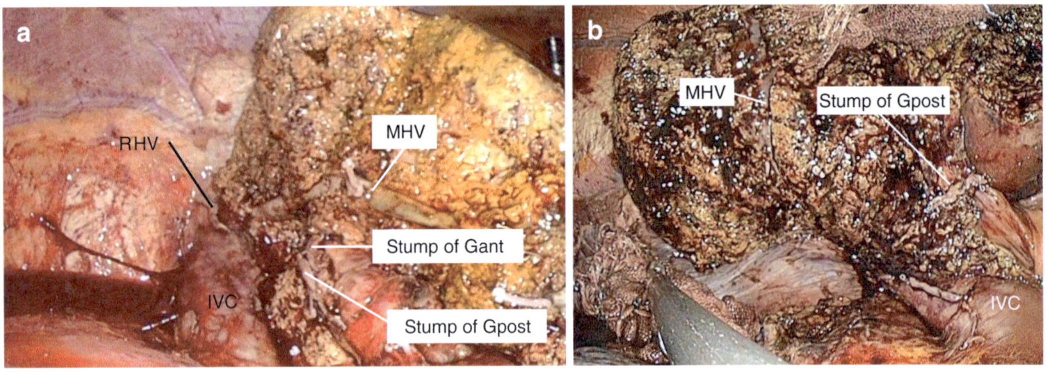

Fig. 5.15 Completion of the liver resection. (**a**) Right hemihepatectomy, (**b**) right posterior sectionectomy

aspect of Gpost is continuously exposed toward the periphery by detaching the caudate process from it. The Glissonean branch of the caudate process is divided. Following parenchymal transection between S6 and the caudate process, the ramifications of G6 and G7 can be identified from the dorsal side (Fig. 5.18b). G7 alone is successfully isolated and divided.

After the division of G7, the liver is divided along the demarcation line, and the RHV is continuously exposed from the root side toward the periphery with a laparoscopic good caudodorsal view (Fig. 5.19). The liver parenchyma between the RHV and the demarcation line on the liver surface is divided by moving the tip of the CUSA® from the RHV toward the demarcation line (Fig. 5.20).

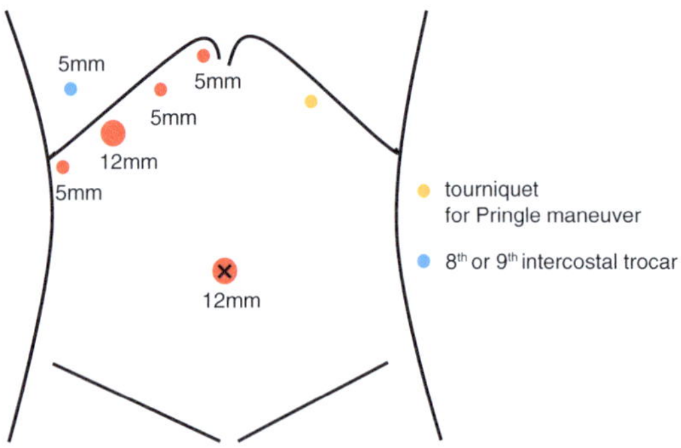

Fig. 5.16 Trocar placement

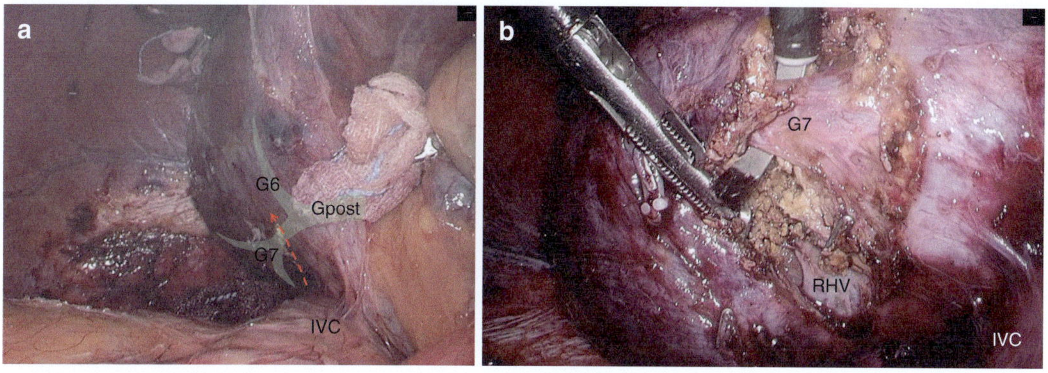

Fig. 5.17 Intrahepatic Glissonean approach to G7 from the dorsal side. (**a**) Initial cutting line, (**b**) isolation of G7

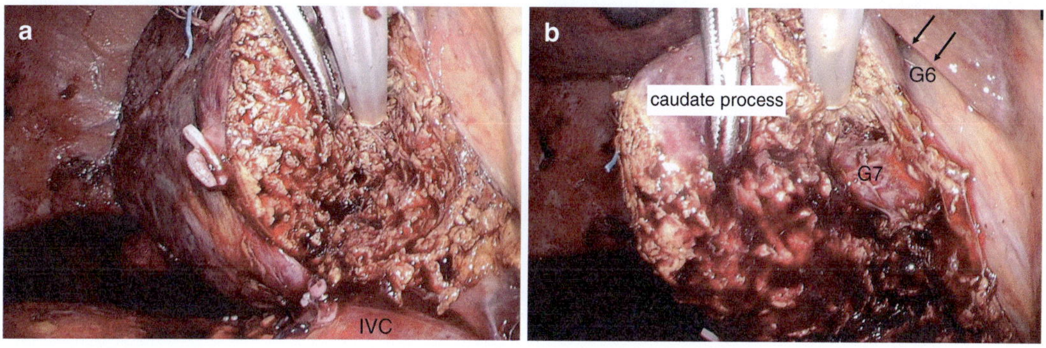

Fig. 5.18 Intrahepatic Glissonean approach to G7 using caudate lobe-first approach. (**a**) Division of the caudate lobe, (**b**) exposure of G7

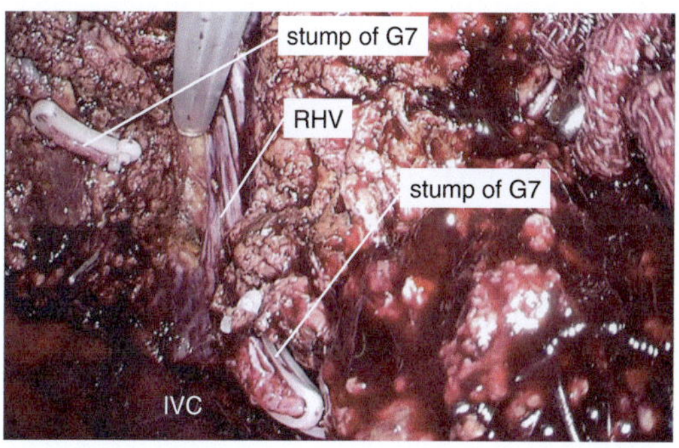

Fig. 5.19 Exposure of the RHV

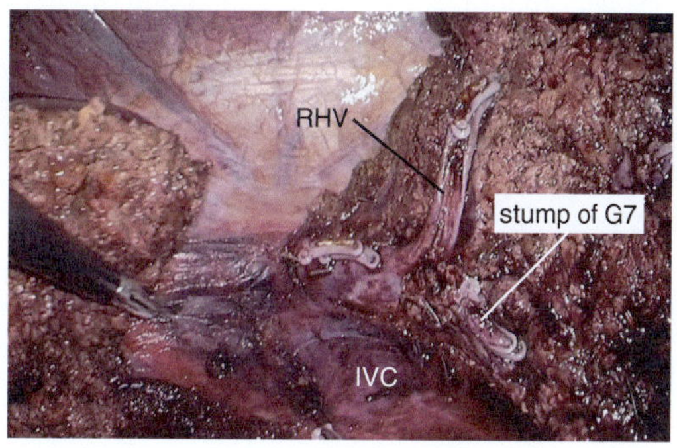

Fig. 5.20 Completion of LALR of S7

5.6 Laparoscopic Unique Approach Utilizing Other MIS Benefits: Intrahepatic Glissonean Approach in LALR of S8 [12]

Since a laparoscope can look into a deep and narrow space, there is an effective approach that makes use of it in addition to the approach utilizing a laparoscopic caudodorsal view. LALR of S8 is one of the most challenging procedures. S8 is the superior area surrounded by the diaphragm and ribs. There is diversity in the branching pattern of G8. Additionally, it is necessary to expose the MHV and RHV in LALR of S8. We standardized the intrahepatic Glissonean approach to G8, exposing the MHV and RHV continuously from the root without dissection around the hepatic hilum. In our method, G8 is successfully approached, regardless of the branching pattern of G8.

The patient is placed in the same position as shown in Fig. 5.8. The trocar placement is illustrated in Fig. 5.21. In LALR of S8, only slight mobilization of the right liver is required. The roots of the MHV and RHV are visualized only after dissection of the falciform and part of the coronary ligaments. The branching point of G8 is marked on the liver surface, referring to IOUS (intraoperative ultrasound). Liver parenchymal dissection is initiated from the cranial side along the major hepatic fissure, which is estimated by the position of the MHV, exposing the MHV from the root side toward the periphery (Fig. 5.22). In intrahepatic approach to G8, intercostal trocars are useful and essential. Since S8 is the most superior area in the right subphrenic cavity, the instruments inserted through the trocars below the costal arch cannot be manipulated at a good angle (Fig. 5.23a). Using CUSA® via an intercostal trocar enables safe exposure of the MHV and RHV trunk from the cranial side because the device can approach those veins in the nonparallel direction (Fig. 5.23b). A flex-tip scope inserted through the trocar placed beneath the right costal arch provides a better view. The hepatic vein branches flowing into the MHV from S8, including the anterior fissure vein (AFV), are cut at confluence. After the division of the major hepatic fissure, the root of G8 is identified at the deeper portion on the right side of the MHV (Fig. 5.24). The parenchyma is divided 1–2 cm toward the right side along the boundary between S8 and S5 after the cutting plane along the MHV reaches the border between S8 and S5 to safely expose G8 at the deepest por-

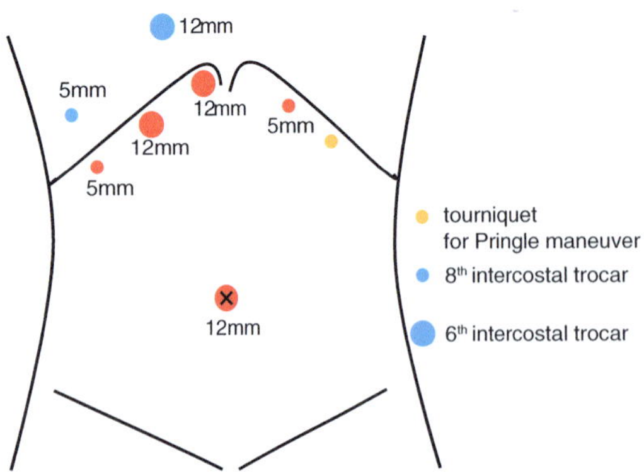

Fig. 5.21 Trocar placement

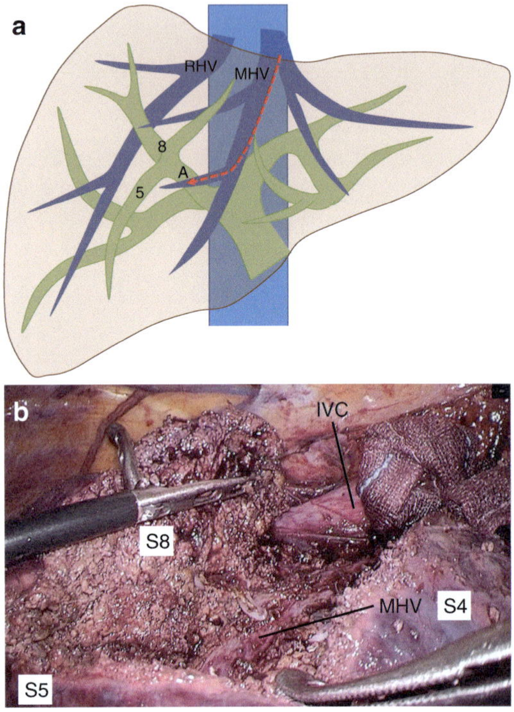

Fig. 5.22 Liver parenchymal dissection along the major hepatic fissure. (**a**) Initial cutting, (**b**) exposure of the MHV

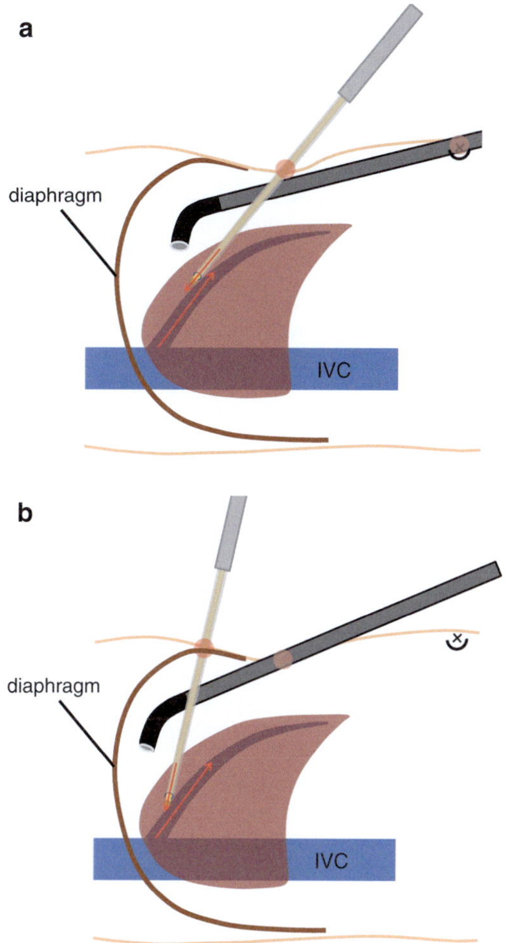

Fig. 5.23 Usefulness of intercostal trocars. (**a**) Approach without intercostal trocars, (**b**) approach using intercostal trocars

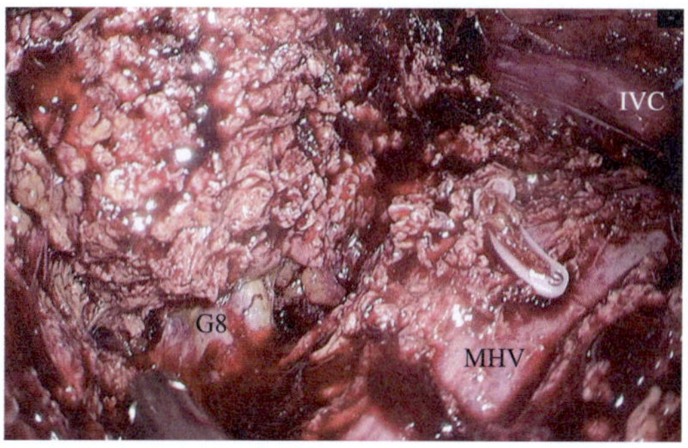

Fig. 5.24 Exposure of G8

tion in a good view. A hepatic vein branch, which joins the MHV running along the intersegmental

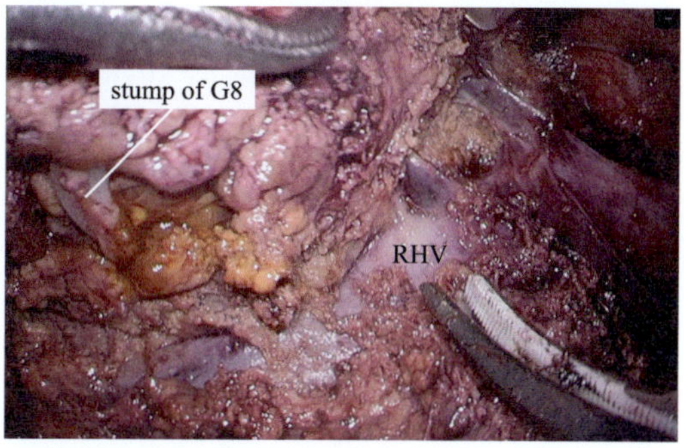

Fig. 5.25 Exposure of the RHV

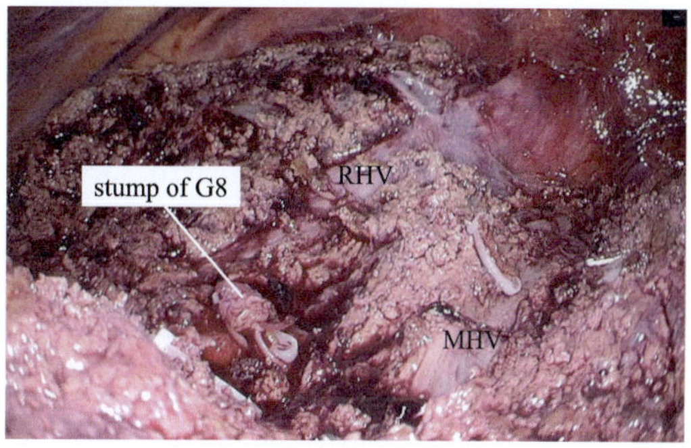

Fig. 5.26 Completion of LALR of S8

plane between S8 and S5, can often be identified, and parenchymal dissection is advanced along the vein. The border between S8 and S5 is also estimated by referring to the preoperative 3D-CT images. G8 is isolated, and S8 is recognized as an ischemic area by clamping the G8. The number and branching patterns of G8s vary, and multiple G8s have to be divided in some cases. After obtaining sufficient space around G8 by dissecting the liver parenchyma between S8 and S5, G8 is divided.

The parenchyma between S8 and S7 is also divided from the cranial side, exposing the RHV from the root side toward the periphery (Fig. 5.25). The liver parenchyma between S8 and the caudate lobe is dissected on the plane between the stump of G8, ventral aspect of the suprahepatic vena cava, and the RHV trunk, holding up S8 toward the ventral side. Between S8 and S5, the liver parenchyma is dissected by moving the tip of the CUSA® from the G8 stump side toward the demarcation line. After the RHV is enough exposed on the right side cutting plane, the remnant liver parenchyma is divided by moving the tip of the CUSA® from the RHV side toward the demarcation line (Fig. 5.26).

This approach can be applied to anatomic resection of the ventral or dorsal areas of S8. AFV runs between the ventral and dorsal areas of S8 and joins the MHV or RHV. During the anatomic resection of the ventral or dorsal area of S8, the AFV is referred to and exposed instead of the RHV or MHV, and only the ventral or dorsal branch of G8 is divided.

5.7 Postoperative Management

Complications that should be cared for after liver resection include postoperative hemorrhage, bile leak, pleural and peritoneal effusion, edema, and liver failure. General conditions, vital signs, blood tests, and drainage properties and volume should be checked for residual liver function and biliary leakage. When drainage fluid is normal, the drain should be removed early (3–4 days postoperatively). Since ascites sometimes increases postoperatively in patients with liver cirrhosis, patients should be assessed by their weight or ultrasonography, and if necessary, diuretics should be used to control ascites.

5.8 Conclusion

We described the basic and advanced techniques for LALR. Our standardized procedures for LALR are feasible and advantageous, utilizing a unique laparoscopic approach that can be useful for surgeons.

Disclosures The authors have no conflicts of interest or financial ties to disclose.

References

1. Buell JF, Thomas MT, Rudich S, et al. Experience with more than 500 minimally invasive hepatic procedures. Ann Surg. 2008;248:475–86.
2. Kaneko H, Takagi S, Otsuka Y, et al. Laparoscopic liver resection of hepatocellular carcinoma. Am J Surg. 2005;189:190–4.
3. Nguyen KT, Gamblin TC, Geller DA. World review of laparoscopic liver resection-2,804 patients. Ann Surg. 2009;250:831–41.
4. Sasaki A, Nitta H, Otsuka K, et al. Ten-year experience of totally laparoscopic liver resection in a single institution. Br J Surg. 2009;96:274–9.
5. Wakabayashi G, Cherqui D, Geller DA, et al. Recommendations for laparoscopic liver resection: a report from the second international consensus conference held in Morioka. Ann Surg. 2015;261:619–29.
6. Tomishige H, Morise Z, Kawabe N, et al. Caudal approach to pure laparoscopic posterior sectionectomy under the laparoscopy-specific view. World J Gastrointest Surg. 2013;5:173–7.
7. Okuda Y, Honda G, Kurata M, et al. Dorsal approach to the middle hepatic vein in laparoscopic left hemihepatectomy. J Am Coll Surg. 2014;219:e1–4.
8. Okuda Y, Honda G, Kobayashi S, et al. Intrahepatic Glissonean pedicle approach to segment 7 from the dorsal side during laparoscopic anatomic hepatectomy of the cranial part of the right liver. J Am Coll Surg. 2018;226:e1–6.
9. Maeda K, Honda G, Kurata M, et al. Pure laparoscopic right hemihepatectomy using the caudodorsal side approach (with videos). J Hepatobiliary Pancreat Sci. 2018;25:335–41.
10. Homma Y, Honda G, Kurata M, et al. Pure laparoscopic right posterior sectionectomy using the caudate lobe-first approach. Surg Endosc. 2019;33:3851–7.
11. Li H, Honda G, Ome Y, et al. Laparoscopic extended anatomical resection of Segment 7 by the caudate lobe first approach: a video case report. J Gastrointest Surg. 2019;23:1084–5.
12. Ome Y, Honda G, Doi M, et al. Laparoscopic anatomic liver resection of segment 8 using intrahepatic Glissonean approach. J Am Coll Surg. 2020;230:e13–20.
13. Ome Y, Honda G, Kawamoto Y. Laparoscopic left hemihepatectomy by the Arantius-first approach: a video case report. J Gastrointest Surg. 2020;24:2180–2.
14. Ome Y, Honda G, Kawamoto Y, et al. Minimally invasive liver resections for malignancies: where is the limit? Laparosc Surg. 2020; https://doi.org/10.21037/ls-20-59.
15. Makuuchi M, Kosuge T, Takayama T, et al. Surgery for small liver cancers. Semin Surg Oncol. 1993;9:298–304.
16. Okuda Y, Honda G, Kurata M, et al. Useful and convenient procedure for intermittent vascular occlusion in laparoscopic hepatectomy. Asian J Endosc Surg. 2013;6:100–3.
17. Kobayashi S, Honda G, Kurata M, et al. An experimental study on the relationship among airway pressure, pneumoperitoneum pressure, and central venous pressure in pure laparoscopic hepatectomy. Ann Surg. 2016;263:1159–63.

18. Yoneda G, Katagiri S, Yamamoto M. Reverse Trendelenburg position is a safer technique for lowering central venous pressure without decreasing blood pressure than clamping of the inferior vena cava below the liver. J Hepatobiliary Pancreat Sci. 2015;22:463–6.
19. Otsuka Y, Katagiri T, Ishii J, et al. Gas embolism in laparoscopic hepatectomy: what is the optimal pneumoperitoneal pressure for laparoscopic major hepatectomy? J Hepatobiliary Pancreat Sci. 2013;20:137–40.
20. Honda G, Kurata M, Okuda Y, et al. Totally laparoscopic hepatectomy exposing the major vessels. J Hepatobiliary Pancreat Sci. 2013;20:435–40.
21. Takasaki K. Glissonean pedicle transection method for hepatic resection: a new concept of liver segmentation. J Hepatobiliary Pancreat Surg. 1998;5:286–91.
22. Yamamoto M, Katagiri S, Ariizumi S, et al. Glissonean pedicle transection method for liver surgery (with video). J Hepatobiliary Pancreat Sci. 2012;19:3–8.
23. Honda G, Ome Y, Yoshida N, et al. How to dissect the liver parenchyma. Excavation with cavitron ultrasonic surgical aspirator. J Hepatobiliary Pancreat Sci. 2020;27:907–12.

Minimally Invasive Surgery for Pancreatic Cancer

6

Anna Caterina Milanetto, Niccolò Napoli, Emanuele Federico Kauffmann, Francesca Menonna, Claudio Pasquali, and Ugo Boggi

Abstract

Minimally invasive pancreatic surgery (MIPS) was first described in the 1990s as laparoscopic pancreatoduodenectomy and, a little later, as laparoscopic distal pancreatectomy. Then, at the beginning of the new millennium, the robot-assisted approach made it possible to overcome some of the limitations of laparoscopy. Minimally invasive pancreatic surgery should allow the same oncologic and clinical outcomes as open pancreatic surgery, with some advantages regarding surgical incision, postoperative pain, and postoperative recovery. Initially, MIPS was applied for benign diseases and low-grade malignant pancreatic neoplasms, while instead, in recent years, the indication for laparoscopic and robot-assisted approaches has been extended to pancreatic cancer, even with associated vascular resection and reconstruction. This chapter details the indications, operative techniques, postoperative outcomes, and personal experience.

Keywords

Laparoscopic pancreatic surgery · Robot-assisted pancreatic surgery · Distal pancreatectomy · Pancreato-duodenectomy · Total pancreatectomy

6.1 Distal Pancreatectomy

6.1.1 Brief History of the Procedure

Laparoscopic distal pancreatectomy (LDP) was first described in 1996 by Cuschieri et al. [1] for chronic pancreatitis and by Gagner et al. [2] for pancreatic neuroendocrine tumors. According to some retrospective case reports, LDP appears to be noninferior to open distal pancreatectomy (ODP) with regard to oncologic outcomes; however, a prospective study comparing the two approaches has not yet been published [3, 4]. In 2014, Lee et al. [5] presented the so-called "Yonsei criteria" to select patients for LDP. The authors recommended that LDP should be used only in the case of a tumor confined to the pancreas, where there is a distance of at least 1 cm from the celiac trunk and the fascia layer between the pancreas and the left adrenal gland is intact [6]. In 2003, Melvin first described a robotic dis-

Supplementary Information The online version contains supplementary material available at https://doi.org/10.1007/978-981-97-7059-5_6.

A. C. Milanetto (✉) · C. Pasquali
Pancreatic and Digestive Endocrine Surgical Unit – Department of Surgery, Oncology and Gastroenterology, University of Padua, Padua, Italy
e-mail: acmilanetto@unipd.it

N. Napoli · E. F. Kauffmann · F. Menonna · U. Boggi
Division of General and Transplant Surgery, University of Pisa, Pisa, Italy

M. Tewari (ed.), *Minimally Invasive Surgery in Cancer*,
https://doi.org/10.1007/978-981-97-7059-5_6

tal pancreatectomy (RDP) performed for a neuroendocrine tumor [7].

Minimally invasive distal pancreatectomy (MIDP) is expected to achieve the same clinical and oncologic outcomes as ODP and also to allow some additional advantages regarding, for example, surgical incision, postoperative pain, and postoperative recovery. From a technical point of view, thanks to the da Vinci robotic surgical system (Intuitive Surgical, Sunnydale, CA, USA), it is possible to overcome some limitations of laparoscopy and improve the approach to the distal pancreas, for example, by reducing tremor due to the rigid lever-fulcrum system by improving the ergonomics of the surgeon, who is no longer forced to prolonged standing or limited two-dimensional vision [8, 9].

6.1.2 Operating Room Setup and Patient Positioning

In the LDP, the patient is positioned supine, in 30° right lateral decubitus, with the hip at the table break and the feet and head tilted 20° [10]. In order to place the patient in the reverse Trendelenburg position, supports must be placed at the level of the rib cage in the right axillary area, at the right hip, and against the patient's feet [11]. The surgical team is arranged as follows: the scrub nurse on the right side near the patient's feet, the surgeon between the patient's lower limbs, the first assistant on the right side, and the second assistant on the left side [12]. The pneumoperitoneum is established at the level of the umbilicus, where the first trocar (11 mm) is placed. Keeping the pneumoperitoneum at 12 mmHg, a 30° laparoscope and three more trocars are inserted under vision, as follows: the first trocar (12 mm) on the left pararectal line, the second trocar (5 or 10–12 mm) on the left anterior axillary line 3–5 cm below the costal margin, and the last trocar (5 or 12 mm) on the right pararectal line slightly cranial to the umbilicus [10].

Robotic DP is performed with the da Vinci robotic surgical system (Intuitive Surgical, Sunnydale, CA, USA) (Si or Xi models). Two surgical specialists are required: the operating surgeon and the assistant surgeon, who stand at the console and operating table, respectively, and work closely together [13]. The patient is placed supine in the reverse Trendelenburg position at 20° with the legs spread apart (Fig. 6.1). Surgery with the Xi system is performed with four 8-mm robotic ports and one 12-mm assistant port. The 12-mm port is placed on the right pararectal line, while the robotic ports are placed along the transverse umbilical line about 6–8 cm apart (Fig. 6.2), and the camera can be inserted through all the ports. If the HDSi system is used, instead, the camera is inserted through an 11-mm umbilical port, the 12-mm assistant port is placed on the pararectal line, and the three robotic ports are placed in a smiling fashion along the left and right anterior axillary lines and along the left pararectal line. After docking the robot, the robotic instruments are inserted under vision.

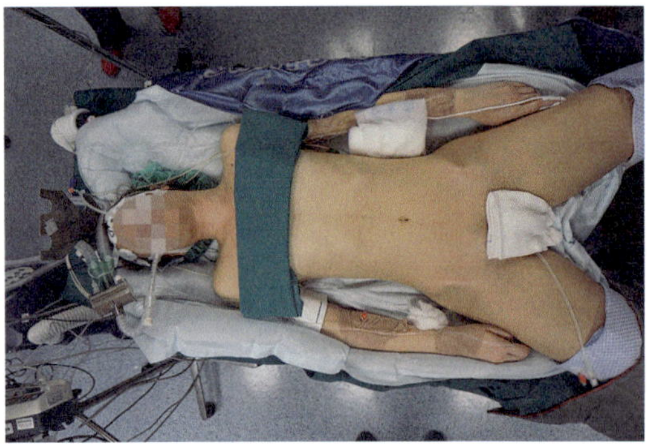

Fig. 6.1 Patient positioning for robotic pancreatic surgery

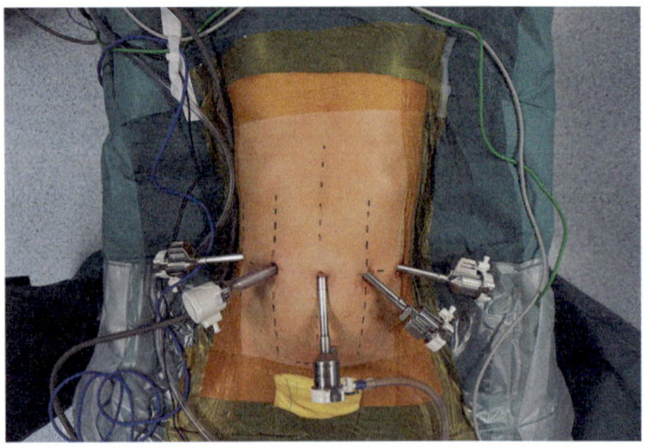

Fig. 6.2 Port placement for robotic distal pancreatectomy

6.1.3 List of Specific Instruments/Gadgets Used

In LDP, the surgeon uses an atraumatic forceps in the nondominant hand for both the pancreas and bowel, and the assistant also uses an atraumatic forceps, through the 5-mm left lateral trocar [11]. The surgeon uses with the dominant hand a bipolar energy or ultrasound dissection instrument, or a combination of both [11]. Pancreatic resection is preferably performed with a mechanical stapler [10]. For closure of large vessels, clip applicators (5–10 mm) or Hem-o-lok (Teleflex Medical, Research Triangle Park, North Carolina, USA) are used, while polypropylene and linen stitches are used for ligation of lymphatic vessels.

In RDP, a Maryland forceps (Intuitive Surgical, Sunnyvale, CA, USA for dissection and coagulation) and a curved scissor with monopolar energy are used for dissection [13]. For adipose tissue section and small vessel hemostasis, an ultrasonic dissector can be used, while mechanical vascular staplers or Hem-o-lok endoclips (Teleflex Medical, Research Triangle Park, North Carolina, USA) should be used for large vessels, and polypropylene and linen sutures can be used for ligation of lymphatic vessels [13]. An intraoperative ultrasound probe must be available in every surgery [64]. Resection of the pancreatic parenchyma can be performed with a mechanical stapler, such as the Signia Stapling System (Covidien, Medtronic Parkway, Minneapolis, USA) [13]; alternatively, an ultrasonic dissector for the pancreatic parenchyma and scissors for the main pancreatic duct can be used.

6.1.4 The Detailed and Stepwise Operative Technique

In minimally invasive surgery performed for pancreatic cancer, for complete lymphadenectomy and adequate oncologic margin, splenectomy is recommended [14], with an *en bloc* resection of the spleen, the tail of the pancreas, and perivascular, and splenic hilum lymph nodes [15]. To improve oncologic radicality in resection of pancreatic body-tail tumors, Strasberg et al. introduced in 2003 a surgical approach called "radical antegrade modular pancreatosplenectomy" (RAMPS) [15]. The RAMPS approach applied to MIDP appears to allow increased overall and disease-free survival and also seems to provide good results as negative posterior margin and lymphadenectomy [16]. Indeed, with this technique, the dissection plane going horizontally from right to left allows radical resection of regional lymph nodes, enhanced by the magnified view of the correct anatomical plane obtained by laparoscopy [17].

Laparoscopic Distal Pancreatectomy

Keeping the pneumoperitoneum at 12 mmHg, visual exploration of the abdominal cavity is performed to exclude the presence of any distant metastases [13]. First, the left flexure of the colon is mobilized and by pulling the colon medially, the lateral peritoneal fold (Toldt's white line) is opened [11]. To access the anterior aspect of the pancreas, the superficial part of the splenocolic ligament is divided and colo-epiploic detachment is performed to the opening of the gastrosplenic ligament [11]. The stomach is lifted anteriorly by inserting a suture needle that passes first through the abdominal wall beside the xiphoid process, along the posterior wall of the stomach and then back through the abdominal wall [11]. This provides better access to the celiac trunk and upper pancreatic border.

To identify the origin of the hepatic and splenic artery, first identify and follow the left gastric artery in a proximal direction, taking care not to injure the left gastric vein, and then excise the lymph nodes along the common hepatic artery toward the celiac trunk [11]. At this point, it is possible to isolate the splenic artery at its origin with a dissector and surround it with a rubber band. Before dissecting the splenic artery, the splenic vein must also be isolated, because the latter is easier to dissect when it is full rather than collapsed [11].

Lifting the peritoneum with a curved dissector, the transverse mesocolon is mobilized with an energy device from the inferior border of the pancreas [11]; with an atraumatic forceps, the surgeon exerts light pressure on the pancreas in the anterior-cranial direction, while the assistant surgeon pulls the transverse mesocolon in the posterior-caudal direction [11]. The dissection of the tiny branches directed from the pancreas to the splenic vein is carried out with the energy device, without using any clips or ligatures [11]; after isolating the splenic vein, the splenic artery is closed with locking clips and divided.

A rubber band is placed around the pancreas, lifting the gland to allow the dissection of the top and back side and to place a stapler around it with the shortest/lowest height possible[11]. After closing the stapler and before activating it, one must visualize the celiac trunk entirely, to avoid its possible inclusion in the stapling line [11]. The Signia Stapling System (Covidien, Medtronic Parkway, Minneapolis, USA) is used; activating gradually compresses the pancreatic tissue and reduces the risk of pancreatic rupture along the staple line [11]. At this point, the splenic vein is dissected with a vascular stapler; the vein can also be dissected together with the pancreas if it is difficult to separate the two structures [11].

The dissection then continues from right to left. The pancreas is released posteriorly, following the plane of Gerota's fascia to perform a complete lymphadenectomy. Proceeding with the dissection to the left, the deepest part of the splenocolic ligament and the splenorenal ligament is dissected from the bottom up [11]. The specimen is then removed *en bloc* and placed in a pouch introduced through the umbilical trocar. A drain is placed along the division line of the pancreas, the subcostal trocar is removed, the stomach is released, and the cranial incision is extended to the umbilicus (or a Pfannenstiel incision, in case of large tumors or splenomegaly), to extract the specimen into the pouch. Finally, the incisions are sutured, with closure of the fascia in the case of larger incisions.

Robot-Assisted Radical Antegrade Modular Pancreatosplenectomy (RAMPS)

We describe here the technique developed in Pisa [18]. The pneumoperitoneum is maintained at 10 mmHg. The trocar for the robotic camera (8 mm) is placed at the level of the umbilicus, so that it is approximately 10–15 cm from the nearest border of the target anatomy, and the abdominal cavity is explored with the robotic laparoscope to exclude any distant metastases [18]. All trocars are placed along the transverse umbilical line, approximately 4 cm apart: the assistant port (12 mm) is located along the right pararectal line, and the other robotic ports are placed along the left pararectal line and along the left and right anterior axillary lines [18]. The patient is placed in the reverse Trendelenburg position (15–20°) and tilted to the right side (5–8°). First, the laser arm sight is aligned on the camera port to begin the docking, and the camera is docked and directed toward the operative anatomy; then, the other arms are also docked and the robotic instruments are placed under vision [18].

By dividing the colon and omentum reflection, the lesser sac is opened, and the dissection is begun in the middle of the transverse mesocolon, proceeding in both directions until the right and left colic flexures are fully mobilized [18].To allow mobilization of the left part of the pancreas, dissection of the peritoneum along the lower margin of the pancreas is begun [18]. Having identified the superior mesenteric vein (SMV), a tunnel is created behind the isthmus of the pancreas, and along its superior margin one resects lymph node 8A to make the common hepatic artery visible and then surrounds it with a rubber band, after identifying its course [18]. To expose the portal vein (PV), it is important to separate the lymphatic tissue that lays between the artery and the superior margin of the isthmus [18]. Since energetic devices can cause thermal damage to vessel walls, each dissection is performed near the major arteries using cold scissors to reduce the risk of late hemorrhage [19].

The splenic artery is divided with ligatures or clips and, when possible, is divided before the splenic vein to reduce blood pooling in the spleen. To adequately remove the retroperitoneal soft tissue *en bloc* with the specimen, dissection is begun in a posterior plane in the mid-lateral direction, identifying the left adrenal gland (Fig. 6.3) and removing *en bloc* the Gerota's fascia covering the upper pole of the left kidney [18]. A transfixed suture is placed on the inferior margin of the pancreas to close the transverse pancreatic artery before dissecting the gland [18].

The main pancreatic duct is identified and electively dissected, and the section surface is closed with single stitches of expanded polytetrafluoroethylene (e-PTFE) 4/0 (Gore, W. L. Gore & Associates, USA) in a fish-mouth configuration [18]. One can also dissect the pancreas using the Signia Stapling System (Covidien, Medtronic Parkway, Minneapolis, USA) or Harmonic scissors (Ethicon Endo-Surgery, Johnson & Johnson, Somerville, NJ, USA). At this point, the pancreatic margin is sent for frozen section. The splenic vein and short gastric vessels are divided and the spleen is mobilized [18]. The round and falciform ligaments of the liver are transposed to cover the retroperitoneal vessels [18]. A 14 Fr pigtail drain is placed near the section line of the pancreas, and the specimen is extracted into a bag through a 5-cm-long Pfannenstiel incision [18].

6.1.5 Postoperative Course and Management

The nasogastric tube is removed at the end of surgery. On the first postoperative day the patient can start taking oral fluids and oral physiological feeding starts from the third day, depending on the patient's clinical condition [13]. On the third and fifth postoperative days, drain amylase is sampled, and the drain is removed on the fifth postoperative day if the amylase of the drain fluid is less than three times the serum amylase and the output is less than 200 ml. The patient is stimulated to move immediately after surgery, but will not have to lift heavy loads for 6 weeks [11].

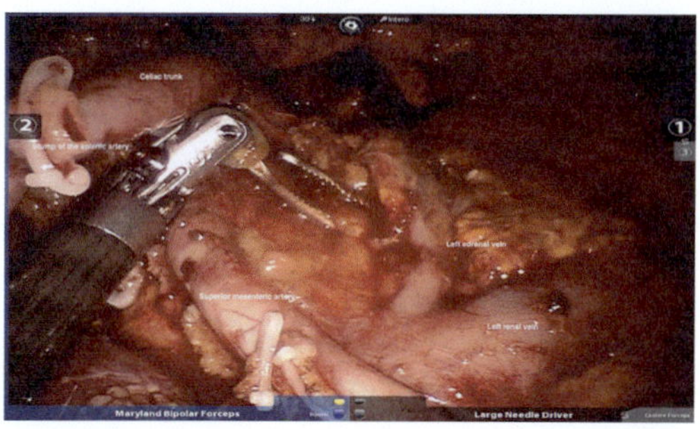

Fig. 6.3 Robot-Assisted Radical Antegrade Modular PancreatoSplenectomy (RAMPS): in order to remove the retroperitoneal soft tissue with the specimen, dissection is begun in a posterior plane in the mid-lateral direction, identifying the left adrenal gland

6.1.6 Complications

As in open surgery, postoperative pancreatic fistula (POPF) after LDP/RDP may occur in 0–34% of cases [6]. Several pancreatic stump closure modalities (i.e., duct ligation, ultrasound and stapler closure, fibrin glue occlusion, mesh, and pancreatic-jejunal anastomosis) are described in the literature [20, 21], but there are still no guidelines or recommendations supported by scientific evidence for the proper management of the pancreatic stump and for the reduction of POPF occurrence [22].

Antibiotics and possibly percutaneous drainage to avoid bacterial and/or fungal infection of drained fluids are the preferred approach for the conservative treatment of POPF, whereas a reoperation may be necessary only in rare cases, due to vascular or septic complications [13].

Early postoperative hemorrhage may occur in 5% of patients, due to pancreatic stump hemorrhage or severe acute pancreatitis. In the former case, it can be easily managed laparoscopically by placing a suture or clip, while in the latter case it may require complex reoperations [13].

Abdominal fluid collections are common and are self-limiting and indolent. Occasionally, placement of percutaneous radiologic or endoscopic drainage may be necessary to treat symptomatic pseudocysts [13]. Bowel or gastric perforation and late hemorrhage caused by splenic artery stump pseudoaneurysm represent other rare complications, which should be treated laparoscopically or by angiographic embolization.

Finally, there are possible late consequences of splenectomy, such as increased exposure to infection and persistent thrombocytosis (14% of patients), so to reduce the risk of infection with capsulated bacteria, vaccination against Haemophilus influenzae, pneumococcus, and meningococcus is mandatory [23]. In cases of persistent thrombocytosis, salicylic acid (100 mg) is indicated to reduce platelet aggregation [24].

6.1.7 Personal Experience

From 2015 to 2019, we performed 35 LDPs. The median age of the patients was 71 years (range, 58–76) and the median ASA score was 3 (range, 2–3). The median BMI was 24.1±4.1 kg/m^2. The median operative time was 312.3 ± 91.5 min, and 20% of patients required intraoperative blood transfusions. Conversion occurred in 2.9% of operations. Final histology showed pancreatic ductal adenocarcinoma in 22 (62.9%) cases, the median number of lymph nodes harvested was 29 (22–41), and the R0 rate in the malignant group was 60.6%. Postoperative complications occurred in 24 out of 35 (68.6%) patients. Postoperative pancreatic fistula occurred in 31.4% of cases; of these, 6 (54.5%) were grade B POPFs, and no grade C POPFs were detected. No patients underwent reoperation, and 90-day mortality was nihil.

From 2008 to 2019, we performed 115 RDPs, of which 54 (47%) with spleen preservation. The patients' median age was 60 years (range, 48–67) and the median ASA score was 2 (range, 2–3). The median BMI was 24.6 ± 4.03 kg/m^2. The median operative time was 297.8 ± 90.9 min, and 7.8% of patients required intraoperative blood transfusions. Conversion occurred in 1.7% of operations. Final histology showed 25 (21.7%) cases of pancreatic ductal adenocarcinoma, with a median number of harvested lymph nodes of 16 (range, 7–30), and the R0 rate was 94.6% in the malignant group. Postoperative complications occurred in 71 out of 115 (61.7%) patients. Postoperative pancreatic fistula occurred in 51.3% of cases; of these, 34 (57.6%) were grade B POPFs, while no grade C POPFs were observed. Four patients were reoperated for postoperative hemorrhage, and 90-day mortality was nihil.

6.2 Pancreatoduodenectomy

6.2.1 Brief History of the Procedure

The first laparoscopic pancreatoduodenectomy (LPD) was described by Gagner and Pomp in 1994 [25], and only 10 years later the first large case series of patients undergoing LPD was published [26]. Most authors [27, 28] still exclude LPD in the case of large or borderline resectable tumors, concomitant chronic pancreatitis, or in obese patients who have already undergone abdominal surgery [29]. Laparoscopic PD is a very complex surgery, both because of the first part of the operation, which involves dissection near vital arterial and venous vessels, and the reconstructive part, which involves making three anastomoses on three different and vital organs [30]. Laparoscopic PD has never achieved widespread popularity given the significant technical difficulties due particularly to the reconstructive part, which requires a longer learning curve than other surgical procedures [30]. In 2019, the LEOPARD-2 trial, which compared LPD and open PD for pancreatic or periampullary tumors, was prematurely discontinued due to unexpected and troubling safety issues [31]. In fact, LPD was associated with higher complication-related mortality than open PD (10% vs. 2%, respectively), and no difference between the groups was observed regarding functional recovery time [31, 32].

The first robotic pancreatoduodenectomy (RPD) was performed by Giulianotti in Italy, in 2001 and reported in 2003 [33]. Robotic surgery provides a stable platform with an enlarged, high-definition, three-dimensional view of the operative field; in addition, since the surgical instruments have a greater freedom of movement and the tremor is suppressed, the surgical dexterity is increased and accuracy and safety in performing an RPD are both improved [34]. As surgeon experience increases, patient selection criteria should progressively include patients with pancreatic cancer and at higher medical risk [34]. According to a recent systematic review of minimally invasive PD, RPD was associated with a shorter hospital stay and less blood loss than LPD, and notably with a lower incidence of conversion to laparotomy [35].

Patients who undergo conversion to laparotomy have a higher rate of complications and worse oncologic outcomes, so it is the low conversion rate demonstrated for RPD that may allow for faster recovery after surgery and thus earlier initiation of adjuvant chemotherapy in patients with cancer [35]. In addition, compared with LPD it appears that robotic assistance may increase the reproducibility of the procedure and probably reduce the learning curve [35]. Since up to 30% of patients have suspected SMV/PV involvement, the value of RPD will also need to be evaluated in cases of resection and reconstruction of these vessels [36]. We also pursue RPD when tumor adhesion to the SMV/PV is an incidental finding during surgery, or when contact between the tumor and veins is limited ($\leq 180°$ in circumference and ≤ 2 cm in length) on preoperative imaging studies [34].

Because RPD has made it possible to overcome some limitations of laparoscopy, in this section on minimally invasive PD we will focus on the robotic approach.

6.2.2 Operating Room Setup and Patient Positioning

The patient is supine with legs spread apart in the reverse Trendelenburg position and tilted to the left [34]. The console with the operating surgeon and the scrub nurse is placed at the patient's feet, and the assistant surgeon is placed between the patient's legs (Fig. 6.4) [34]. When using the Si system, the robotic tower is positioned at the patient's head and the ports are placed along a smiling line [34]. The optical port (11 mm) is placed along the right midclavicular line at the level of the umbilicus and the assistant port (12 mm) at the supra- or subumbilical location [37]. An 8-mm robotic port is placed along the right anterior axillary line 3–4 cm above the optic port, while the other two robotic ports (8 mm) are placed in a mirror-image fashion on the left side [37]. When the Xi system is used instead, the robotic tower is placed on the left side of the patient and the ports are placed along a straighter line [34]. The assistant port (12 mm) is placed immediately below or above the umbilicus, and four robotic ports (8 mm) are placed on the right and left pararectal line and the right and left anterior axillary line, respectively (Fig. 6.5) [37].

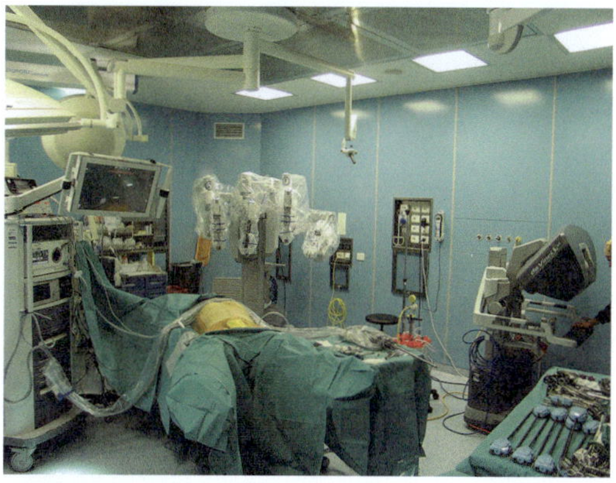

Fig. 6.4 Operating room setup for robotic pancreatic surgery

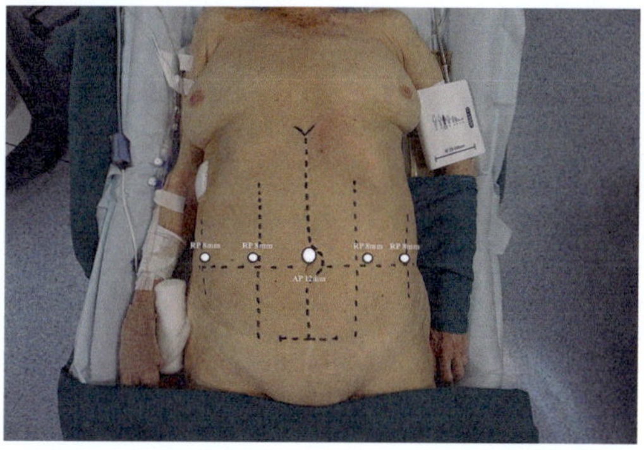

Fig. 6.5 Port placement for robotic pancreatoduodenectomy

6.2.3 List of Specific Instruments/Gadgets Used

Surgical resectability must be assessed with high-quality radiological imaging, and the gold standard of imaging is computed tomography with three-dimensional vascular reconstruction, which allows detection of vascular anatomic variants and relationships of the neoplasm with the SMV/PV and arteries [34]. The most common cause of conversion to open surgery is unexpected adhesions of the tumor with the SMV/PV and anatomic variants, so carefully evaluating preoperative imaging can reduce unplanned conversions [38]. Monopolar scissors, Maryland-type bipolar forceps (Intuitive Surgical, Sunnyvale, CA, USA), a fenestrated forceps used as a retractor, and Harmonic scissors (Ethicon Endo-Surgery, Johnson & Johnson, Somerville,

NJ, USA) are used for RPD [34]. Laparoscopic or robotic staplers, laparoscopic bulldogs, and vascular loops should also be available.

6.2.4 The Operative Technique in a Detailed and Stepwise Manner

Robotic Pancreatoduodenectomy

We describe here the technique developed in Pisa [34, 37, 39]. After confirming the absence of distant metastases, some sutures are used to suspend the liver to the anterior abdominal wall: a trans-parietal suture at the level of the round ligament of the liver, an intracorporeal suture between the fundus of the gallbladder and the right diaphragmatic dome to elevate liver segments 5 and 6, and a final suture between segment 3 and the left diaphragmatic dome [34].

Dissection starts from the hepatoduodenal ligament, and the gallbladder is not removed until the end of surgery, as it is used to retract the liver. The common bile duct, PV and common hepatic artery are identified, after removal of the station 8A lymph nodes, and they are isolated on a rubber band [34]. Both the gastroduodenal artery and the main biliary duct are identified and dissected between linen 0 ligatures, after taking the margin from the duct for frozen section and a bile culture swab [34].

Proceeding from the left to the right, the gastrocolic ligament is opened until the mobilization of the right flexure of the colon is completed [39]. The fourth robotic arm lifts the gastric antrum thus opening the dissection plane, and the right gastroepiploic vessels are dissected after closure with Hem-o-lok (Teleflex Medical, Research Triangle Park, North Carolina, USA). To perform a pylorus-preserving RPD, one dissects the duodenum just beyond the pylorus with a laparoscopic stapler loaded with a vascular cartridge [34].

The isthmus of the pancreas is then separated from the SMV/PV and hemostatic sutures are placed along the superior and inferior margins of the pancreas [34]. With the Harmonic scalpel (Ethicon Endo-Surgery, Johnson & Johnson, Somerville, NJ, USA), the first few centimeters of the gland are dissected, and when approaching the location of the main pancreatic duct instead, robotic scissors are used to visualize and divide it [34]. The pancreatic section margin is sent for frozen section. With the fourth robotic arm, the duodenum is handled to perform the Kocher maneuver, and suspended on the right side during dissection of the posterior margin, so that the uncinate process is pulled away from the SMV/PV and the resection line along the right side of the superior mesenteric artery (SMA) is exposed [34].

The posterior peritoneal layer is then opened and the first jejunal loop is retracted on the right side of the SMV/SMA. The jejunal mesentery is divided on this side with a Harmonic scalpel (Ethicon Endo-Surgery, Johnson & Johnson, Somerville, NJ, USA), but the bowel will be dissected later so that it can easily rotate around the superior mesenteric vessels during the reconstructive phase [40].

Proceeding along the periadventitial plane of the SMA, pancreaticoduodenal arteries and veins are identified and dissected between ligatures or clips, minimizing the use of energetic devices to avoid a thermal injury to large-caliber vessels' walls [18]. The retroperitoneal large lymphatic vessels are dissected after closure with clips to reduce the occurrence and amount of retroperitoneal fluid collections [34]. It is critically important from an oncologic point of view to remove *en bloc* the peripancreatic lymph node stations (12a–c, 8a, 8p, 9, 14a–d) and extrapancreatic nerve plexus tissue [34].

A single jejunal loop is used for reconstruction, which is transposed to the supramesocolic site by passing behind the superior mesenteric vessels or by the transmesocolic route. Typically, a pancreatic-jejunal anastomosis is preferred with a duct-to-mucosa technique according to modified Blumgart [41], which consists of 2 or 4 U-shaped transfixed stitches of 4-0 ePTFE (Gore, W. L. Gore & Associates, USA) passed to wrap the pancreas with the intestine, avoiding the duct [34]. The duct-to-mucosa anastomosis is then performed with interrupted sutures of 5-0 polydioxanone, and only at this point all sutures are tied. When the duct is small (<4 mm), an internal stent is used to facilitate suturing. Approximately 10 cm downstream of the pancreatic anastomosis, the end-to-side hepatic-jejunal anastomosis is made in a double layer with 5-0 polydioxanone sutures [34]. Finally, at a distance of 10–15 cm from the biliary anastomosis, the duodenal-jejunal anastomosis in double layer is performed [34]. The specimen is extracted in an endoscopic pouch through a small transverse incision at the suprapubic site. To protect the stump of the gastroduodenal artery, we use to mobilize and wrap the round and falciform ligaments of the liver around the hepatic artery [34]. Two 14 Fr pigtail drains are placed: one posterior to the hepatic-jejunal anastomosis, the other one anterior to the pancreatic-jejunal anastomosis [34].

Robotic Pancreatoduodenectomy with Resection and Reconstruction of the Superior Mesenteric/Portal Vein

We now present some details of the additional surgical maneuvers employed for resection and reconstruction of the SMV/PV [39, 40, 42, 43]. By artery-first approach to both the SMA and the celiac trunk, it can be determined whether the tumor is resectable by approaching the SMA through different routes [44]. The generally feasible approach is the anterior one, combined with a medial approach to the uncinated process [40]. After dividing the pancreas at the isthmus, one surrounds with a rubber band and lifts the splenic vein. A dissection of the SMA is performed caudal-cranially to the aortic plane and along the right side to the celiac trunk, dissecting between ligatures or clips the pancreaticoduodenal arteries [43]. To increase the likelihood of achieving an R0 resection, the head of the pancreas is mobilized *en bloc* with the involved vein segment and the lympho-neural tissue that lies between the SMA and the celiac trunk ("mesopancreas") [43, 45, 46]. At this point, the right side of the SMA and celiac trunk are skeletonized to gain a clear view of the inferior vena cava and left renal vein [43]. The vessels are then cross-clamped with laparoscopic bulldog forceps, first the SMA and then the SMV to reduce intestinal congestion [42].

Typically, a segmental resection of the vein is performed, and the vein may be reconstructed by direct end-to-end anastomosis (type III vein resection) or by an interposition graft (type IV vein resection); this choice will depend on the length of the resected segment [43, 47]. If a tangential resection of a large lateral wall has been performed, a peritoneal patch or autologous vein patch [43, 48], usually the internal jugular vein, is used to repair the vein [42]. Alternative options for reconstruction may be vascular prostheses [49], which are not used in our center because of the infectious risk in the context of gastrointestinal surgery, or a cold-preserved vein segment from deceased organ donors [50].

If the SMV/PV junction is included in the resected segment, after completing the cranial anastomosis to the PV the splenic vein is always restored, either on the reconstructed portal-mesenteric vein or on the inferior vena cava [42, 43]. Vascular anastomoses are performed with two half-running sutures of 6/0-7/0 ePTFE (Gore, W. L. Gore & Associates, USA) of 10-12 cm in length, and before knotting the last suture, heparinized saline solution is used to flush the SMV/PV [40, 42, 43]. All clamps are then released, starting with the cranial clamp placed on the PV to check at a low pressure the integrity of the vascular anastomoses and, if necessary, place single stitches in addition.

6.2.5 Postoperative Course and Management

The amylase in the drain fluid is routinely measured on days 3 and 5. The drainage tube is usually removed around day 5 if drainage fluid amylase is less than three times serum amylase and output is less than 200 ml. Total parenteral nutrition is initially given, then around postoperative day 1 liquid diet usually starts and semifluid diet around day 3. Mobilization begins on postoperative day 1.

6.2.6 Complications

In our recent report of 112 RPDs, in the last 72 consecutive patients we observed no grade C POPF and an overall 90-day mortality rate of 3.6% [51]. In addition, we showed a surprisingly low conversion rate of 2.7% (3 out of 112). Conversion was required because of factors unrelated to robotic assistance (intolerance to pneumoperitoneum or vascular injury after port insertion), and never due to technical problems [51]. Peng et al. [52] published a systematic review and meta-analysis of nine nonrandomized observational clinical trials with a total of 680 patients undergoing RPD and open PD. The comparison showed that RPD was associated with higher margin negativity ($P = 0.006$), lower overall complication rate ($P = 0.012$), and shorter length of hospital stay ($P = 0.002$) than open PD, while regarding the number of harvested lymph nodes, operative time, reoperation rate, complication rate (delayed gastric emptying, biliary fistula, and global and clinically relevant POPF), and mortality, there were no statistically significant differences between RPD and open PD [52].

6.2.7 Personal Experience

Regarding RPD, from June 2008 to June 2020, we performed 213 operations. The postoperative course was uneventful in 22% of patients, while serious complications (Clavien-Dindo >III) occurred in 12.7% of patients. Clinically relevant POPF occurred in 15% of patients (grade C POPF was 4.2%). Delayed gastric emptying (grade B and C) occurred in 39% of patients. The conversion rate was 1.9% and 90-day mortality was 4.7%. Reoperation was required in 11.3% of cases. Final histology showed pancreatic cancer in 165 (78.9%) patients, and the mean number of harvested lymph nodes was 42 ± 14.

Despite restrictive criteria in patient selection, RPD with *en bloc* resection and SMV/PV reconstruction remains a difficult operation, which we decided to perform after an experience of more than 400 open PDs with vascular resection and extensive experience with vascular procedures in thousands of solid organ transplants [42]. According to our latest report [43], from 2011 to 2019, 184 patients underwent RPD, and 22 (12.0%) of them received RPD with isolated vein resection (splenic-mesenteric junction in ten cases, and SMV in nine cases). Based on the International Study Group on Pancreatic Surgery classification [47], these procedures were classified as follows: one (4.5%) type I (partial venous excision with direct venorrhaphy), three (13.6%) type II (partial venous excision with patching), ten (45.5%) type III (segmental resection with primary venous-venous anastomosis), and eight (36.4%) type IV (segmental resection with interposed venous conduit). All but one operation were completed with robotic assistance (conversion rate 1 out of 22 cases), with median intraoperative blood loss of 900 ml (up to 1430 ml) [43]. Postoperative complications occurred in 16 patients, found to be grade ≥III according to Clavien-Dindo in five patients (22.7%) [43]. Only one patient had a POPF (grade B), four patients required a reoperation, and two patients died within 90 days [43]. Regarding final histology, 18 patients had a pancreatic ductal adenocarcinoma; microscopic residual tumor ≤1 mm was found in 11 patients, and vascular infiltration was confirmed in 13 out of 22 patients [43]. At the longest available follow-up, the reconstructed vein is patent in 19 out of 22 patients, the median overall survival is 39.7 months, and the median disease-free survival 32.9 months [43].

6.3 Total Pancreatectomy

6.3.1 Brief History of the Procedure

Robotic total pancreatectomy (RTP) has limited indications compared with other pancreatic resections, including: extension of PD or DP when in the pancreatic stump the margins are persistently positive, hereditary pancreatic tumors (e.g., familial adenomatous polyposis, hereditary nonpolyposis colon cancer), multifocal neuroendocrine neoplasms, intraductal papillary mucinous neoplasm or adenocarcinoma involving the entire gland, and chronic pancreatitis with refractory pain [53]. When surgery is performed in case of chronic pancreatitis and low-grade malignancy tumors, both the spleen and splenic vessels can be preserved [54].

Total pancreatectomy lies somewhere between PD and DP as technical difficulty, and since it still has some delicate steps such as dissection of the uncinate process and posterior margin and the reconstructive phase, it may represent a pancreatic resection in which the advantages of robotic assistance become apparent [40]. However, considering the rarity of indications for TP, the learning curve may be longer for this surgical operation [40].

6.3.2 Operating Room Setup and Patient Positioning

The patient is supine with legs spread, in the reverse Trendelenburg position at 20° and slightly prone on the left side [40]. The da Vinci robotic tower (Intuitive Surgical, Sunnydale, CA, USA) is docked as previously described for RPD. The robotic surgeon operates from the da Vinci console (Intuitive Surgical, Sunnydale, CA, USA), and the assistant surgeon stands between the patient's legs [40]. As previously described for RPD, five ports are positioned [40].

6.3.3 List of Specific Instruments/Gadgets Used

As robotic instruments, monopolar scissors, Maryland bipolar forceps (Intuitive Surgical, Sunnyvale, CA, USA), Harmonic scissors (Ethicon Endo-Surgery, Johnson & Johnson, Somerville, NJ, USA), and a fenestrated forceps are used [34].

6.3.4 The Operative Technique in a Detailed and Stepwise Manner

We describe here the technique developed in Pisa [40]. In some patients, the surgery starts as in RPD and is converted to TP because of intraoperative findings and/or frozen section [40].

Typically, after exploration of the abdominal cavity, the greater omentum is incised along the margin of the transverse colon, the lesser sac is entered, and the left gastric vein is identified, which is released and preserved to avoid gastric venous congestion if splenectomy is planned [40, 55, 56]. The left pancreas is then mobilized *en bloc* with the spleen, or cautiously separated from the splenic vessels [40]. The first duodenal portion will be dissected only after completing the dissection of the body-tail of the pancreas to keep the left hypochondrium free [40]. After mobilizing the right flexure of the colon, the right gastroepiploic vessels are identified and dissected between Hem-o-lok clips (Teleflex Medical, Research Triangle Park, North Carolina, USA) [40]. To expose the hepatoduodenal ligament and retract the liver, the gallbladder is drawn cranially and upward [40].

The first part of the duodenum is dissected with a laparoscopic stapler, after division between ligatures of the right gastric vessels [40]. The gastroduodenal artery and bile duct are divided after ligation (with 0 linen thread for the artery) [40]. Then, the duodenum is lifted and retracted toward the left side, and a Kocher maneuver is performed to free the first jejunal loop and transpose it to the right side of the superior mesenteric vessels [40]. At this point, we dissect the jejunal mesentery with the Harmonic scalpel (Ethicon Endo-Surgery, Johnson & Johnson, Somerville, New Jersey, USA), but not the small intestine, to make its rotation around the superior mesenteric vessels easier during the reconstructive phase [40]. Without having to reposition the patient or the robot, one can mobilize the third duodenal portion and divide the ligament of Treitz from the right side of the mesenteric vessels [40]. If *en bloc* splenectomy is planned, the splenic vessels should be ligated and divided now, so that the SMV/PV is mobilized and dissected along the right margin of the SMA, closing all vessels with ligature or clips avoiding energy devices as much as possible [40]. After dissecting the first jejunal loop, the specimen is placed in an endoscopic bag and excised through a suprapubic incision.

The reconstructive phase involves the use of a single jejunal loop: double-layer end-to-side hepatic-jejunal anastomosis is first performed, using 6/0 or 5/0 polydioxanone half-running sutures, and then 10–15 cm downstream, a double-layer duodenal-jejunal (or gastro-jejunal) anastomosis is made [40]. Two 12 Fr drains are then placed: one from the right side, posterior to the biliary anastomosis, and the other from the left side in the bed of the spleen [40].

6.3.5 Postoperative Course and Management

Total pancreatectomy induces diabetes characterized by both complete insulin deficiency and absence of functional glucagon [57]. These patients typically have lower daily insulin requirements than other diabetic patients [58], and episodes of even severe hypoglycemia after meals may frequently occur after insulin administration [59]. Postprandial hypoglycemia can be prevented by the combined use of long-acting insulin and during meals short-acting insulins [60]. In addition, pumps for continuous subcutaneous insulin infusion [61] and, in cases of late postprandial hypoglycemia, glucagon injections [62] can be used. Finally, in selected cases and in adequate centers, pancreatic *insulae* auto-transplantation can be performed [63].

Postoperative management after TP is also burdened by complete exocrine insufficiency, and to avoid steatorrhea, replacement therapy with high doses of pancreatic enzymes (up to 120,000 IU of pancrelipase per meal) is required, to be administered in combination with a proton pump inhibitor to prevent gastric acid juices from inactivating the enzymes prematurely [64]. These patients may need a caloric intake of up to 5000 kcal/day, given the malabsorption of fats and sugars [65], and a complex carbohydrate diet with vitamin and calcium supplementation to prevent weight loss and osteoporosis, and to control postprandial blood glucose changes [60].

6.3.6 Complications

Apart from POPF, the complications that may occur after TP are the same as those observed after PD and DP: delayed gastric emptying, biliary fistula, and post-pancreatectomy hemorrhage. In a recent case series with 25 patients undergoing open and planned TP, intra-abdominal hemorrhage, biliary fistula, and surgical reoperation were 4% [66]. Specific vaccinations are mandatory to avoid the risk of infection after splenectomy.

6.3.7 Personal Experience

We previously reported a series of 11 patients undergoing RTP, providing a case-by-case comparison with open surgery [40]. Two patients underwent resection and reconstruction of the SMV/PV, but no RTP was converted to laparoscopy or open surgery [40]. Robotic TP was associated with longer operative time but less blood loss than open surgery [40]. Postoperative complications occurred in similar rates after RTP and open TP, but those that occurred after RTP were mostly (five out of seven) minor complications (Clavien-Dindo grade I and II) [40]. Two patients required reoperation for an abdominal collection and hemorrhage that could not be alternatively treated, respectively, and no postoperative deaths occurred [40].

Patients undergoing RTP were able to mobilize and received their first full liquid and oral diet earlier than patients undergoing open surgery, also reporting better pain scale scores and less need for analgesics in the early postoperative days [40]. At final histology, all resection margins were negative, and the mean number of lymph nodes examined, all resected *en bloc* with the specimen, was higher in RTP than in open TP (45 vs. 36, respectively) [40]. The results of RTP should also be evaluated in the long term and especially in patients with benign disease or low-grade malignant tumors, which are the predominant indication for this type of surgical procedure [40].

References

1. Cuschieri A, Jakimowicz JJ, van Spreeuwel J. Laparoscopic distal 70% pancreatectomy and splenectomy for chronic pancreatitis. Ann Surg. 1996;223(3):280–5.
2. Gagner M, Pomp A, Herrera MF. Early experience with laparoscopic resections of islet cell tumors. Surgery. 1996;120(6):1051–4.
3. Bjornsson B, Sandstrom P. Laparoscopic distal pancreatectomy for adenocarcinoma of the pancreas. World J Gastroenterol. 2014;20(37):13402–11.
4. Jin T, Altaf K, Xiong JJ, et al. A systematic review and meta-analysis of studies comparing laparoscopic and open distal pancreatectomy. HPB (Oxford). 2012;14(11):711–24.
5. Lee SH, Kang CM, Hwang HK, et al. Minimally invasive RAMPS in well-selected left-sided pancreatic cancer within Yonsei criteria: long-term (>median 3 years) oncologic outcomes. Surg Endosc. 2014;28(10):2848–55.
6. de Rooij T, Klompmaker S, Abu Hilal M, et al. Laparoscopic pancreatic surgery for benign and malignant disease. Nat Rev Gastroenterol Hepatol. 2016;13(4):227–38.
7. Melvin WS, Needleman BJ, Krause KR, et al. Robotic resection of pancreatic neuroendocrine tumor. J Laparoendosc Adv Surg Tech A. 2003;13(1):33–6.
8. Damoli I, Butturini G, Ramera M, et al. Minimally invasive pancreatic surgery—a review. Wideochir Inne Tech Maloinwazyjne. 2015;10(2):141–9.
9. Wright GP, Zureikat AH. Development of minimally invasive pancreatic surgery: an evidence-based systematic review of laparoscopic versus robotic approaches. J Gastrointest Surg. 2016;20(9):1658–65.
10. Casadei R, Ricci C, Taffurelli G. Minimally invasive distal pancreatectomy for pancreatic cancer. In: Boggi U, editor. Minimally invasive surgery of the pancreas. 1st ed. Milan: Springer; 2018. p. 169–78.
11. Björnsson B, Sandström P. Laparoscopic distal pancreatectomy: how I do it. In: Tewari M, editor. Surgery for pancreatic and periampullary cancer. 1st ed. Singapore: Springer; 2018. p. 195–202.
12. Hu M, Zhao G, Wang F, et al. Laparoscopic versus open distal splenopancreatectomy for the treatment of pancreatic body and tail cancer: a retrospective, mid-term follow-up study at a single academic tertiary care institution. Surg Endosc. 2014;28:2584–91.
13. Butturini G, Giardino A, Damoli I. Robotic distal pancreatectomy with en bloc splenectomy. In: Boggi U, editor. Minimally invasive surgery of the pancreas. 1st ed. Milan: Springer; 2018. p. 211–8.
14. Edwin B, Sahakyan MA, Abu Hilal M, et al. Laparoscopic surgery for pancreatic neoplasms: the European Association for Endoscopic Surgery clinical consensus conference. Surg Endosc. 2017;31(5):2023–41.
15. Strasberg SM, Drebin JA, Linehan D. Radical antegrade modular pancreatosplenectomy. Surgery. 2003;133(5):521–7.
16. Kim EY, Hong TH. Initial experience with laparoscopic radical antegrade modular pancreatosplenectomy for left-sided pancreatic cancer in a single institution: technical aspects and oncological outcomes. BMC Surg. 2017;17(1):2.
17. Coppola A, Caputo D, Giuliante F. Laparoscopic distal pancreatectomy with en bloc splenectomy. In: Boggi U, editor. Minimally invasive surgery of the pancreas. 1st ed. Milan: Springer; 2018. p. 195–202.
18. Napoli N, Kauffmann EF, Menonna F, et al. Robot-assisted radical antegrade modular pancreatosplenectomy including resection and reconstruction of the spleno-mesenteric junction. J Vis Exp. 2020;(155). https://doi.org/10.3791/60370.
19. Emam TA, Cuschieri A. How safe is high-power ultrasonic dissection? Ann Surg. 2003;237(2):186–91.
20. Blansflied JA, Rapp MM, Chokshi RJ, et al. Novel method of stump closure for distal pancreatectomy with a 75% reduction in pancreatic fistula rate. J Gastrointest Surg. 2011;16(3):524–8.
21. Diener MK, Seiler CM, Rossion I, et al. Efficacy of stapler versus hand-sewn closure after distal pancreatectomy (DISPACT): a randomized, controlled multicentre trial. Lancet. 2011;377(9776):1514–22.
22. Reeh M, Nentwich MF, Bogoeversuski D, et al. High surgical morbidity following distal pancreatectomy: still an unsolved problem. World J Surg. 2011;35(5):1110–7.
23. Hammerquist RJ, Messerschmidt KA, Pottebaum AA, et al. Vaccinations in asplenic adults. Am J Health Syst Pharm. 2016;73(9):e220–8.
24. Barbui T, Barosi G, Grossi A, et al. Practice guidelines for the therapy of essential thrombocythemia. A statement from the Italian Society of Hematology, the Italian Society of Experimental Hematology and the Italian Group for Bone Marrow Transplantation. Haematologica. 2004;89(2):215–32.
25. Gagner M, Pomp A. Laparoscopic pylorus-preserving pancreatoduodenectomy. Surg Endosc. 1994;8:408–10.
26. Dulucq JL, Wintringer P, Mahajna A. Laparoscopic pancreaticoduodenectomy for benign and malignant diseases. Surg Endosc. 2006;20:1045–50.
27. Delitto D, Luckhurst CM, Black BS, et al. Oncologic and perioperative outcomes following selective application of laparoscopic pancreaticoduodenectomy for periampullary malignancies. J Gastrointest Surg. 2016;20:1343–9.
28. Dokmak S, Ftériche FS, Aussilhou B, et al. Laparoscopic pancreatico-duodenectomy should not be routine for resection of periampullary tumors. J Am Coll Surg. 2015;220:831–8.
29. Corcione F, Cuccurullo D, Angelini P. Laparoscopic pancreatoduodenectomy. In: Boggi U, editor.

Minimally invasive surgery of the pancreas. 1st ed. Milan: Springer; 2018. p. 219–30.
30. Giulianotti PC, Mangano A, Bustos RE, et al. Operative technique in robotic pancreaticoduodenectomy (RPD) at University of Illinois at Chicago (UIC): 17 steps standardized technique. Lessons learned since the first worldwide RPD performed in the year 2001. Surg Endosc. 2018;32:4329–36.
31. van Hilst J, de Rooij T, Bosscha K, et al. Laparoscopic versus open pancreatoduodenectomy for pancreatic or periampullary tumours (LEOPARD-2): a multicentre, patient-blinded, randomised controlled phase 2/3 trial. Lancet Gastroenterol Hepatol. 2019;4:199–207.
32. Gharios J, Hain E, Dohan A, et al. Pre- and intraoperative diagnostic requirements, benefits and risks of minimally invasive and robotic surgery for neuroendocrine tumors of the pancreas. Best Pract Res Clin Endocrinol Metab. 2019;33:101294.
33. Giulianotti PC, Coratti A, Angelini M, et al. Robotics in general surgery: personal experience in a large community hospital. Arch Surg. 2003;138:777–84.
34. Boggi U, Perrone VG, Vistoli F. Robotic pancreatoduodenectomy. In: Boggi U, editor. Minimally invasive surgery of the pancreas. 1st ed. Milan: Springer; 2018. p. 241–54.
35. Kamarajah SK, Bundred J, Saint Marc O, et al. Robotic versus conventional laparoscopic pancreatico-duodenectomy: a systematic review and meta-analysis. Eur J Surg Oncol. 2020;46:6–14.
36. Hidalgo M. Pancreatic cancer. N Engl J Med. 2010;362:1605–17.
37. Napoli N, Kauffmann EF, Menonna F, et al. Indications, technique, and results of robotic pancreatoduodenectomy. Updates Surg. 2016;68:295–305.
38. Wellner UF, Küsters S, Sick O, et al. Hybrid laparoscopic versus open pylorus-preserving pancreatoduodenectomy: retrospective matched case comparison in 80 patients. Langenbecks Arch Surg. 2014;399:849–56.
39. Boggi U, Signori S, De Lio N, et al. Feasibility of robotic pancreaticoduodenectomy. Br J Surg. 2013;100:917–25.
40. Boggi U, Palladino S, Massimetti G, et al. Laparoscopic robot-assisted versus open total pancreatectomy: a case-matched study. Surg Endosc. 2015;29:1425–32.
41. Fujii T, Sugimoto H, Yamada S, et al. Modified Blumgart anastomosis for pancreaticojejunostomy: technical improvement in matched historical control study. J Gastrointest Surg. 2014;18:1108–15.
42. Boggi U, Lombardo C, Napoli N. Robotic pancreatoduodenectomy for pancreatic cancer with superior mesenteric/portal vein resection and reconstruction. In: Boggi U, editor. Minimally invasive surgery of the pancreas. 1st ed. Milan: Springer; 2018. p. 255–64.
43. Kauffmann EF, Napoli N, Menonna F, et al. Robot-assisted pancreaticoduodenectomy with vascular resection: technical details and results from a high-volume center. Laparosc Surg. 2020;4:37.
44. Sanjay P, Takaori K, Govil S, et al. 'Artery first' approaches to pancreatoduodenectomy. Br J Surg. 2012;99:1027–35.
45. Inoue Y, Saiura A, Yoshioka R, et al. Pancreatoduodenectomy with systematic mesopancreas dissection using a supracolic anterior artery-first approach. Ann Surg. 2015;262:1092–101.
46. Chowdappa R, Challa VR. Mesopancreas in pancreatic cancer: where do we stand—review of literature. Indian J Surg Oncol. 2015;6:69–74.
47. Bockhorn M, Uzunoglu FG, Adham M, et al. Borderline resectable pancreatic cancer: a consensus statement by the International Study Group of Pancreatic Surgery (ISGPS). Surgery. 2014;155:977–88.
48. Dokmak S, Aussilhou B, Calmels M, et al. Laparoscopic pancreaticoduodenectomy with reconstruction of the mesentericoportal vein with the parietal peritoneum and the falciform ligament. Surg Endosc. 2018;32:3256–61.
49. Liao K, Wang H, Chen Q, et al. Prosthetic graft for superior mesenteric-portal vein reconstruction in pancreaticoduodenectomy: a retrospective, multicenter study. J Gastrointest Surg. 2014;18:1452–61.
50. Meniconi RL, Santoro R, Guglielmo N, et al. Pancreaticoduodenectomy with venous reconstruction using cold-stored vein allografts: long-term results of a single center experience. J Hepatobiliary Pancreat Sci. 2016;23:43–9.
51. Kauffmann EF, Napoli N, Menonna F, et al. Robotic pancreatoduodenectomy with vascular resection. Langenbecks Arch Surg. 2016;401:1111–22.
52. Peng L, Lin S, Li Y, et al. Systematic review and meta-analysis of robotic versus open pancreaticoduodenectomy. Surg Endosc. 2017;31:3085–97.
53. Coratti A, Annecchiarico M. Minimally invasive total pancreatectomy. In: Boggi U, editor. Minimally invasive surgery of the pancreas. 1st ed. Milan: Springer; 2018. p. 265–76.
54. Giulianotti PC, Addeo P, Buchs NC, et al. Early experience with robotic total pancreatectomy. Pancreas. 2011;40:311–3.
55. Sandroussi C, McGilvray ID. Gastric venous reconstruction after radical pancreatic surgery: case report and review of the literature. J Gastrointest Surg. 2010;14:1027–30.
56. Rebibo L, Chivot C, Fuks D, et al. Three-dimensional computed tomography analysis of the left gastric vein in a pancreatectomy. HPB. 2012;14:414–21.
57. Andreou A, Klein F, Schmuck RB, et al. Incidence and oncological implications of previously undetected tumor multicentricity following pancreaticoduodenectomy for pancreatic adenocarcinoma in patients undergoing salvage pancreatectomy. Anticancer Res. 2017;37:5269–75.
58. Vigili de Kreutzenberg S, Maifreni L, Lisato G, et al. Glucose turnover and recycling in diabetes secondary to total pancreatectomy: effect of glucagons infusion. J Clin Endocrinol Metab. 1990;70:1023–9.

59. Slezak LA, Andersen DK. Pancreatic resection: effects on glucose metabolism. World J Surg. 2001;25:452–60.
60. Heidt DG, Burant C, Simeone DM. Total pancreatectomy: indications, operative technique, and postoperative sequelae. J Gastrointest Surg. 2007;11:209–16.
61. Radermecker RP, Scheen AJ. Continuous subcutaneous insulin infusion with short-acting insulin analogues or human regular insulin: efficacy, safety, quality of life, and cost-effectiveness. Diabetes Metab Res Rev. 2004;20:178–88.
62. Heptulla RA, Rodriguez LM, Bomgaars L, et al. The role of amylin and glucagon in the dampening of glycemic excursions in children with type 1 diabetes. Diabetes. 2005;54:1100–7.
63. Galvani CA, Rodriguez Rilo H, Samamé J, et al. Fully robotic-assisted technique for total pancreatectomy with an autologous islet transplant in chronic pancreatitis patients: results of a first series. J Am Coll Surg. 2014;218:e73–8.
64. Kahl S, Malfertheiner P. Exocrine and endocrine pancreatic insufficiency after pancreatic surgery. Best Pract Res Clin Gastroenterol. 2012;18:947–55.
65. Dressler CM, Fortner JG, McDermott K, et al. Metabolic consequences of (regional) total pancreatectomy. Ann Surg. 1991;214:131–40.
66. Crippa S, Tamburrino D, Partelli S, et al. Total pancreatectomy: indications, different timing, and perioperative and long-term outcomes. Surgery. 2011;149:79–86.

Minimally Invasive Surgery for Colon Cancer

7

Swapnil Patel and Avanish Saklani

Abstract

There is no one best approach for laparoscopic surgery for colon cancers. Various surgeons have standardized the procedure to provide the best outcomes in their ambient operative set-up. This chapter provides an overview of the basic tenets of laparoscopic approach to colon cancer surgery focusing on principles of complete mesocolic excision with central vascular ligation and D3 lymphadenectomy. The video supplement highlights the technical nuances of laparoscopic right and left hemicolectomy in a case requiring total colectomy for colonic adenocarcinoma.

Keywords

Laparoscopic colectomy · Complete mesocolic excision · Central vascular ligation · D3 lymphadenectomy · Minimally invasive surgery

Supplementary Information The online version contains supplementary material available at https://doi.org/10.1007/978-981-97-7059-5_7.

S. Patel
Department of Surgical Oncology, MPMMCC & Homi Bhabha Cancer Hospital, Tata Memorial Centre, Varanasi, Uttar Pradesh, India

A. Saklani (✉)
Colorectal Division, Department of GI & HPB Surgery, Tata Memorial Centre, Mumbai, Maharashtra, India

7.1 Introduction

Minimally invasive surgery for early colon cancers is close to becoming the standard of care, when performed in experienced hands. Various surgeons have proposed various modifications of the procedure over time, each standardized in their own way. One common underlying principle is the concept of complete mesocolic excision (CME) with central vascular ligation (CVL) with D-3 lymphadenectomy as proposed by Hohenberger [1]. Efficacy of minimally invasive surgery (MIS) approach to colectomy has been established both for laparoscopic and robotic platforms. COST, COLOR, and CLASSIC trials have well established the superiority of laparoscopic-assisted colectomy over open approach with regard to short-term outcomes along with equivalent long-term oncological adequacy [2–5]. Robotic colectomy has been shown to have equivalent outcomes as laparoscopic colectomy, albeit with higher expenditures [6]. In this chapter we describe the tenets for conduct of a laparoscopic colectomy, focusing on technical aspects for conduct of an oncologically safe colectomy.

1. *Patient selection*: Oncological adequacy of laparoscopic approach for a colectomy has been well established for early colon cancers (cT1–3 with limited regional nodal burden), as reflected by the patients randomized in the

M. Tewari (ed.), *Minimally Invasive Surgery in Cancer*,
https://doi.org/10.1007/978-981-97-7059-5_7

trials listed above. The adequacy of laparoscopy for advanced lesions, i.e., more than cT3 or cancers with heavy nodal burden has not been established. However, studies albeit not randomized have shown that select locally advanced tumors should not be excluded from laparoscopic surgery [7]. Conduct of surgery in lesions with obstructed gut is technically difficult [8].

2. *Patient positioning and operating room setup*: Appropriate patient positioning in the background of adequate arrangement in operating room (OR) goes a long way in an easy surgery. The common adopted OR setups are as shown in Fig. 7.1. Various operative setups have been proposed for a laparoscopic right colectomy, most commonly the French position and the supine positions. For a left-sided colonic resection or a rectal resection, the OR arrangement is more constant with the laparoscopic cart near left leg.
3. *Preoperative understanding of the vascular anatomy around superior mesenteric axis*: It is imperative to have a good quality contrast-enhanced computed tomography scan (CECT) of abdomen prior to surgery and discuss regarding the vascular pedicles to anticipate during the laparoscopic surgery. This becomes more important when operating a right colon cancer as the anatomy of branches of superior mesenteric artery and vein (SMA and SMV) is more variable than the vasculature of the left colon [9, 10]. Presurgery knowledge regarding vascular anatomy helps in an easy conduct of the surgery with possible decrease in vascular complication. The vascular anatomy with variations has been detailed in the video supplement.
4. *Port placement*:

   The position of ports depends on the approach undertaken for colectomy as detailed below. Authors usually approach a laparoscopic right colectomy using a combination of caudal to cranial and medial to lateral approach in supine position. The port position utilized by authors is detailed in Fig. 7.2.
5. *Approaches for conduct of laparoscopic right colectomy*:

   Laparoscopic right colectomy has been traditionally approached in three ways as described below.

   (a) *Medial to lateral approach (MtL)*:

      (I) Serial ligation of the vascular pedicles at the root of the superior mesenteric axis, starting from ileocolic, then right colic pedicle, and then middle colic pedicle.

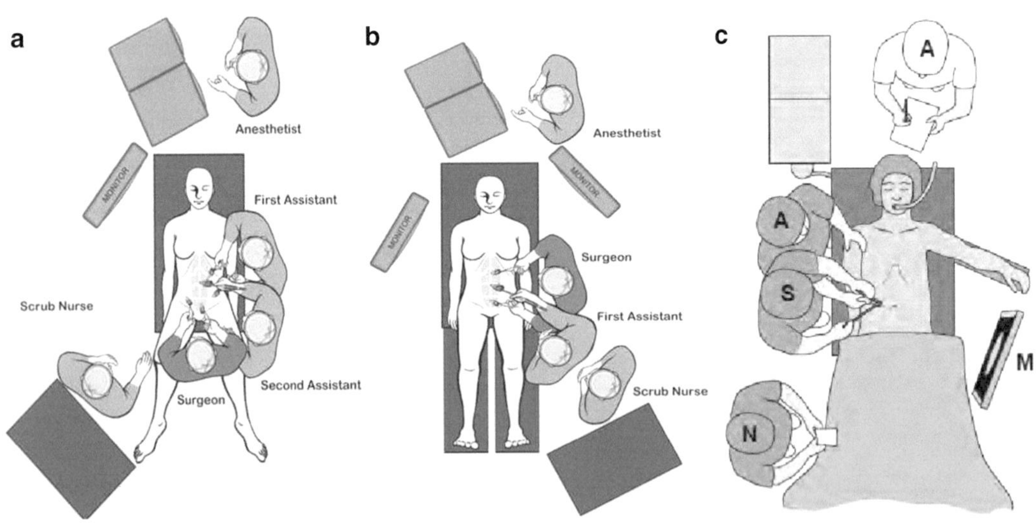

Fig. 7.1 Operating room setup for a laparoscopic colectomy for (**a**) right colectomy in French position, (**b**) right colectomy in supine position, (**c**) left colectomy

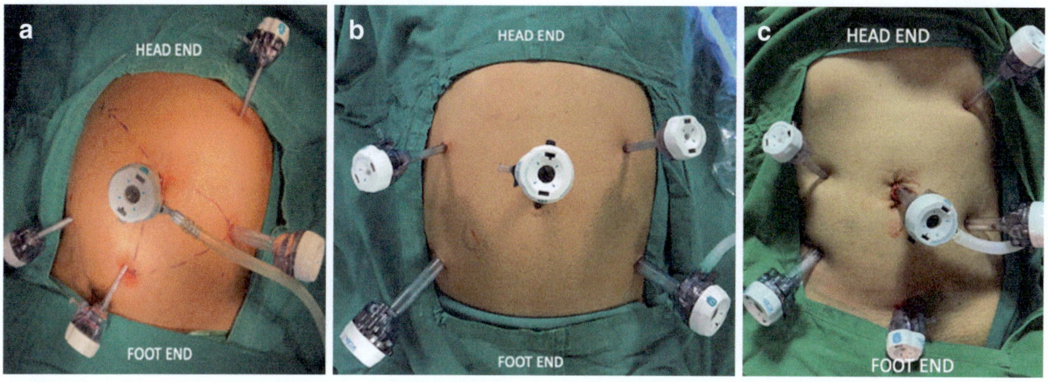

Fig. 7.2 Position of laparoscopic ports (**a**) right colectomy—combination of medial to lateral and caudal to cranial approach, (**b**) left colectomy—medial to lateral approach, (**c**) total colectomy

(II) Mobilization of the mesocolon off the retroperitoneum.
(III) Lateral peritoneal cut.
(IV) Dissection in lesser sac and releasing hepatic flexure [11, 12].

(b) *Lateral to medial approach (LtM)*: Proponents of this approach cite early reproducibility of the technique, especially in the training module.
(I) Mobilizing the colon from the lateral abdominal wall first.
(II) Detachment of colon from the stomach and duodenum by dissection in lesser sac.
(III) Dissection and ligation of the vascular pedicles.
(IV) Mobilization of mesocolon off the retroperitoneum [13].

(c) *Caudal to cranial approach (CtC)*:
(I) Initial dissection is done by the scoring over the root of mesentery to lift the mesocolon and root of mesentery off the retroperitoneum.
(II) Separating the mesocolon from the duodeno-pancreatic fascia (Fredet's fascia) to completely lift the mesocolon off the posterior attachments while maintaining its integrity, called complete mesocolic excision (CME) [14].
(III) Serially dissecting and ligating the vascular pedicles at the root of the superior mesenteric axis.
(IV) Lastly, the dissection separating the right colon from the stomach and along the line of Toldt [15, 16].

All three approaches fare equally in terms of oncological outcomes with equivalent postoperative outcomes [17, 18].

The authors follow a combined caudal to cranial and medial to lateral approach for conduct of laparoscopic right colectomy. This technique has been detailed in the video supplement.

6. *Anastomosis following laparoscopic right colectomy*:

   Ileo-colic anastomosis, either intracorporeal or extracorporeal and either hand-sewn or stapled does not result in any clinically relevant difference in perioperative outcomes following a laparoscopic right hemicolectomy [19].

7. *Approach to a laparoscopic left colectomy*:

   Laparoscopic approach to a left colectomy is relatively more fixed when compared to that for right colonic resection. The conduct of the surgery is divided into the following reproducible steps:

   (a) Dissection below Inferior mesenteric vein.
   (b) Dissection and ligation of Inferior mesenteric artery.
   (c) Medial to lateral dissection.
   (d) Lateral peritoneal cut.
   (e) Splenic flexure mobilization.

(f) Specimen transection and delivery.
(g) Intra-corporeal colo-colic or colo-rectal anastomosis.

The conduct of the surgery has been detailed in the attached video supplement.

8. *Instrument and machinery requirement*:

   The entire surgery is conducted using a laparoscopic monopolar electrosurgical unit in combination with a vessel sealing device at standard operating settings.

   During the course of the surgery, the patient is subjected to various positions to facilitate the desired bowel positioning and dissection. Prior to start of the surgery, the position is confirmed in the extremes of positions that may be needed. During the dissection of the left colon, the patient is placed in 45° Trendelenberg position with a maximum right tilt. During the dissection of the right colon (employing medial to lateral technique), the patient is positioned in a 30° reverse Trendelenberg position with a maximum left tilt.
9. Postoperative management:

   Enhanced recovery after surgery (ERAS) is followed strictly in the author's unit for all elective colorectal surgeries. After a standard right or a left colectomy, the nasogastric tube is removed on postoperative day 0. The patient is allowed liquid diet on postoperative day 1 and then on soft diet subsequently depending on resumption of bowel movements.
10. Operating experience of the authors' unit:

    At the Tata Memorial Hospital, approximately 200 right colectomies are performed every year. Among these 30% cases are elective, 30% are semi-emergency, and the remaining 40% cases are emergency.

    While the emergency cases are always done using an open approach, the majority of elective cases are done using minimally invasive approach (mainly, laparoscopic).

    Annual morbidity rate is around 3% (clavein dindo grade 3b and above) and the mortality rate is less than 1% for all the colectomies (elective and emergency).

7.2 Video Supplement

7.2.1 Case Description

A 45-year gentleman diagnosed with splenic flexure adenocarcinoma and colonic polyposis was planned for laparoscopic total colectomy with ileo-rectal anastomosis. Sequential dissection of left colon followed by right colon was done ensuring CME, CVL with D3 lymphadenectomy. Anastomosis was done using Knight-Griffin technique using a 4 cm utility incision. Surgery was performed over 4 h with 200 mL blood loss. The patient went home on day 6.

This video demonstrates left colonic dissection followed by right colonic dissection (caudal-cranial with medial-lateral approach used). Beginning with left colonic mobilization facilitates easy splenic flexure mobilization.

The procedure was carried out in the steps as detailed below:

1. Dissection of left colon:
   (a) Dissection of inferior mesenteric artery and ligation at the root (Fig. 7.3a)
   (b) Dissection of inferior mesenteric vein and ligation at the root (Fig. 7.3b, c)
   (c) Medial to lateral dissection of descending colon (Fig. 7.3d)
   (d) Splenic flexure mobilization (Fig. 7.3e, f)
   (e) Upper rectal dissection in TME plane
   (f) Distal specimen transection
2. Changing the position of operating room setup
3. Dissection of right colon
   (a) Dissection of mesocolon off the retroperitoneum along Toldt's fascia and Fredet's fascia (Fig. 7.4a, b)
   (b) Dissection along the SMV (Fig. 7.5a)
   (c) Ligation of ileo-colic pedicle, right colic pedicle, and middle colic pedicle (Fig. 7.5b–d)
   (d) Dissection in lesser sac and along lateral peritoneal attachment (Fig. 7.6a, b)
4. Specimen delivery and extracorporeal anastomosis

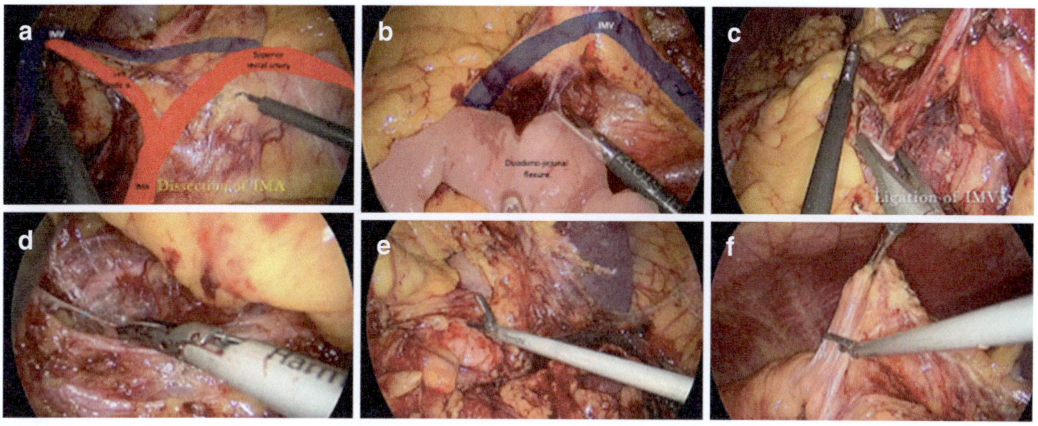

Fig. 7.3 (**a**–**f**) Dissection of left colectomy: (**a**) dissection of inferior mesenteric artery, (**b**, **c**) dissection and ligation of inferior mesenteric vein, (**d**) medial to lateral dissection, (**e**, **f**) splenic flexure dissection

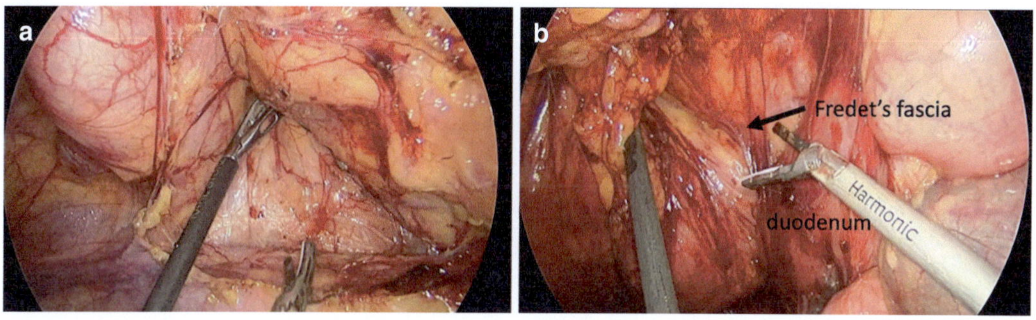

Fig. 7.4 (**a**, **b**) Dissection of right colon in the retroperitoneal fascial planes (**a**) Toldt's fascia, (**b**) Fredet's fascia

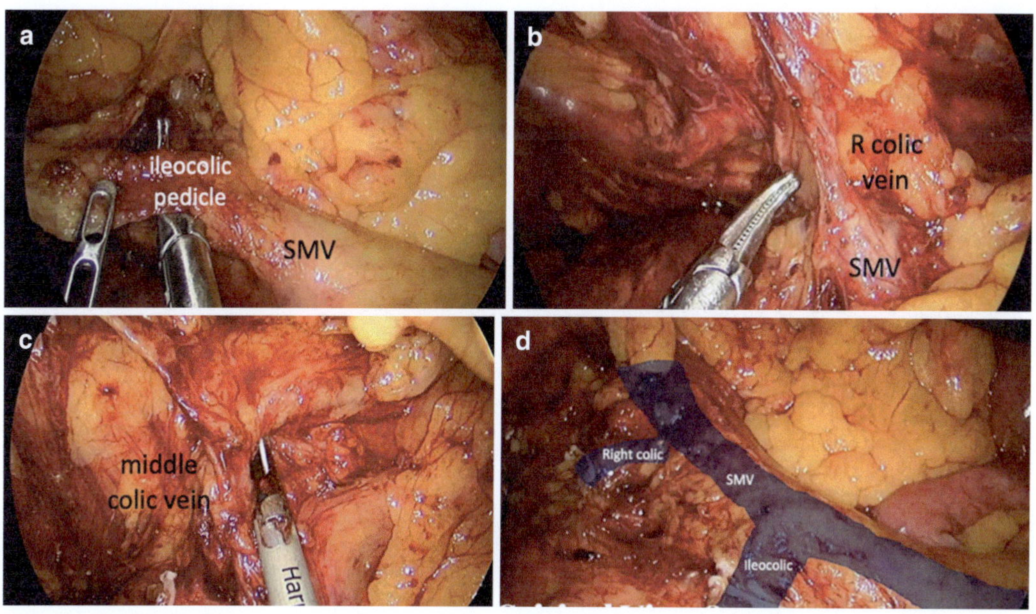

Fig. 7.5 (**a**–**d**) Dissection along the superior mesenteric vein (**a**) ileocolic vein, (**b**) right colic vein, (**c**) middle colic vein, (**d**) dissected SMV

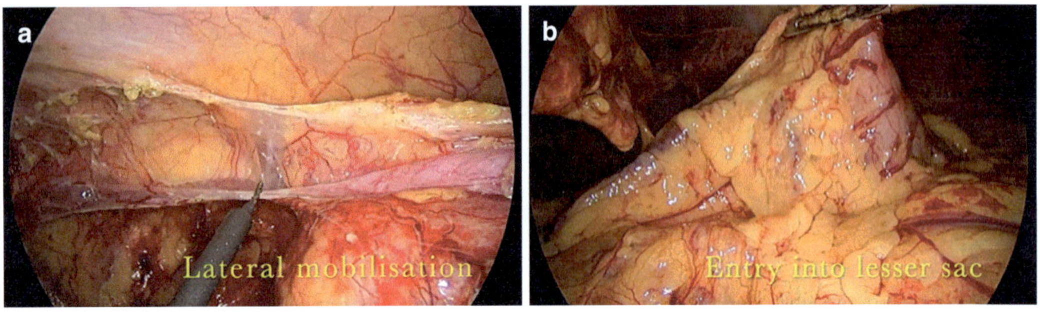

Fig. 7.6 (**a**, **b**) Mobilization of the right colon (**a**) along the lateral peritoneal attachment, (**b**) in the lesser sac

References

1. Hohenberger W, Weber K, Matzel K, Papadopoulos T, Merkel S. Standardized surgery for colonic cancer: complete mesocolic excision and central ligation—technical notes and outcome. Colorectal Dis. 2009;11(4):354–64.
2. A comparison of laparoscopically assisted and open colectomy for colon cancer. N Engl J Med. 2004;350(20):2050–9.
3. Laparoscopically assisted vs open colectomy for colon cancer: a meta-analysis. Arch Surg. 2007;142(3):298.
4. On Behalf of the COLOR (COlon cancer Laparoscopic or Open Resection) Study Group, Deijen CL, Vasmel JE, de Lange-de Klerk ESM, Cuesta MA, Coene P-PLO, et al. Ten-year outcomes of a randomised trial of laparoscopic versus open surgery for colon cancer. Surg Endosc. 2017;31(6):2607–15.
5. Guillou PJ, Quirke P, Thorpe H, Walker J, Jayne DG, Smith AM, et al. Short-term endpoints of conventional versus laparoscopic-assisted surgery in patients with colorectal cancer (MRC CLASICC trial): multicentre, randomised controlled trial. The Lancet. 2005;365(9472):1718–26.
6. Park JS, Kang H, Park SY, Kim HJ, Woo IT, Park I-K, et al. Long-term oncologic after robotic versus laparoscopic right colectomy: a prospective randomized study. Surg Endosc. 2019;33(9):2975–81.
7. Yamanashi T, Nakamura T, Sato T, Naito M, Miura H, Tsutsui A, et al. Laparoscopic surgery for locally advanced T4 colon cancer: the long-term outcomes and prognostic factors. Surg Today. 2018;48(5):534–44.
8. van Dalen ASHM, Ali UA, Murray ACA, Kiran RP. Optimizing patient selection for laparoscopic and open colorectal cancer resections: a national surgical quality improvement program-matched analysis. Am Surg. 2019;85(2):206–13.
9. Kuzu MA, İsmail E, Çelik S, Şahin MF, Güner MA, Hohenberger W, et al. Variations in the vascular anatomy of the right colon and implications for right-sided colon surgery. Dis Colon Rectum. 2017;60(3):290–8.
10. Wu C, Ye K, Wu Y, Chen Q, Xu J, Lin J, et al. Variations in right colic vascular anatomy observed during laparoscopic right colectomy. World J Surg Oncol. 2019;17(1):16.
11. Mohanty S. Laparoscopic right hemicolectomy (medial-to-lateral approach). In: Karamanos E, editor. Common surgeries made easy [Internet]. Cham: Springer; 2020. p. 95–8. [cited 25 Sept 2021] Available from: http://link.springer.com/10.1007/978-3-030-41350-7_15.
12. Franklin Jr ME. Right colon cancer: medial to lateral [Internet]. Available from: https://www.youtube.com/watch?v=NlD4ZnfIQKM
13. Young-Fadok TM. Laparoscopic lateral-to-medial dissection—a safer approach? [Internet]. Available from: https://youtu.be/zAz_XdSceh8
14. Garcia-Granero A, Pellino G, Frasson M, Fletcher-Sanfeliu D, Bonilla F, Sánchez-Guillén L, et al. The fusion fascia of Fredet: an important embryological landmark for complete mesocolic excision and D3-lymphadenectomy in right colon cancer. Surg Endosc. 2019;33(11):3842–50.
15. Li H, He Y, Lin Z, Xiong W, Diao D, Wang W, et al. Laparoscopic caudal-to-cranial approach for radical lymph node dissection in right hemicolectomy. Langenbecks Arch Surg. 2016;401(5):741–6.
16. Li H. A novel technique for laparoscopic right hemicolectomy with CME: the caudal-to-cranial approach [Internet]. Available from: https://www.youtube.com/watch?v=0PvQ6WjkAtk
17. Li F, Zhou X, Wang B, Guo L, Wang J, Wang W, et al. Comparison between different approaches applied in laparoscopic right hemi-colectomy: A systematic review and network meta-analysis. Int J Surg. 2017;48:74–82.
18. Hussain A, Mahmood F, Torrance AW, Tsiamis A. Impact of medial-to-lateral vs lateral-to-medial approach on short-term and cancer-related outcomes in laparoscopic colorectal surgery: A retrospective cohort study. Ann Med Surg. 2018;26:19–23.
19. Allaix ME, Degiuli M, Bonino MA, Arezzo A, Mistrangelo M, Passera R, et al. Intracorporeal or extracorporeal ileocolic anastomosis after laparoscopic right colectomy: a double-blinded randomized controlled trial. Ann Surg. 2019;270(5):762–7.

8 Minimally Invasive Surgery for Rectal Cancer

Kurt A. Melstrom and Andreas M. Kaiser

Abstract

This chapter will touch on the brief history of MIS for rectal cancer. The major preoperative considerations including setup and port placement will follow. In-depth descriptions and depictions of three main operations will be given for both laparoscopic and robotic approaches, using the traditional 2D laparoscopic and the main Intuitive robotic models in use today (da Vinci Xi platform). This includes the low anterior resection (LAR), low anterior resection with coloanal anastomosis or the so-called ultralow LAR (ULAR), and finally the abdominoperineal resection (APR). Major postoperative considerations will be discussed including the most prominent complications and their management.

Finally, we will outline the authors' own experiences with these procedures and provide a perspective of future developments. As several new robotic and hybrid laparoscopic platforms are entering the surgery market, their specific place will yet have to be defined. But unquestionably, this same chapter will probably look very different a decade from now in terms of options.

Keywords

Rectal cancer · Minimally invasive surgery · Laparoscopic surgery · Robotic surgery · Low anterior resection · Ultralow anterior resection · Abdominoperineal resection

8.1 Introduction

Colorectal cancer represents the third most common cancer in the United States in terms of incidence and mortality whereby rectal cancer accounts for about one third or an estimated 46,000 new cases per year [1]. This specific cancer has increasingly been recognized as being a highly complex disease process that benefits from a multimodality approach to carefully weigh the different treatment modalities (chemotherapy, radiation, surgery) and specific protocols. Innovation in the areas of rectal cancer treatment aims at improving both the patient's oncological as well as functional outcomes.

The gold standard for rectal cancer surgery had traditionally been through an open approach [2]. But even that open technique evolved from a rather

The authors have not received any financial support for this manuscript.

Supplementary Information The online version contains supplementary material available at https://doi.org/10.1007/978-981-97-7059-5_8.

K. A. Melstrom · A. M. Kaiser (✉)
Division of Colorectal Surgery, Department of Surgery, City of Hope National Medical Center, an NCI-Designated Comprehensive Cancer Center, Duarte, CA, USA
e-mail: akaiser@coh.org

M. Tewari (ed.), *Minimally Invasive Surgery in Cancer*,
https://doi.org/10.1007/978-981-97-7059-5_8

indiscriminate to a highly sophisticated, anatomical pelvic dissection: total mesorectal excision (TME) had become the standard of care in rectal cancer surgery since its development in the 1980s. But since the 1990s, when minimally invasive techniques entered the market, there has been a veritable revolution—starting with laparoscopic surgery first, followed later by robotic and transanal surgery platforms [3]. However, despite the changes and offering other advantages, the benchmark to achieve the same quality of the TME specimen remained the same [4].

The main drawback to an open procedure is not just the large incision with more pain and a higher chance for a hernia, but also the more extensive trauma to the bowels through mechanical and room air exposure, both of which are associated with increased formation of adhesions and possible future bowel obstructions. Minimally invasive surgery offers the advantage of much smaller incisions, which can translate into less postoperative pain, quicker return of bowel function, and shorter hospital stays. There are many different approaches and hybrid techniques that are employed to each surgeon's training and preference [3, 4].

8.2 History

MIS for rectal cancer has a complex history, which has spanned the last three decades. The advent of laparoscopic surgery in the early 1990s saw the rapid adoption of techniques for cholecystectomy and appendectomy [5]. Colorectal surgery lagged behind and initially was limited to easier segmental colectomies (right hemicolectomy, sigmoid/left hemicolectomy). Factors contributing to the slow adoption included the added complexity of multi-quadrant resections, specimen retrieval, and a need to fashion a reliable anastomosis; furthermore, an early small series reporting a higher than expected incidence of port site recurrences raised concerns about the safety of the approach but was relatively quickly countered by more robust data to the contrary [5]. By the mid-2000s, major randomized controlled trials found laparoscopic colon surgery to be both safe and effective, even though not necessarily better [6]. Laparoscopic surgery for rectal cancer followed with some delay. The MRC CLASICC trial first reported outcomes in its subgroup of rectal cancers. It found a nonsignificant increase in positive circumferential resection margin (CRM) rates in the laparoscopic surgery arm [7], but no measurable negative long-term impact [8]. It took another decade before several major laparoscopic versus open trials were published in 2015. The European COLOR II trial found shorter lengths of stay and quicker bowel recovery in laparoscopic patients [9]. The Australian ALaCaRT and the United States ACOSOG Z6051 trials were launched in a parallel design. A first interim report in 2015 analyzed a pathological composite quality score, and in that regard, laparoscopic surgery failed to prove being noninferior compared to the open approach [10, 11]. Despite this early concern within the surgical community, the long-term data on oncological outcomes a few years later showed no negative impact of the laparoscopic approach on overall or disease-free survival [12, 13].

While laparoscopic surgery for rectal cancer was further being investigated while slowly adopted, robotic surgery was introduced as a refinement to the laparoscopic technique. The first reports of robotic rectal cancer surgery were published in the mid-2000s. The technology and surgical techniques continued to rapidly evolve in parallel with laparoscopic surgery. Even though both platforms ultimately represent the same minimally invasive approach, the largest and most impactful trial elected to compare laparoscopic and robotic surgery primarily in regard to conversion rates rather than oncological outcomes, and it did so without including an open surgery arm. The ROLARR trial from 2017 showed no differences in the primary and secondary end points unless subjected to some subgroup analysis [14]. A smaller Korean trial, which was published the following year, looked at oncologic outcomes and found no differences in the quality of the rectal specimens [15]. Since 2010, there has been a fivefold increase in robotic as compared to only a 1.1-fold increase in laparoscopic oncological procedures [16]. The rapid rise in popularity of the robotic surgery platform is multifactorial in origin but likely relates to the ease of use as compared to laparoscopic surgery, combined with better marketing and a monopoly position of the original manufacturer [3].

Transanal endoscopic microsurgery (TEMS) or transanal minimally invasive surgery (TAMIS) evolved as more sophisticated tools for endoluminal management of rectal lesions [17]. Their indications were limited to precancerous or early cancerous lesions and hence remained rather limited. However, they gave the impetus to develop the transanal approach to a full oncological bottom-up resection of rectal cancer, also referred to as transanal TME (TaTME). Removal of the entire rectum via a transanal MIS approach was described as early as 2010. Major registry and randomized controlled trials on this procedure are still evolving, and smaller studies have shown conflicting results [18, 19]. The rationale behind this approach was to gain better visualization and dissection in the most distal part of the resection, which in the transabdominal approach may be particularly challenging in very obese patients with a narrow pelvis. *For further details on TaTME, please refer to the dedicated chapter elsewhere in the book.*

8.3 Patient and Operating Room Setup

One of the great advantages of MIS surgery for rectal cancer is its flexibility. There are so many areas where techniques can be modified to accommodate the patient's specific circumstances and be optimal to the advantage of the individual surgeon. This chapter is not comprehensive in that aspect but attempts to highlight some of the principles and rationales behind major techniques.

8.3.1 Patient Selection

The first consideration as with any surgery is appropriate patient selection. As the surgeon becomes more familiar and proficient with any of the techniques, patient selection can be expanded [4]. The learning curve for laparoscopic rectal surgery is on the order of 40–90 cases while that of robotic surgery is shorter at 15–44 cases [20]. There really is no absolute contraindication to MIS rectal cancer surgery, but there are many relative contraindications.

One must give pause when considering MIS for patients with known or expected particularly hostile surgical fields [17]. Extensive previous surgeries will make it difficult if not impossible to establish the necessary working spaces. Recurrent or locally advanced cancer often destroys normal tissue planes, which makes it more challenging to define and achieve appropriate tissue margins. The lack of tactile sensation is a known disadvantage of the MIS approach. While the laparoscopic method has at least some physical feedback from the tissue manipulation, the current generation of robots does not provide any physical and at best only some visual "tactile" feedback.

If a combined surgery is indicated (e.g., synchronous metastatic liver resection, or plastics flap closure for pelvic exenteration) that requires an open approach, the benefit of applying MIS may be rather limited [4]. However, we have on occasions been able to avoid a major extension of an incision by using the planned L-shape incision for a liver resection to first carry out a laparoscopic low anterior resection (Fig. 8.1).

Finally, patients with significant comorbidities and limited operability (related to cardiac or pulmonary disease) may sometimes be better suited to a faster open approach. However, one must individually weigh the postoperative advantages of the MIS approach against its longer operating times.

8.3.2 Operating Room Setup

Each operating room setup needs to be tailored to the space and resources available. Every room will need vision screens on both sides of the patient such that "surgeon—pathology—screen" are on a direct line. Ideally, the monitors should be outfitted with a sterile handle for easy repositioning by the surgeon. Every room should be equipped with a colonoscope that has carbon

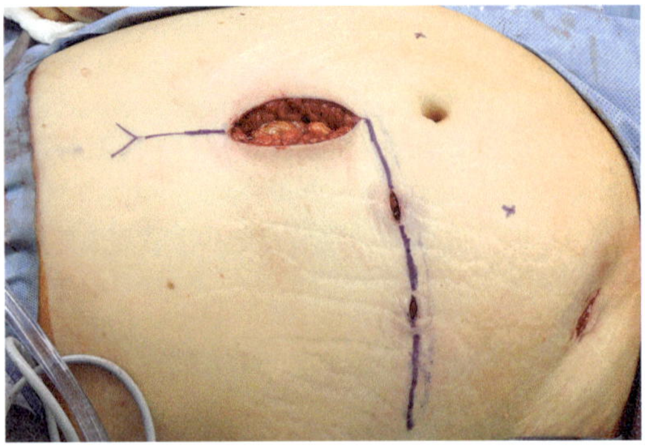

Fig. 8.1 Port and incision layout for combination of hand-assisted laparoscopic surgery (HALS) for low anterior resection and liver resection (through an L-shaped laparotomy)

dioxide insufflation visible to the bedside surgeon and a feed directly connected to the robotic console for a picture-in-picture visualization. This may be crucial for endoscopic confirmation of the tumor location as well as to perform a visually enhanced leak test of the anastomosis at the end.

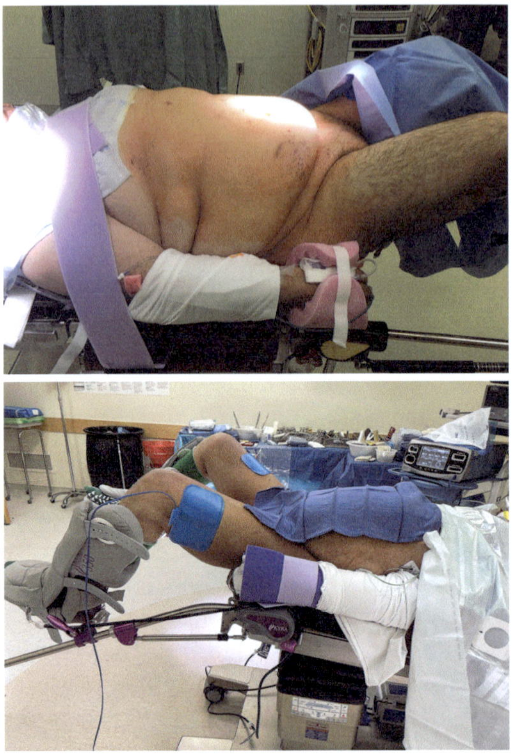

Fig. 8.2 Patient positioning in modified lithotomy with tucked arms (two examples)

8.3.3 Patient Positioning

The patient should be placed on the table in a modified lithotomy position with the legs in stirrups (Fig. 8.2). Arms are routinely tucked alongside the patient for better bedside access. The knee flexure should have an obtuse angle of 110 to 120 degrees. The hip flexure should be kept at zero degrees during the abdominal dissection but changed to 90° for the perineal approach other than simple stapler insertion. This allows access to the pelvis as well as keeps the patient from sliding.

The patient should be secured and prevented from sliding with supportive positioning tools. These include special foam padding, bean bags, shoulder harnesses, and belt straps. The table should be tested prior to draping the patient to ensure it is working and that the patient is properly secured.

One of the MIS strategies for optimizing the surgical field is to reposition the operating table such that the target is best exposed and other structures (e.g., small bowel) follow gravity and fall away. In multi-quadrant surgery, e.g., pelvic surgery plus splenic flexure mobilization, there is a need to shift the position during the procedure. This process is unhindered during laparoscopic surgery. However, one disadvantage of robotic surgery is that the table cannot be moved once the robot is docked. A change in position will require removing the instruments and undocking the arms. However, there are integrated operating tables (Tablemotion®) that are paired with the robot tower and the arms and allow for repositioning without redocking.

8.3.4 Laparoscopic Setup

The laparoscopic setup does not have to vary too much from the open setup, except that the surgeon and the assistant—for portions of the procedure—potentially stand on the same side of the patient in order to work on the opposite site of the patient's body (e.g., lateral and splenic flexure mobilization). Nonetheless, monitors must be arranged on both sides to allow for comfortable viewing if the assistant or technician are on the left side. The scrub technician and instrument table should be positioned such that access to the anus is preserved.

8.3.5 Robot Positioning and Setup

For robotic surgery, the room should be large enough to accommodate the robot; for teaching purposes, a dual console system is desirable. Even though the Xi robot has 360° freedom of rotation for the boom, it is—for a low anterior resection—typically docked from the patient's left side with a lower abdominal setting. This position of the robot from the left allows the bedside assistant better access from the right. Once the ports have been inserted, the patient is positioned in steep Trendelenburg with a tilt toward the right to allow for the small bowel to fall away from the pelvis and the inferior mesenteric vessels.

8.3.6 Port Placement

Port positioning follows some common configuration patterns but by no means is written in stone and may be varied as needed. Prior to deciding on a specific port layout, one should take several specific aspects into consideration:

- Will there be a stoma (colostomy, ileostomy)?
- Where will the specimen be extracted (suprapubic, umbilical, transanal)?
- How is the pneumoperitoneum established (Veress needle, open cut-down technique)?

Sometimes, a stoma marking represents an ideal place for a port, but very often it does not. In those latter instances, the authors prefer to place the ports in an optimal configuration as if no stoma was needed at all. In some situations, however, it may prove very convenient to start by placing a mini-gelport equipped with a port, either at the designated stoma site or the designated extraction site. Doing so allows for placement of specimen extraction or an anvil insertion in midst of the case.

Laparoscopic Ports There is a need for one 10 mm port for the camera, as well as a 12 mm port for a linear stapler. The 2–3 other ports can be 5 mm. The camera is placed near the umbilicus, the stapler port in the right lower quadrant. One 5 mm port is placed in the left hemi-abdomen at the level of the umbilicus, and another one in the right upper quadrant. A third 5 mm port is optional if more retraction is needed (Fig. 8.3).

Robotic Ports Ports for the Xi robot are generally set up in a straight line (Fig. 8.4). The slope of that line is perpendicular to a line that targets the middle of the operative field. For example, if a low anterior resection does not require a splenic flexure mobilization because the sigmoid is very redundant, the operative field would range from the sigmoid to the pelvis, and the middle would be in the left groin. If on the other hand a splenic flexure mobilization was needed, the field would extend from the splenic flexure to the pelvis with the middle being at the distal descending colon. As a result, the slope would be flatter in the first and steeper in the second scenario. If the line is too short to accommodate four ports with a distance between them of 6–8 cm, one of the ports may be chosen off that line (Fig. 8.4, panels d–f). An additional accessory port is placed in the right

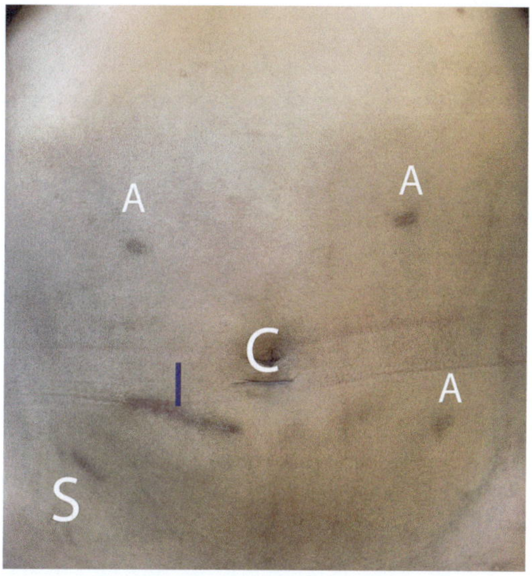

Fig. 8.3 Port layout for laparoscopic low anterior resection: *C* camera (10–12 mm), *S* stapler (12 mm), *A* assistant ports (5 mm), *I* ileostomy site after ultimate takedown

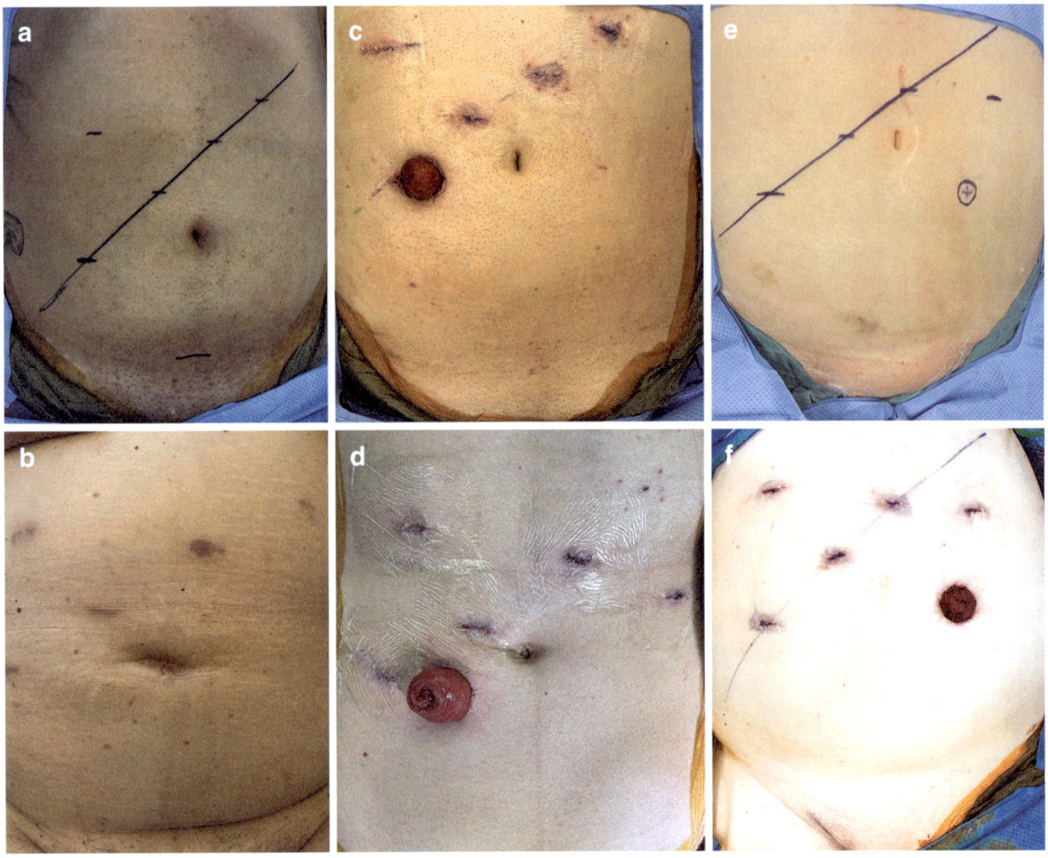

Fig. 8.4 Port layouts for Xi robot: panels **a** and **b**: Low anterior resection with suprapubic extraction site. Panels **c** and **d**: Ultralow anterior resection, coloanal anastomosis, diverting ileostomy. Panels **e** and **f**: Abdominoperineal resection with end colostomy

upper quadrant. Often times, a special type of port is used in that location that allows for a pressure-controlled maintenance of the pneumoperitoneum.

Many systems now include some form of smoke evacuation of the abdominal space via air exchange or electrostatic precipitation. This is key to keeping the field of view clean.

8.3.7 Port Management

All 10 and 12 mm ports should ultimately at the end of the case be closed to the fascia. For the smaller port, closure of the skin may suffice, except if the patient is very skinny.

8.4 Instruments

There are arrays of instruments, too many to individually list. Each surgeon will typically develop a preference list. As a general principle, all procedures require retracting and grasping instruments, dissecting instruments, as well as tools to achieve hemostasis (monopolar, bipolar, advanced-energy). Advanced energy devices have become an instrumental part of safe and hence faster dissection. Suction/irrigators are used to keep the surgical area clean and free of blood or secretions. Staplers come in different lengths, staple heights, and configuration to perform safe transection of named blood vessels or the bowels. Clip appliers serve at safely sealing a tubular structure with either metal or locking plastic clips.

Laparoscopy: Laparoscopic soft bowel graspers come in many different shapes and forms. The instruments should be atraumatic to minimize the risk of bowel injuries. As long as reusable instruments are employed, there is no limitation as to the number of different instruments utilized. The authors' preference is to use single-action micro-fenestrated graspers and an advanced energy device for dissection, and a padded grasper for retraction.

Robotic: There is a tempting variety of dockable instruments. However, in contrast to laparoscopy, the cost of the procedure accumulates with every single instrument connected to a robot arm, regardless of how long or how many times it is used after that. It is therefore recommended to select the basic instruments of choice and to minimize the use of too many others. Typical instruments include the Cadiere or the Prograsp for retraction, monopolar scissors for dissection, and either a bipolar fenestrated grasper or a vessel sealer for hemostasis. For more involved intracorporeal suturing, a needle driver with incorporated scissors (suture-cut) is very practical, but for a single stitch, it might be more cost-effective to use any of the already engaged graspers as a "needle driver."

8.5 Surgical Technique

The concept of the total mesorectal excision (TME) represents the basis for all pelvic dissections for rectal cancer. It requires a solid anatomical knowledge combined with great skills. The dissection must follow the embryological defined anatomical mesorectal fascial plane in order to achieve an oncologically optimal specimen with an intact mesorectum, negative circumferential, proximal, and distal margins while minimizing collateral damage and preserving the pelvic nerves for best postsurgical bowel, bladder, and sexual function.

The proximal margin is typically defined without any problems and either entails the projection of the vascular pedicle to the bowel wall or at least 10 cm proximal to the beginning of the tumor. The distal margin would best entail at least 5 cm of normal rectum below the tumor. However, for tumors in the lower third of the rectum, a closer margin will be acceptable. 2 cm would be optimal, but on occasion, a lesser margin of 1 cm or even less might be acceptable. If an adequate distal margin is not possible, and abdominoperineal resection with complete removal of the anus must be carried out.

8.5.1 Core Steps

8.5.1.1 Exploration and Exposure

Once access has been established, a global exploration of the abdomen is necessary to exclude carcinomatosis or liver disease. The omentum and small bowel are then shifted away from the target field. This is typically achieved by placing the patient in steep Trendelenburg position with a tilt to the right side.

8.5.1.2 Medial to Lateral Development of Retro-Pedicular Window

The procedure starts with identification of the inferior mesenteric artery (IMA). Retraction of the pedicle creates a visual triangle between the grasping instrument, the origin of the pedicle, and the base from retroperitoneum to the sacral promontory (Fig. 8.5, panel a). The serosa is scored along the base of this triangle. That will open the areolar tissue and allow the insufflation to develop the natural plane between the mesentery and the retroperitoneum. Further development within the areolar tissue continues into the space between the presacral and the mesorectal fascia propria (Fig. 8.5, panel b). At this point, the IMA should be mobilized toward its origin, keeping in mind that the main hypogastric plexus runs underneath. Limiting the dissection posterior will help preserve this plexus.

8.5.1.3 Ureteral Identification

Injury to the ureters is a serious and costly complication and should be minimized. It is standard to identify the left ureter and gonadal vessels, but it is prudent to also verify the location of the right ureter. As the medial to lateral dissection underneath the vascular pedicle is continued, the

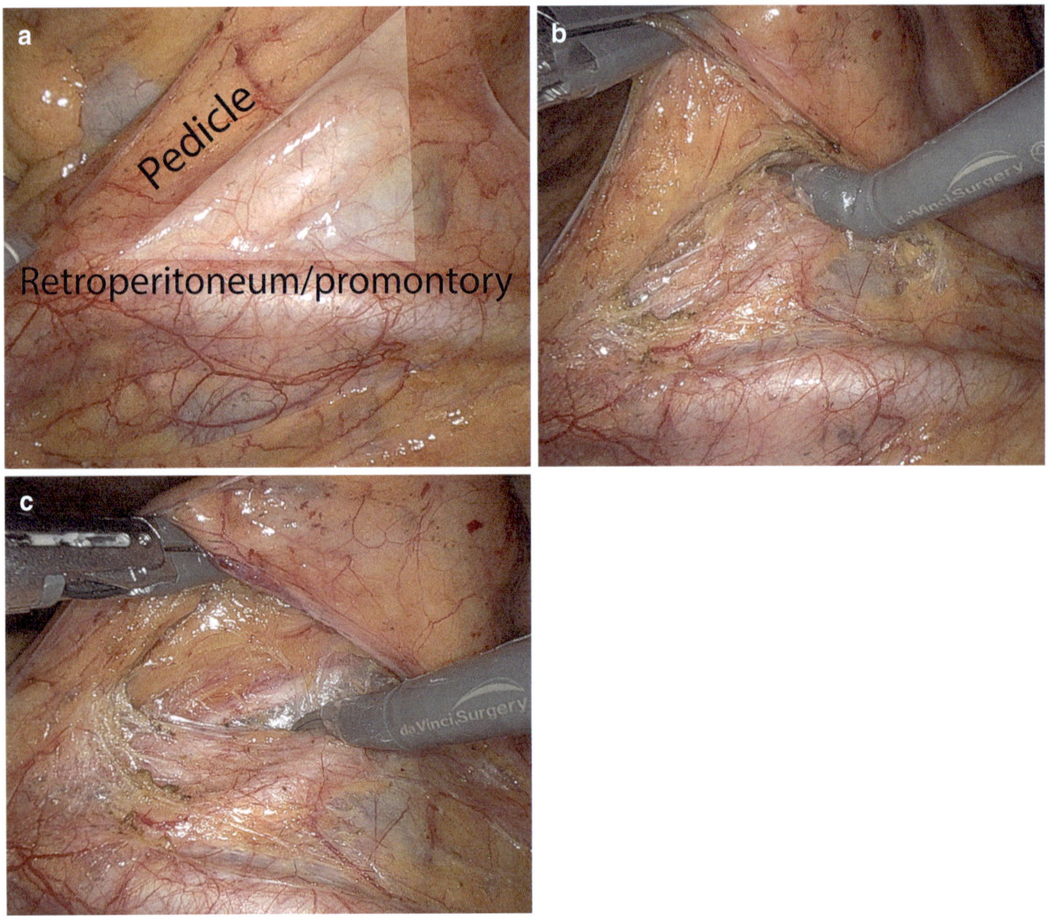

Fig. 8.5 Isolation of vascular pedicle and visualization of ureter. Panel **a**: The "Pedicle triangle" is formed by the pedicle, the extension of retroperitoneum to promontory, and the line between elevating clamp and the promontory. Panel **b**: Incision of serosa. Panel **c**: Identification of the vermiculating left ureter

retroperitoneal tissues are deflected and moved backward. This gentle maneuver will typically lead to the ureter, which is confirmed by its vermiculating contractions (Fig. 8.5, panel c). Dissecting the incorrect plane carries some dangers. Riskier (and also more common) than being too anterior is to get too posterior behind the ureter and gonadal vessels and to lay bare the iliac vessels and/or the psoas muscle.

If identification of the left ureter is difficult, the medial to lateral approach should be complemented by a lateral to medial dissection. In anticipation of difficulties (e.g., redo-surgery, very large tumors, significant inflammation), preoperatively placed ureteral stents are a valuable adjunct. They can either be lighted or injected with indocyanine green (ICG) such that they will fluoresce when viewed under near-infrared light (Fig. 8.6). The Xi robot has built near-infrared capabilities into the system, whereas most laparoscopic systems depend on being complemented by a separate unit.

8.5.1.4 Division of the Vascular Pedicle

The next step is to isolate and divide the pedicle. Artery and vein can either be individually isolated and divided or addressed as one. There are different ways to accomplish that (Fig. 8.7). A great deal of controversy surrounded the question whether a low or a high ligation of the IMA is needed. A high ligation should result in more nodal tissue and increased mobility, but it can injure more nerves. A low ligation, i.e., of the

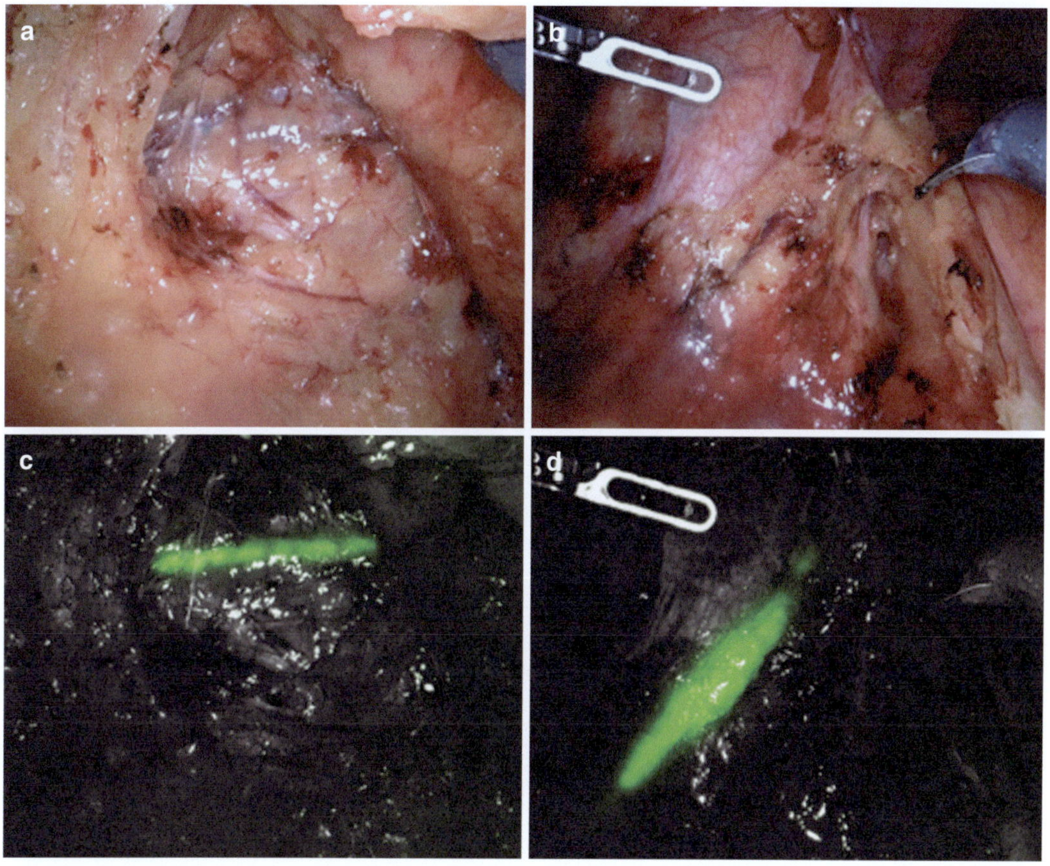

Fig. 8.6 Injection of the ureters with ICG: panels **a** and **b** show the natural lighting, panels **c** and **d** the corresponding fields with ICG fluorescence imaging that nicely visualizes the left ureter

superior rectal artery rather than the IMA, preserves an additional vascular perfusion "charge" but the intact left colic may limit the length and reach for the anastomosis.

Reverification of the ureter's location is strongly advised before dividing any structure. To isolate the artery, the mesentery is opened just below the inferior mesenteric vein (IMV). This will quite easily connect to the prior field of the posterior dissection. The skeletonized vessels can then be divided with an advanced sealing device, between clips (Fig. 8.7, panel a), or by means of a stapler (Fig. 8.7, panel b). If a bleeding occurs, the advanced energy device will likely short out on the staples or clips. In that situation, an endoloop device or a manual suture ligation are useful tools to regain control of the bleeding vessel stump.

8.5.1.5 Medial to Lateral Dissection

Once the pedicle has been divided, it is placed on traction and elevated. A medial to lateral mobilization of the sigmoid and descending colon are done as far lateral and cephalad as possible. The IMV can be followed to the lower edge of the pancreas. It does not have to be divided there, however, doing so may help with getting better mobility. Care should be taken not to damage an arc of Riolan that typically runs close to this area and provides a valuable source of collateral perfusion. The retroperitoneal dissection again follows the natural embryological and largely avascular plane. At the level of the splenic flexure, the pancreas should be expected and stay below. The lesser sac can be entered by dividing the mesentery just above the pancreas.

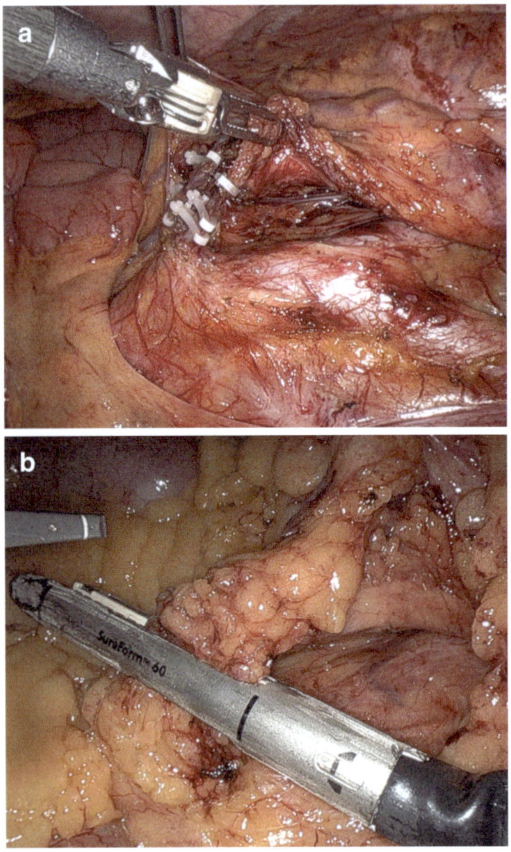

Fig. 8.7 Safe division of the vascular pedicle. Panel **a**: Clipping of vessels. Panel **b**: Stapling of pedicle

8.5.1.6 Mobilization of the Splenic Flexure

Taking down the splenic flexure is an optional maneuver if the proximal bowel length and mobility are otherwise insufficient for a tension-free anastomosis or—in the case of an abdominoperineal resection—a colostomy, respectively. For the mobilization, it is usually helpful to adjust the table to lesser or even reversed Trendelenburg position with maintained tilt to the right. The positional change is seamless in laparoscopy or with integrated robotic tablemotion, but otherwise may require a redocking of the robot.

If the prior retroperitoneal dissection has been carried out far enough, the takedown of the splenic flexure is very straightforward. The omentum is dissected off the distal transverse colon. The cephalad to caudad and the lateral to medial mobilization move toward and around the flexure from the transverse and the sigmoid colon, respectively. As the colon is retracted medially, the line of Toldt is opened and should easily connect with the prior posterior plane of dissection. The lesser sac is then entered from above and the dissection continued beyond the flexure until the colon is completely mobile.

A splenic injury with ensuing bleeding is most commonly caused by excessive traction rather than direct trauma. It is therefore important to avoid undue tension and to continue the dissection close to the colon while steadily and carefully releasing the retroperitoneal and colonic attachments.

8.5.1.7 Managing the Proximal Resection Site

The next step is the identification and management of the proximal bowel resection site. As previously stated, the site is chosen either in continuation of the vascular pedicle to the bowel wall or at least 10 cm proximal to the tumor. The transected vascular pedicle is elevated and the mesocolon divided in stepwise fashion all the way to the bowel (Fig. 8.8, panel a). A band of roughly 1 cm of the bowel wall should be circumferentially cleaned.

The further step depends on whether the surgery ultimately entails (a) a stapled anastomosis, (b) a coloanal pull-through with hand-sewn anastomosis, or (c) an abdominoperineal resection. For (a) and (c), the bowel is proximally transected (Fig. 8.8, panel b) with a linear stapling device (unless the surgeon plans to exteriorize the bowel for resection and anvil placement). For (b), the area is left in continuity as the final trimming is carried out after pulling the specimen and the proximal colon through the pelvic floor. Sometimes it is helpful to place a marking stitch at the designated proximal resection site for easy determination of the complete pull-through.

8.5.1.8 Preparation of Possible Ileostomy

In cases where an ileostomy is planned, it may be desirable to prepare the terminal ileum before diving into the pelvis. The terminal ileum is identified and roughly 15–20 cm proximal to the ileocecal valve, a window is created in the small bowel mesentery. A Penrose is inserted and sutured to itself to serve as a handle. The efferent

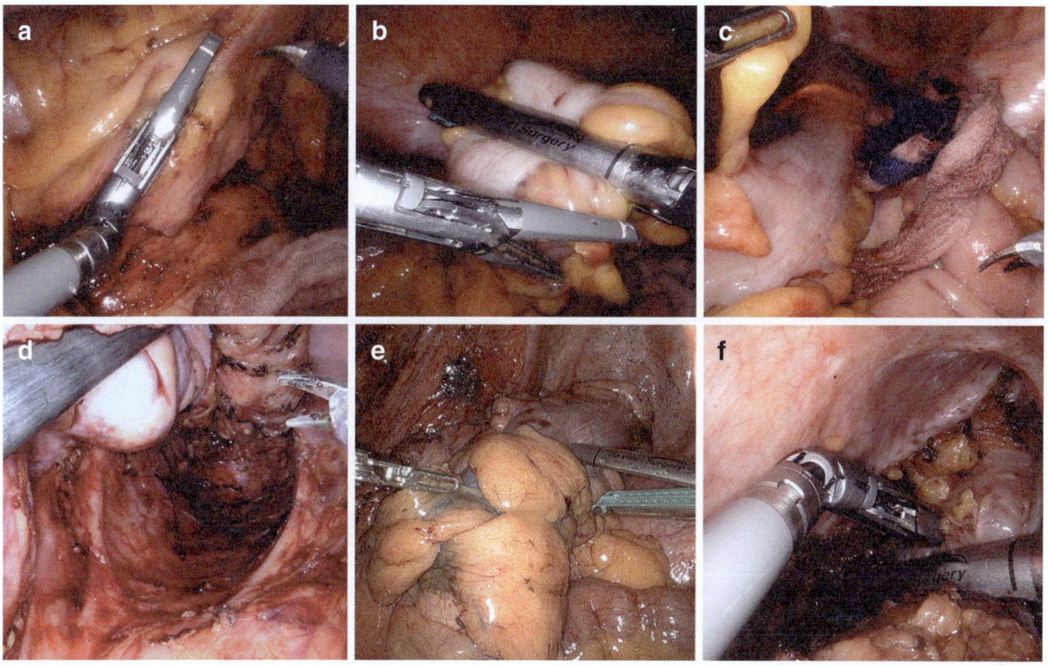

Fig. 8.8 Mobilization and resection of the rectum. Panel **a**: Division of the mesocolon up to the proximal resection site. Panel **b**: Stapler transection of the bowel at the proximal end of the specimen. Panel **c**: Flexible sigmoidoscopy to reverify location of the tumor. Panel **d**: Posterior mobilization along fascial plane. Panels **e** and **f**: Distal stapler division of the bowel

and the afferent limb are marked in an absolute way that will allow for definitive assessment of the correct orientation once the bowel is exteriorized. Prior to releasing the pneumoperitoneum, a locking clamp is placed on that Penrose such that it can ultimately be easily pulled up and exteriorized once a trephine has been created.

8.5.1.9 Pelvic Dissection

Once proper length has been achieved and the proximal resection site managed, the actual core step of the oncological surgery—the pelvic rectal dissection—is carried out. The peritoneum is opened on both sides of the rectum and connected anteriorly along the peritoneal reflection.

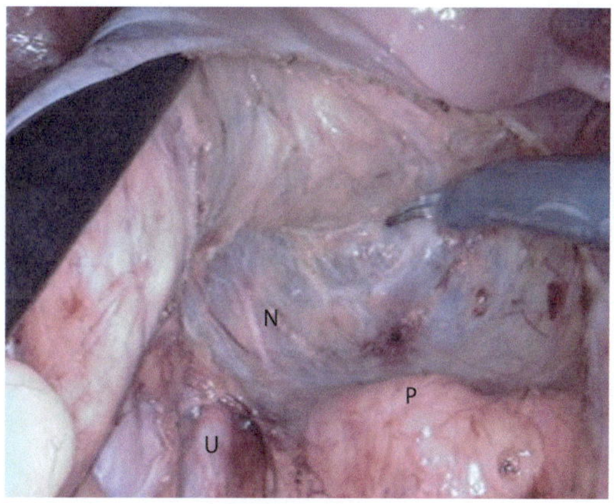

Fig. 8.9 Posterior mobilization in the avascular plane, leaving essential structures behind: *P* promontory, *U* ureter, *N* hypogastric nerve plexus

The posterior rectal mobilization requires gentle traction of the rectum away from the sacrum (Figs. 8.8, panel d and 8.9). The avascular areolar space is developed between the presacral fascia (posterior layer) and the fascia propria of the rectum. The hypogastric nerves, possibly a median sacral artery, as well as the dangerous presacral vein plexus are behind the presacral fascia (Fig. 8.9). Violation of that layer can trigger dramatic events and should be carefully avoided. At the level of S3/S4, the presacral fascia and the mesorectal fascia fuse and form Waldeyer's fascia. If the dissection is to be continued beyond that level, the fascia propria must be actively incised as otherwise the posterior dissection derails into the dangerous presacral space.

The anterior dissection enters at the peritoneal reflection and follows the Denonvilliers fascia. In a male patient, the seminal vesicles and the backside of the prostate serve as landmarks. However, in very obese patients, these structures may be hiding and more difficult to develop. In a female patient, the posterior vaginal wall must be gently separated from the anterior rectal wall whereby excessive energy application should be avoided to minimize collateral tissue damage.

The lateral dissection entails the division of mostly adipose and some connective tissue components that separate the anterior and the posterior dissection plane. Use of an advanced energy device offers a very efficient dissection technique.

As the dissection continues circumferentially toward the pelvic floor, the working area is sequentially switched between posterior, lateral, and anterior. In the deeper section, visualization and mobility become an increasing issue, particularly in a narrow pelvis of an obese patient. The laparoscopic (and occasionally the robotic) dissection with straight instruments may be hindered by the promontory or the pelvic sidewall. While a certain degree of struggle may be inevitable, the surgeon needs to assess whether the ports need adjustments or additional dissection ports may have to be inserted.

Standard TME principles should be followed to the level necessary for the respective choice of distal resection management as outlined in the following sections for the three main categories. Under best of circumstances, a distal margin of 5 cm would be optimal, but 2 cm are generally accepted. This distance, however, can even be shorter than that (1cm or less as long as it is proven negative) if sphincter preservation is among the patient's top priorities.

8.5.2 Low Anterior Resection with Stapled Anastomosis

For this scenario, the distal rectum is divided internally, followed by a stapled anastomosis. The designated level of distal transection (as outlined previously) may potentially have to be verified by flexible sigmoidoscopy (Fig. 8.8, panel c). At that level, the mesorectum must be divided perpendicularly to the bowel wall. Use of an advanced energy device is best suited for that purpose to minimize the risk of a brisk bleeding from the vascular arcade. Care must be taken not to denude the remaining rectal stump of its mesorectum.

The distal stapling of the bowel can be very challenging in a narrow pelvis (Fig. 8.8, panels e, f). There are several brands of 12 mm staplers that can be used for the laparoscopic approach. These are usually best introduced through the right lower quadrant port. Alternatively, a stapler may be introduced through the Pfannenstiel incision that will also be used as the extraction site. The robot has its own stapler arsenal with a length of 30, 45, or 60 mm. The staple height varies; for transection of the bowel, the thicker green load is preferred. The more cartridges are needed, the worse is the statistical outcome with increased risk of anastomotic complications. Ideally, the transection should be carried out with one or at most two loads. While the 60 mm stapler will allow for transection of more tissue per firing, it also requires more working room. In the limited space of the distal rectum, it is therefore sometimes better to use the shorter cartridges. Depending on the subsequent maneuvers, the resected specimen can either be immediately retrieved or parked in the right lower quadrant (ideally within an isolation bag, Fig. 8.10, panel a), allowing for visualization of the empty pelvis and ICG perfusion assessment of the rectal stump (Fig. 8.10, panels b, c).

Performing the stapled anastomosis can be effectuated in different ways. The traditional approach with minimally invasive surgery was an extracorporeal anastomosis (ECA). To that effect, the proximal bowel end is temporarily exteriorized (either around the umbilicus, the left lower quadrant, or through a suprapubic Pfannenstiel incision), and the anvil inserted; the bowel subsequently returned to the peritoneal cavity in order to perform the pelvic anastomosis after reinsufflation of the pneumoperitoneum.

Particularly the use of the robot has allowed for an intracorporeal anastomosis (ICA), which may even be performed without undocking the robot. The anvil is delivered through the eventual extraction site, potentially even at the very beginning of the case before docking the robot

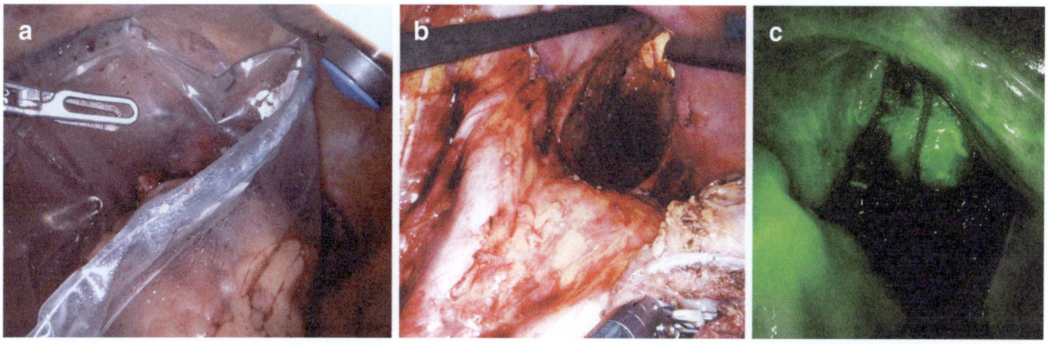

Fig. 8.10 Completed low anterior resection. Panel **a**: Placement of specimen into isolation bag. Panel **b**: Inspection of empty pelvis. Panel **c**: ICG fluorescence for assessment of perfusion of rectal stump

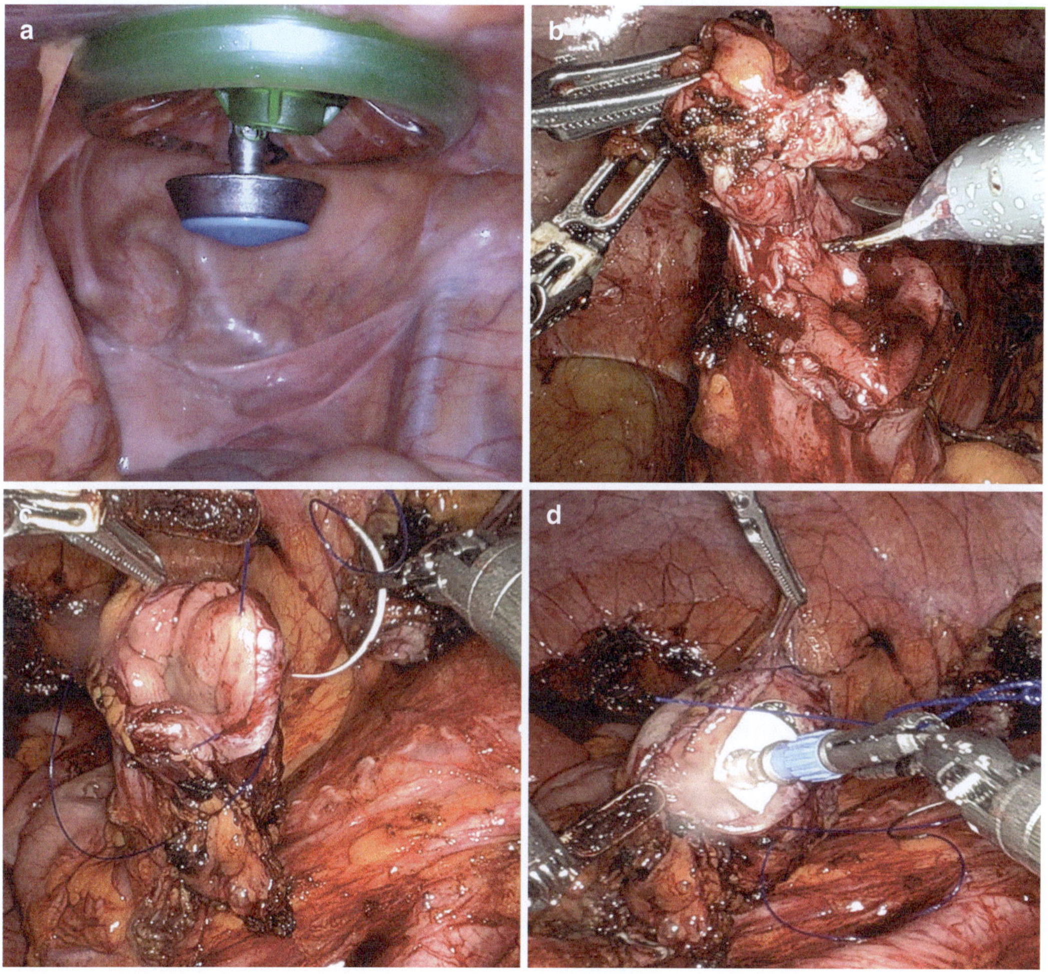

Fig. 8.11 Anvil placement for intracorporeal anastomosis (ICA). Panel **a**: Intraabdominal parking of the EEA anvil (on a string); panel **b**: resection of proximal stapler line up to well-perfused bowel wall; panel **c**: Pursestring suture. Panel **d**: Parachuting the suspended anvil into the proximal bowel end

(Fig. 8.11, panel a). ICG fluorescence imaging can be used to assess the quality of the bowel perfusion (Figs. 8.10, panel c and 8.12, panels a and b). The staple line is removed from the proximal colon and the anvil is sutured in place robotically (Fig. 8.11, panels b–d).

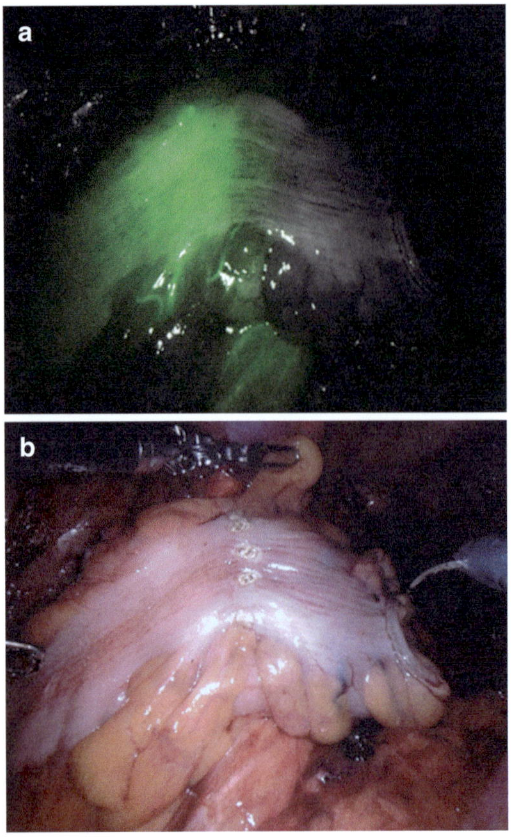

Fig. 8.12 ICG imaging: Intravenous injection of ICG visualizes a demarkation of between well and the poorly perfused end of the proximal colon (panel **a**) and allows to place marks at the demarcation line (panel **b**)

The anastomosis is carried out by passing the EEA stapler through the anus to the end of the rectal stump. The spike should be deployed next but not through the staple line (Fig. 8.13). The anvil is connected, and the correct rotation of the proximal bowel verified. As the stapler is slowly closed, one must make sure that no other structures (vagina, bladder, etc.) are accidentally incorporated into the stapler mechanism. The stapler is fired and subsequently retrieved. The quality and intactness of the stapler donuts will have to be assessed. A digital exam and an air leak test are done (Fig. 8.14). Best is to submerge the anastomosis under water while performing a flexible sigmoidoscopy as it allows to visualize and assess the anastomosis for bleeding while verifying on the abdominal side that no air bubbles escape (Fig. 8.14). If the air leak test turns out to be positive, the area of leakage should be identified and oversewn. It is standard to divert in this case if not planning to do so anyway. If there is enough available bowel length, a complete redoing of the anastomosis should be considered.

8.5.3 Ultralow Anterior Resection/Coloanal Anastomosis

For tumors of the lower third of the rectum, the entire rectum must be resected. As long as the anal sphincter complex is not involved, a primary anastomosis is still an option. A complete removal of the rectum will require precise visualization and mobility in a deep and narrow space.

In contrast to an APR, the dissection automatically narrows as the mesorectum naturally thins out in the last section above the sphincter complex. The levator complex and sphincter muscles need to be kept intact. The more work that can be done from the abdominal side, the easier becomes the transanal portion.

After this, the operation switches to the perineal dissection. A Lonestar retractor with eight retracting hooks is placed (Fig. 8.15). One might close the distal rectum with a mucosal pursestring suture to avoid cancer contamination of the field. The mucosa is incised at the dentate line. If the internal muscle is preserved, the mucosa is carefully dissected off the sphincter complex before transitioning to full-thickness above the sphincter complex. If an intersphincteric dissection is carried out, the intersphincteric groove is exposed and the full bowel wall dissected off the external anal sphincter and the puborectalis muscle. As the internal sphincter muscle represents the extension of the muscularis propria of the rectum, this dissection is actually easier to pursue.

Once the transanal dissection has connected with the abdominal dissection and the distal rectum is circumferentially freed up, the entire specimen can be pulled through until the previously mentioned marking stitch has been visualized (Fig. 8.15, panel a). A good blood supply should

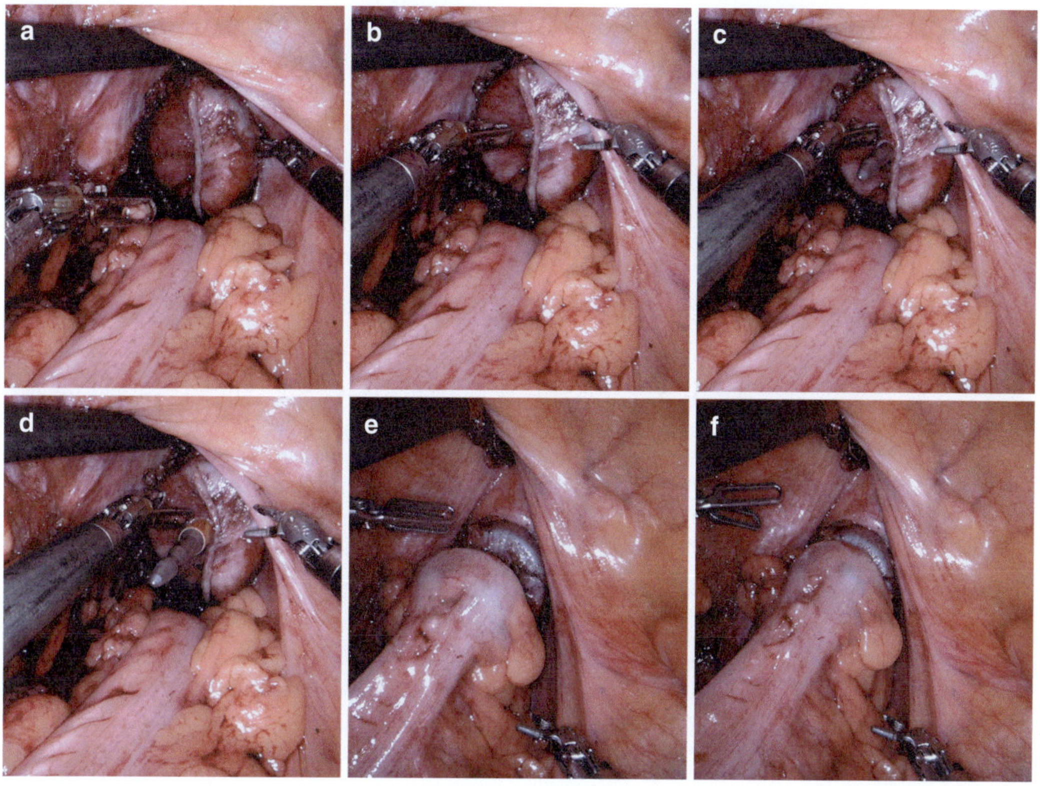

Fig. 8.13 Stapled anastomosis. Panel **a**: Stapler inserted to the end of the rectal stump. Panel **b–d**: Advancing the spear next to the staple line. Panel **e**, **f**: Closure of the stapler

be obvious. The pulled-through rectum is anchored to the pelvic floor musculature with circumferential seromuscular stitches. The specimen is then resected and sent for pathology for assessment of the distal margins. The pulled-through tissue is trimmed to appropriate length and the handsewn anastomosis is fine-tuned (Fig. 8.15, panel b). The Lone Star retractor may now be removed.

An alternative to a straight coloanal anastomosis is to perform a colonic J-pouch anal anastomosis. In that case, the terminal end of the colon is folded and a roughly 5–6 cm J-pouch created. The apex of it will subsequently be sutured as described above for the straight anastomosis.

After completion of the anastomosis, the surgeon returns to the abdomen to pull out the previously prepared small bowel loop for the ileostomy. The maturation of the ileostomy will be carried out in standard fashion once all ports have been closed and should result in a symmetric and well-perfused nipple of 2.5–3.5 cm (Fig. 8.16).

8.5.4 Abdominoperineal Resection

When the sphincter complex is involved with tumor or if there are other, for example, functional reasons against restoration of continuity, a complete abdominoperineal resection with permanent stoma and closure of the pelvic floor are carried out. In the case of a cancer, that typically involves removal of the sphincter complex and perianal skin. In contrast, if the rationale is more based on functional aspects, an intersphincteric resection with complete deepithelialization of the anal canal may suffice.

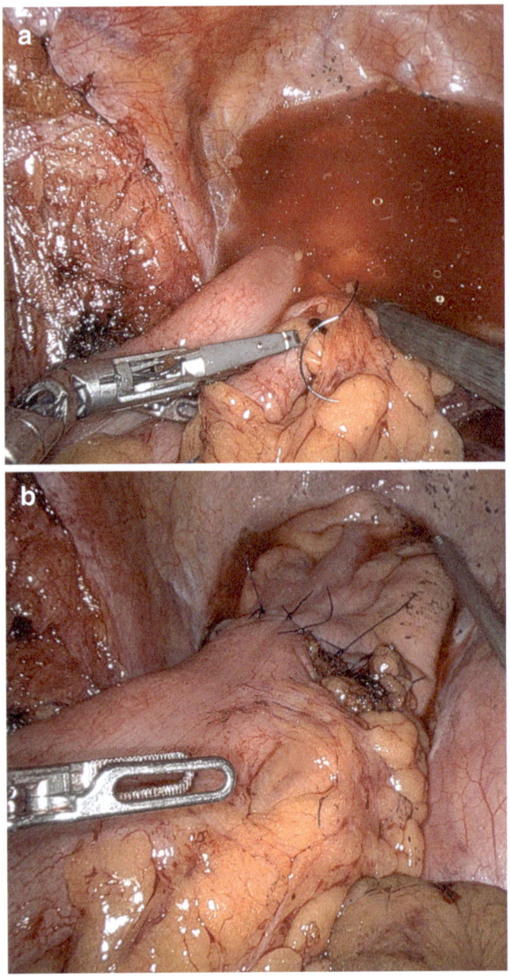

Fig. 8.14 Anastomosis testing/finetuning. Panel **a**: Air leak test by submerging anastomosis under water and insufflating pressured air through flexible sigmoidoscope. Panel **b**: Optional oversewing of the anastomosis

Similar to the coloanal pull-through procedure, a major advantage of the MIS approach is that no abdominal extraction site is needed as the tumor bearing specimen will be retrieved via the perineal defect. It should be noted though that sometimes a major defect within heavily radiated tissue will require a tissue transfer for closure. If a transabdominal VRAM flap is chosen, the entire surgery would be naturally carried out as an open rather than an MIS approach.

The TME portion again runs in a similar fashion until one reaches the pelvic floor. At this point, further dissection along the rectum should stop as it will cause a "coning" of the specimen. The robotic portion can stop at this point; however, that will leave a significant amount of work to be done from the perineum. Alternatively, the perineal dissection can be started from the abdomen. The levators are incised and divided posteriorly. Cautery or the vessel sealer can be used here. The dissection can then be continued laterally. Ideally the entire levator complex can be divided to the ischiorectal fat. This fat can also be divided as caudad as possible. Again, the more work is carried out from above, the easier the perineal portion.

Before switching to the perineal approach, the proximal end of the colon - that will need to be guided out through the abdominal wall at the designated stoma site to fashion the colostomy - is internally secured with a locking grasper.

The surgeon switches to the perineal approach (Fig. 8.17). The anus is closed with two concentric sutures (Fig. 8.17, panel a). An elliptic incision is drawn around the anus (Fig. 8.17, panel b). In a female patient with an anterior tumor, that elliptic incision continues directly into the posterior vagina and encompasses part of the posterior vaginal wall. As the skin is incised, the two sides of the skin are brought together and clamped with a few Kocher clamps that further serve as the traction handle. The dissection is continued through the ischioanal fat. The ischioanal ligament is divided and the pelvic floor musculature divided with the advanced energy device. Once the posterior hemicircumference is opened up and connected with the abdominal dissection, the specimen is eviscerated, and the anterior dissection com-

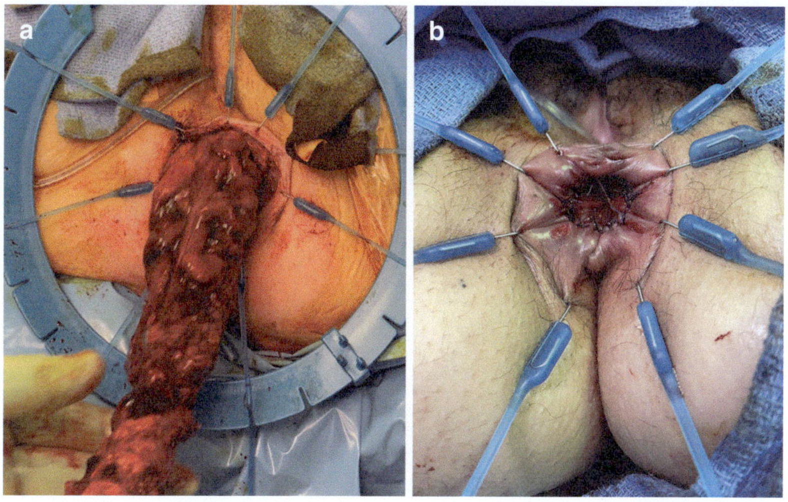

Fig. 8.15 LoneStar retractor for exposure during coloanal anastomosis. Panel **a**: Transanal extraction of the specimen. Panel **b**: Completed coloanal anastomosis

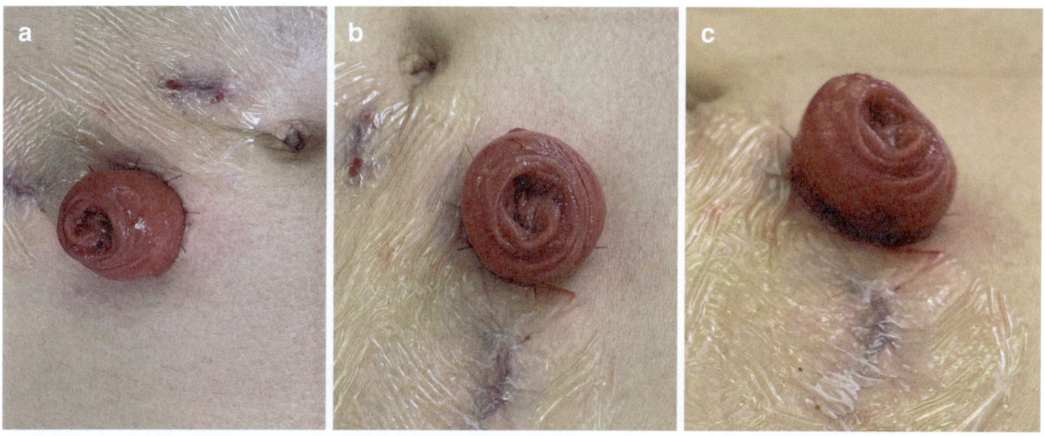

Fig. 8.16 Diverting loop ileostomy from different angles (panels **a**–**c**): The efferent limb should be buried at the base of the afferent limb such that it is almost not visible

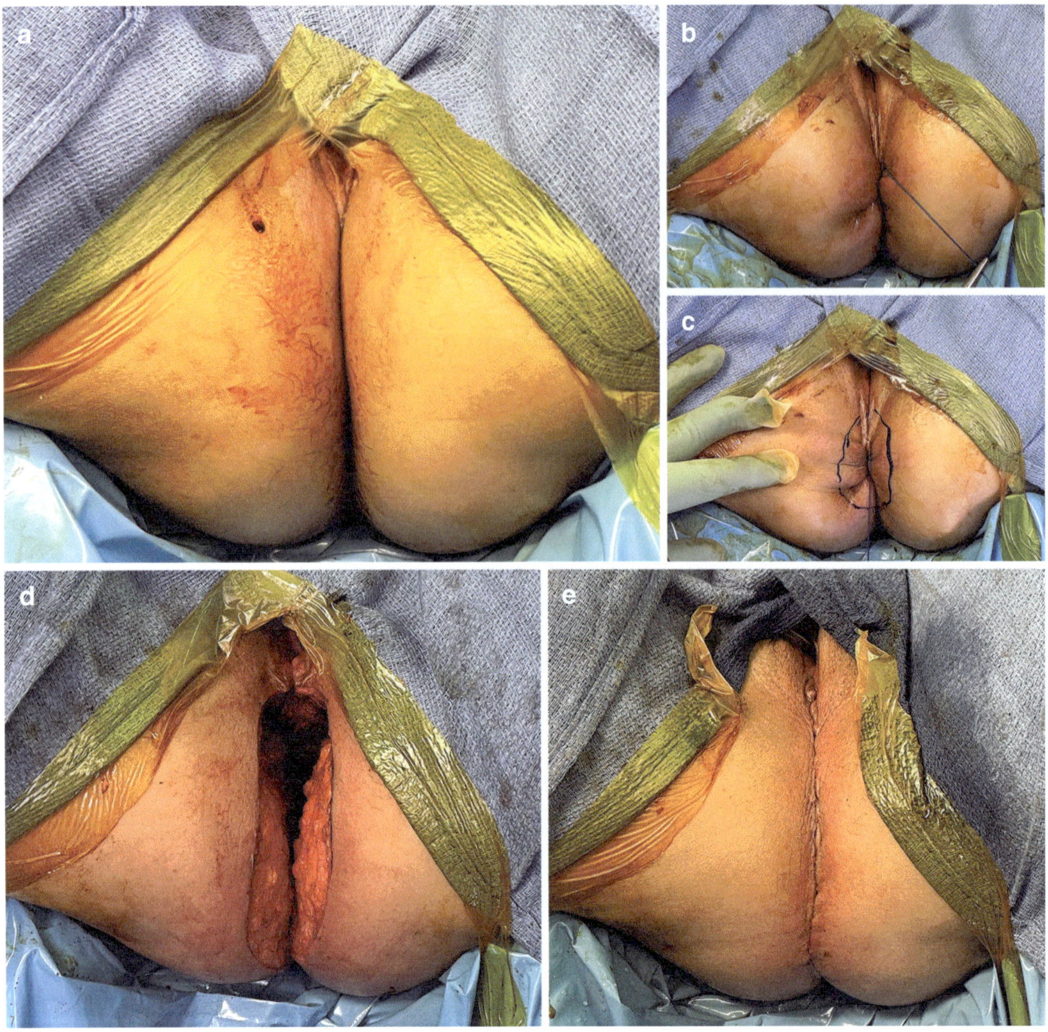

Fig. 8.17 Abdominoperineal resection. Panel **a**: Appearance before the perineal resection. Panel **b**: Suture closure of the anus. Panel **c**: Marking of elliptic incision around the suture-closed anus. Panel **d**: Resulting defect after removal of the specimen. Panel **e**: Closed anus

pleted with bi-digital guidance. The transverse perineal muscles serve as anterior landmark. Care must be taken to avoid injuring anterior structures by staying posterior to that muscle on one hand and to accidentally open the distal rectum by staying too posterior on the other hand. The specimen is retrieved. The perineal wound and defect (Fig. 8.17, panel c) are irrigated and subsequently closed in a layered fashion (Fig. 8.17, panel d).

8.6 Postoperative Care

Patients who undergo a MIS rectal cancer surgery are ideally suited for an enhanced recovery (ERAS) protocol. Major surgery societies have published multiple guidelines on this approach [21]. While wound care is not different than in other circumstances, the standard tenets of these protocols include: early feeding, early ambulation, limited use of drains, early removal of the foley catheter, alternative pain medications to narcotics, and techniques to control high ileostomy output. Administration of a peripherally acting mu-opioid receptor antagonist has been shown to provide a modest improvement in return of bowel function. C-reactive protein (CRP) levels alone or in combination with procalcitonin levels are promising adjunct tests to predict anastomotic leaks before symptoms arise, or—when the respective levels are low—to serve as a negative predictive test.

8.7 Complications

8.7.1 Intraoperative Complications

Bleeding, injury to adjacent structures (ureters, vagina, bladder/prostate), bowel ischemia, and small bowel injury are the most common intraoperative complications and have been addressed in the respective sections.

8.7.2 Short-Term Complications

The major short-term complications with a proctectomy include wound infection and anastomotic leaks. Major trials did not show any difference in wound infection rates in MIS versus open cases with rates in both of about 10% [7]. A wound infection is treated with opening of the wound, assessing for a fascial dehiscence and antibiotics as clinically necessary. An anastomotic leak is the most feared complication. Leak rates have not shown a correlation with the surgical platform (open, laparoscopic, or robotic). Commonly accepted leak rates range from 2 to 10% depending on the study [10, 15], but higher incidences have been reported, particularly after preceding radiation treatment. A clinical suspicion for a leak needs to be confirmed with a computed tomography with rectal contrast unless the patient is obviously septic. For patients who are already diverted with an ileostomy, the signs of a leak are much more subtle. Urinary retention and pelvic pressure may give a hint of a leak. Depending on the magnitude of a leak and the clinical symptomatology, the management may range from antibiotic treatment, prolonged diversion to more aggressive approaches with possible reoperation and potential takedown of the anastomosis.

An inadvertent bowel injury caused by trocar and instrument placement is in the differential diagnosis of an anastomotic complication and may be one of the more specific complications associated with the minimally invasive approach. Great care must be emphasized time and again to avoid these types of injury especially with the robotic approach where all tactile sensation is lost. If such an injury has not been recognized at the time of surgery, progressive septic signs will usually evolve with typical symptoms of peritonitis in the first 48 h. The patient will need to be brought back to the operating room for surgical correction of the problem.

Dehiscence, infection, and delayed wound healing are very common complications of the perineal wound after an abdominoperineal resection and affect at least 25% of the patients. The risk is higher if there is evident radiation injury to the perineal tissue, and if the perineal excision has to be very wide as a result of the tumor presentation. Most of these infections ultimately heal with conservative measures. But in a small group of patients, further surgery including transfer of myocutaneous muscle flaps may be needed.

8.7.3 Long-Term Complications

Any abdominal surgery carries a risk of incisional hernias, whereby the minimally invasive approach scores favorably compared to an open approach. One of the major advantages of MIS surgery is that the port site incisions are very small, and that the extraction site can be placed off midline. The incidence of extraction site hernias was reported as 10% for midline incisions, 3.7% for transverse left lower quadrant incisions, and 0.9% for Pfannenstiel incisions [22].

Any pelvic procedure may negatively impact the pelvic innervation even if the major branches of the hypogastric nerves have been preserved.

The triple impact of surgery, radiation, and chemotherapy aggravates that neurological impairment. Studies have failed to show any difference in rates of dysfunction based on the surgical modality [14, 23]. Urinary dysfunction entails urinary retention or incontinence. Sexual dysfunction in males involves retrograde ejaculation and erectile dysfunction, whereas women are affected by vaginal dryness, dyspareunia, or reduced vaginal dimensions. While most patients regain full function in the first year, problems do persist.

Low anterior resection syndrome (LARS) is an umbrella term for functional manifestations associated with a restorative proctectomy. Those may entail urgency, frequency, incontinence, or stool clustering. For ultralow anterior resections, formation of a colonic J-pouch has been associated with reduced symptomatology in the first 1–2 years; in the longer run, however, the differences level out, and stool clustering becomes more prevalent in patients with a colonic J-pouch. Adjuncts in the management apart from dietary and habit modifications include physical therapy and biofeedback training, sacral nerve stimulation, antimotility agents, support groups, and scheduled evacuation enemas. Ultimate surgical options include conversion to an ostomy or reconstruction of the anastomosis if a structural problem is evident. The role of sacral nerve stimulation specifically for LARS has not been fully investigated but on occasion has been found to alleviate some of the patients' symptoms.

8.8 Personal Experience and Conclusion

The authors are seasoned enough to have obtained a solid training in open rectal cancer surgery, but also to witness the evolution of minimally invasive surgery from skepticism to embracement. At our institution, we have—despite versatility in pure laparoscopic surgery—over time largely switched to the robotic approach for most primary surgeries that are performed in the hundreds every year.

But the old truth should be remembered that proficiency in a solid decision-making and "old-fashioned" technique may achieve better results than a pre-proficient sloppy modern technique, particularly in absence of a mature oncological thought process. Key for continued success is therefore to achieve the same or a better dissection while using the less invasive approach. Teaching, education, and monitoring are essential. Increased familiarity with the minimally invasive platforms has unquestionably resulted in more versatile surgeons' skills. Complementing human limitations by technical innovations and artificial intelligence is not limited to surgery but visible in nearly all areas of our lives (cars, homes, etc.). There are numerous competing systems entering or about to enter the surgical market. Competition has always been a driver of innovation and pushed down the costs. But the exact role each individual system will be able to play is hard to predict.

In conclusion, MIS surgery for rectal cancer provides a viable, safe, and effective alternative to the open approach—as long as the long-established principles of oncological surgery are followed throughout the decision-making and the procedure [4].

References

1. American Cancer Society. Cancer facts & figures 2024. Atlanta; 2024. Available from: https://www.cancer.org/research/cancer-facts-statistics/all-cancer-facts-figures/2024-cancer-facts-figures.html.
2. Kaiser AM. McGraw-Hill manual: colorectal surgery. New York: McGraw-Hill Medical; 2009. Available from: https://accesssurgery.mhmedical.com/book.aspx?bookID=425
3. Melstrom KA, Kaiser AM. Role of minimally invasive surgery for rectal cancer. World J Gastroenterol. 2020;26(30):4394–414.
4. Zelhart M, Kaiser AM. Robotic versus laparoscopic versus open colorectal surgery: towards defining criteria to the right choice. Surg Endosc. 2018;32(1):24–38.
5. Kaiser AM, Corman ML. History of laparoscopy. Surg Oncol Clin N Am. 2001;10(3):483–92.
6. Nelson H, Sargent DJ, Wieand HS, Fleshman J, Anvari M, Stryker SJ, et al. A comparison of laparoscopically assisted and open colectomy for colon cancer. N Engl J Med. 2004;350(20):2050–9.

7. Guillou PJ, Quirke P, Thorpe H, Walker J, Jayne DG, Smith AM, et al. Short-term endpoints of conventional versus laparoscopic-assisted surgery in patients with colorectal cancer (MRC CLASICC trial): multicentre, randomised controlled trial. Lancet. 2005;365(9472):1718–26.
8. Green BL, Marshall HC, Collinson F, Quirke P, Guillou P, Jayne DG, et al. Long-term follow-up of the Medical Research Council CLASICC trial of conventional versus laparoscopically assisted resection in colorectal cancer. Br J Surg. 2013;100(1):75–82.
9. Bonjer HJ, Deijen CL, Abis GA, Cuesta MA, van der Pas MH, de Lange-de Klerk ES, et al. A randomized trial of laparoscopic versus open surgery for rectal cancer. N Engl J Med. 2015;372(14):1324–32.
10. Fleshman J, Branda M, Sargent DJ, Boller AM, George V, Abbas M, et al. Effect of laparoscopic-assisted resection vs open resection of stage II or III rectal cancer on pathologic outcomes: the ACOSOG Z6051 Randomized Clinical Trial. JAMA. 2015;314(13):1346–55.
11. Stevenson AR, Solomon MJ, Lumley JW, Hewett P, Clouston AD, Gebski VJ, et al. Effect of laparoscopic-assisted resection vs open resection on pathological outcomes in rectal cancer: the ALaCaRT Randomized Clinical Trial. JAMA. 2015;314(13):1356–63.
12. Fleshman J, Branda ME, Sargent DJ, Boller AM, George VV, Abbas MA, et al. Disease-free survival and local recurrence for laparoscopic resection compared with open resection of stage II to III rectal cancer: follow-up results of the ACOSOG Z6051 Randomized Controlled Trial. Ann Surg. 2019;269(4):589–95.
13. Stevenson ARL, Solomon MJ, Brown CSB, Lumley JW, Hewett P, Clouston AD, et al. Disease-free survival and local recurrence after laparoscopic-assisted resection or open resection for rectal cancer: the Australasian Laparoscopic Cancer of the Rectum Randomized Clinical Trial. Ann Surg. 2019;269(4):596–602.
14. Jayne D, Pigazzi A, Marshall H, Croft J, Corrigan N, Copeland J, et al. Effect of robotic-assisted vs conventional laparoscopic surgery on risk of conversion to open laparotomy among patients undergoing resection for rectal cancer: the ROLARR Randomized Clinical Trial. JAMA. 2017;318(16):1569–80.
15. Kim MJ, Park SC, Park JW, Chang HJ, Kim DY, Nam BH, et al. Robot-assisted versus laparoscopic surgery for rectal cancer: a Phase II Open Label Prospective Randomized Controlled Trial. Ann Surg. 2018;267(2):243–51.
16. Stewart CL, Ituarte PHG, Melstrom KA, Warner SG, Melstrom LG, Lai LL, et al. Robotic surgery trends in general surgical oncology from the National Inpatient Sample. Surg Endosc. 2019;33(8):2591–601.
17. Devaraj B, Kaiser A. Impact of technology on indications and limitations for transanal surgical removal of rectal neoplasms. World J Surg Proced. 2015;5(1):1–13.
18. Larsen SG, Pfeffer F, Kørner H, Norwegian Colorectal Cancer Group. Norwegian moratorium on transanal total mesorectal excision. Br J Surg. 2019;106(9):1120–1.
19. European Society of Coloproctology (ESCP) Collaborating Group. An international multicentre prospective audit of elective rectal cancer surgery; operative approach versus outcome, including transanal total mesorectal excision (TaTME). Colorectal Dis. 2018;20(Suppl 6):33–46.
20. Matsuyama T, Kinugasa Y, Nakajima Y, Kojima K. Robotic-assisted surgery for rectal cancer: Current state and future perspective. Ann Gastroenterol Surg. 2018;2(6):406–12.
21. Carmichael JC, Keller DS, Baldini G, Bordeianou L, Weiss E, Lee L, et al. Clinical practice guidelines for enhanced recovery after colon and rectal surgery from the American Society of Colon and Rectal Surgeons and Society of American Gastrointestinal and Endoscopic Surgeons. Dis Colon Rectum. 2017;60(8):761–84.
22. Lee L, Abou-Khalil M, Liberman S, Boutros M, Fried GM, Feldman LS. Incidence of incisional hernia in the specimen extraction site for laparoscopic colorectal surgery: systematic review and meta-analysis. Surg Endosc. 2017;31(12):5083–93.
23. Andersson J, Abis G, Gellerstedt M, Angenete E, Angerås U, Cuesta MA, et al. Patient-reported genitourinary dysfunction after laparoscopic and open rectal cancer surgery in a randomized trial (COLOR II). Br J Surg. 2014;101(10):1272–9.

9 Transanal Total Mesorectal (taTME) Excision in Rectal Cancer

A. Caycedo-Marulanda, M. Dean, and M. Chand

Abstract

Transanal total mesorectal excision (taTME) constitutes a novel approach for the radical removal of the rectum. The procedure was designed to take advantage of the natural orifice surgery concept; it allows for the bottom-up dissection of the rectum through the insertion of either a flexible or rigid transanal platform.

Historically, removal of the rectum represents a technical challenge due to the anatomical constraints posed by the rigid pelvis. The procedure gathered great interest from surgeons across the world; this ultimately met significant scrutiny after the publication of a local moratorium from Norway.

The procedure is done by either a sequential or a synchronous approach with single or dual teams, respectively. Surgeons can use specifically designed equipment or adapt laparoscopic instruments for this procedure. Standardization of the procedure for the learning and safe implementation of the procedure have not been agreed upon. Despite having mastered the technique, the authors recognize that taTME has the potential for devastating and otherwise infrequent complications; therefore extreme caution is recommended if a decision is made to embark in the implementation of taTME. We present our perspective and experience on this complex intervention.

Keywords

Transanal · TME · Rectal cancer · Natural orifice surgery

9.1 History and Evolution of taTME

Total mesorectal excision (taTME) was initially described by Sylla et al. in 2010 [1]. Accessing the distal pelvis has always posed a technical challenge for surgeons, and this has remained constant even with the evolution of laparoscopic surgery. Even though the procedure was initially conceived as an advancement of natural orifice surgery (NOTES), surgeons rapidly realized it could also provide an approach to overcome the technical difficulties of accessing the pelvis. The precursor of taTME is the transanal endoscopic surgery (TEMS) procedure created and developed by Professor Buess in the 1980s in Germany as a method to locally resect large rectal polyps that were difficult or impossible to remove

---

Supplementary Information The online version contains supplementary material available at https://doi.org/10.1007/978-981-97-7059-5_9.

A. Caycedo-Marulanda (✉)
Queen's University, Kingston Health Sciences Centre, Kingston, ON, Canada

M. Dean · M. Chand
University College London Hospital, London, England

M. Tewari (ed.), *Minimally Invasive Surgery in Cancer*,
https://doi.org/10.1007/978-981-97-7059-5_9

through conventional endoscopic methods [2]. The TEMS procedure encountered early and sustained opposition before it was widely accepted.

taTME, as most novel procedures, was preceded by the work of different surgeons that contributed to the evolution of surgery; perhaps one of the most relevant contributions included the seminal work on cadaveric models by Whiteford et al. [3]. One vital concept that is supported by the proponents of taTME is the ability to control the distal margin, which has been argued to be uncertain when using other approaches. The idea of having the opportunity to adequately control the distal margin by using a bottom-up approach was first solidified by Gerald Marks with the transanal-transabdominal proctosigmoidectomy (TATA) in the 1980s [4].

Removal of the rectum has always been particularly difficult, not only because of the challenge presented by the rigid confines of the pelvis, but in addition the need to stay on the correct embryologic plane as described by Professor Heald [5]. It is also vital to preserve function. Patient selection is of crucial importance, and while there are no standard criteria, most surgeons would exclude T4 tumors, high tumors (>10 cm), and emergency presentations including obstruction. taTME may be the preferred approach for male patients, obese patients, or any patients with a narrow and/or deep pelvis.

Surgeons have been eager to adopt the technique of taTME and its popularity rapidly increased with the development of the flexible platform for transanal minimally invasive surgery (TAMIS) in 2009, as it was more affordable than the TEMS approach and required instruments conventionally used in laparoscopy. As the eagerness to learn and implement the procedure continued, multiple courses and workshops were offered around the globe; simultaneously a multitude of publications and case series were presented in scientific journals and surgical meetings [6–9]. As more experience was acquired, many began to realize the technical difficulties of the technique and the potential for serious complications that this novel procedure could pose for surgeons and ultimately to patients [10]. taTME remains an innovative surgical technique, and patients should be counseled about the risks and benefits as part of the consent process. This includes the present limitations on long-term oncological data and functional outcomes.

9.2 Controversies

One particular concern surrounding any approach for cancer surgery is the oncologic safety. In early 2019, authors from Norway [11] published results showing an unusual pattern of early multifocal local recurrence (LR) in the pelvis, with rate close to 10% LR at a median of 11 months. Complete data showed the LR to 7.6% on 157 patients [12]. The results were alarming considering the historical LR in the country was 3.4%. As a consequence, a local moratorium on taTME was issued in Norway. Criticism surrounding the Norwegian data arises from the low volume of cases per center and the lower than expected rate of neoadjuvant therapy those patients received, as well as the high incidence of R1 resections (13%) perhaps suggesting a technical issue. The Norway results have led many to exercising extreme caution and even abandoning the procedure, for instance, the Association of Coloproctology of Great Britain and Ireland (ACPGBI) has recommended a pause for reflection [13], suggesting that only sites with experience and good outcomes continue to offer taTME in the UK and halting the training of further surgeons until the safety concerns are resolved.

In contrast, there have been a large number of publications from various authors providing excellent results, which include large cohorts with local recurrence rates well in line with those from laparoscopic and open literature [6, 14–18]. In addition to these, there has been great interest in providing adequate guidance in regard to the criteria for selecting patients for this procedure and the methods to achieve adequate training to reach proficiency [20].

9.3 Patient Positioning and Operating Room Setup

As in any other surgical approach for rectal surgery, patients are placed in Lloyd Davis position with both arms tucked and secured in

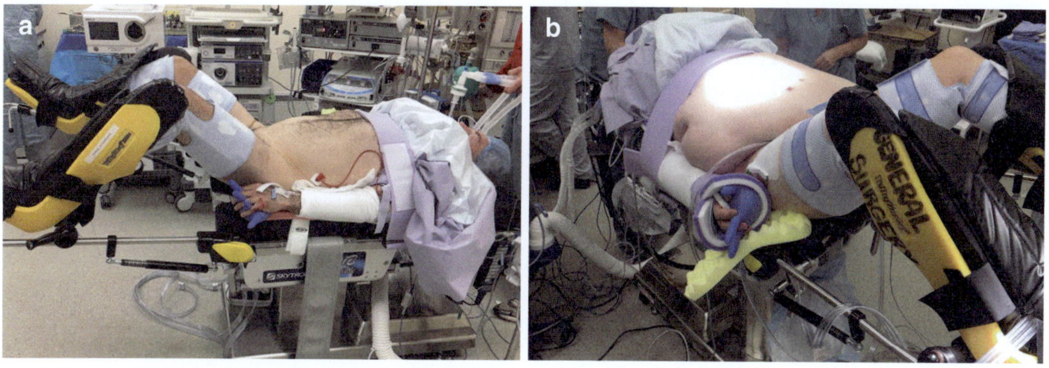

Fig. 9.1 Patients in lithotomy position on a memory pad, with both arms tucked

a way that prevents patient movement during positioning in steep Trendelenburg and table tilt positions. It is our preference to use the Pink-Pad® patient positioning system and avoid other pieces of equipment like a bean-bag or shoulder retainers that could potentially cause harm (Fig. 9.1a, b). The abdominal team stand on the patients' right side with the monitor and insufflation tower on the patients' left. The transanal team sit between the patients' legs, with the instrument table to the patients' left.

9.4 List of Specific Instruments

The literature reports different transanal platforms (TEM/TEO/glove port/TAMIS platform), single team versus two team operating, abdominal dissection techniques (laparoscopic/robotic) and specimen extraction techniques (transanal/transabdominal). In this chapter, the authors have restricted the description to those cases performed with conventional laparoscopic equipment using the TAMIS® platform, with either one or a two team approach.

In addition to the conventional laparoscopic equipment for the transabdominal dissection, the required additional tools for the transanal portion includes:

- Airseal® Insufflation System (Fig. 9.2)
- GelPOINT® Path Transanal Access Platform (aka TAMIS platform)
- Laparoscopic needle drivers x 2, laparoscopic monopolar coagulation suction R.Wolff®, 5 mm Cobra-teeth grasper)
- Lonestar retractor® with 6–8 stay hooks
- 29 mm EEA stapler, 0 prolene x2

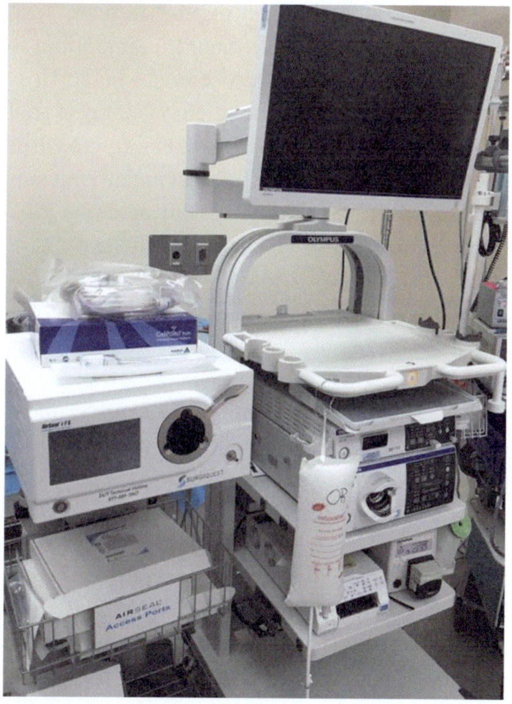

Fig. 9.2 Valveless inssuflation device (Airseal (r), endo tower for the transanal visualization Endoeye (r) Olympus

Two separate instrument sets and video towers are required, one for each approach (transabdominal and transanal, respectively). It is also necessary to have two individual insufflators; for the transanal approach we recommend to use an insufflating system that incorporates continuous smoke evacuation and provides a stable pneumo-space. The latter recommendation is of vital importance to prevent bellowing, as it would significantly impair visualization.

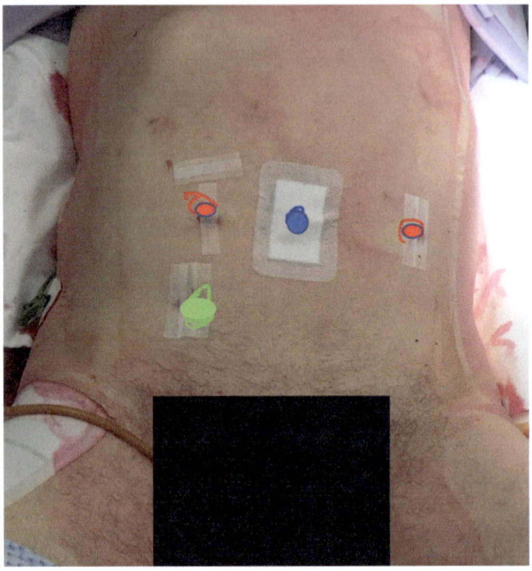

Fig. 9.3 Position of trocars. Blue: Hasson 10–12 mm, red: 5 mm, green: 10–12 mm

9.5 The Operative Technique in a Detailed Stepwise Manner

9.5.1 Abdominal Phase

It is our practice to start via a transabdominal approach by using conventional laparoscopic instruments with four ports, including a 10–12 Hassan umbilical port (Fig. 9.3). Abdominal dissection is conducted in a regular fashion, with multiport colonic mobilization. It is important to decide early during the procedure whether it is necessary to takedown the splenic flexure, if so it should be done before the transanal approach is commenced. The only step that remains a must is the division of the mesentery starting at the inferior mesenteric artery pedicle toward the point of division at the colon (5:21′ video). This is followed by a perfusion assessment of the colonic remnant preferably with indocyanine green (ICG) (5:34′ video) .

As previously stated, either one team (sequential) or two team (synchronous) approaches are possible. In case a two team approach is taken, one team should persist during the transabdominal dissection in reaching as low as possible depending on both the tumor location and anatomical conditions. In the case of a two team approach, judgment regarding the moment to start the transanal dissection needs to be applied as well as continuous communication between the teams while the two-sided dissection progresses. It is feasible to start the transanal portion right at the moment the colonic dissection (6:38′ video) has been finalized and the surgeon is ready to undertake the upper rectum dissection or will approach the peritoneal reflection. Transillumination can be used to guide the transanal team to the upper dissection plane. Once both dissection planes meet, the abdominal team can continue to assist the transanal team by retracting the rectum upward.

9.5.2 Transanal Phase

The transanal dissection requires a stepwise approach. Our recommendations are as follows:

- Placement of the transanal port: This might require the use of the Lonestar retractor® in order to efface the anal canal and facilitate introduction of the TAMIS® platform (Fig. 9.4).
- Identification of the lower edge of the tumor and placement of purse-string suture using 0-Prolene below (0:20″ video) the level of the tumor, ensuring a negative distal margin. This part of the procedure requires even stitches to

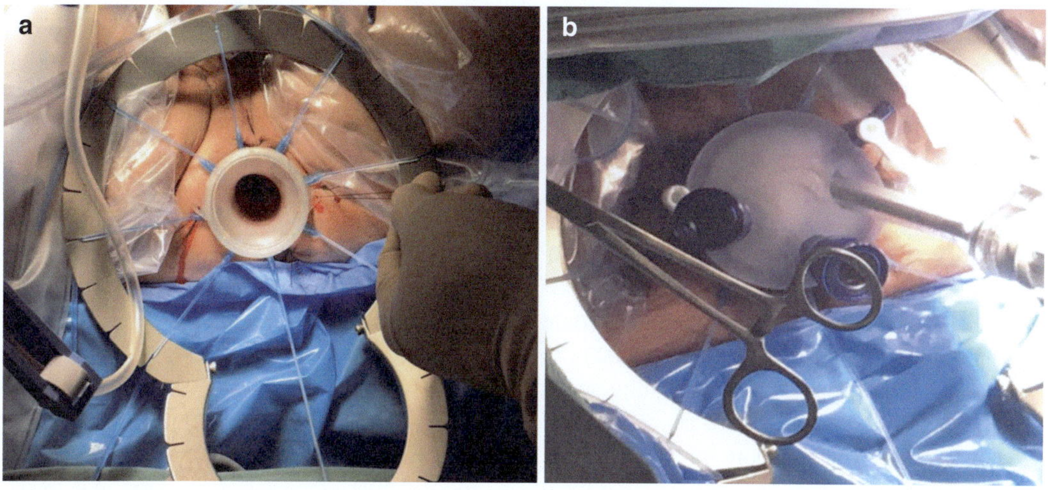

Fig. 9.4 (**a**) TAMIS platform inserted transanally with Lone Star®. (**b**) Gelpoint® path with trocars

be placed very close to one another with particular avoidance of the following:
  - Spiraling up or down.
  - Encompassing neighboring structures (vagina, prostate, muscle, or vascular structures).
- For low-mid rectal tumors, the purse string suture might be placed directly through the GelPOINT with the cap removed. The surgeon usually changes gloves immediately after tying up the purse string, since it requires the GelPOINT® path to be removed and direct contact with the rectal lumen.
- Cleansing the rectum with Povidone® is done followed by a washout with abundant saline until the iodine is clear out (1:03′ Video).
- The GelPOINT Cap is pierced with two 10 mm cannulas and a 10–12 mm cannula for the AirSeal Insufflation System®. Pneumorectum is maintained with carbon dioxide at a pressure of 12–15 mmHg and low flow of 5 L/min.
- A circumferential "tattoo" is made by scoring the mucosa with the electrocautery hook, in order to demarcate the transection (rectotomy) site. This can be determined by either staying 1 cm out of the center of the purse string or the equivalent, which is staying right at the outer edge of the radial folds (1:14′ video). One should avoid a limited rectotomy at one location since that will cause significant anatomical distortion; instead, it is ideal to create a circular and even full thickness rectal wall division at a 90° angle to the bowel wall (1:37′ video). As the circumferential dissection is performed, one can recognize a full thickness rectotomy as there is no evidence of any radial muscle fibers and perirectal fat is identified.
- The real bottom-up dissection of the mesorectum starts at this point, and the surgeon must recognize the mesorectal edge in order to progress cephalad toward the peritoneal cavity (2:30′ video). It is crucial to keep in mind the concept of even dissection and avoidance of "digging" a hole in one point.
- Circular dissection is usually started at the 12 o'clock position followed by the 6 o'clock. The mesorectum anteriorly is usually thin. Conscious identification of the anterior structures (prostate or vagina) can be achieved relatively easier with a combination of blunt and sharp dissection of the tissue, followed by extending it toward the sides.
- This "frontal to lateral" dissection is recommended as moving from the sides toward the front will lead to dissecting behind prostate (3:46′ video), which could lead to catastrophic complications such as urethral injuries. In a situation in which the dissection is moving from the lateral aspects toward the front, the

surgeon will encounter a paired neurovascular structure located at the 11 and 1 o'clock, those correspond to the neurovascular bundles of Walsh. Bleeding at these locations is serious warning to stop and reassess the plan of dissection before further proceeding.

- The neurovascular bundles of Walsh are commonly known to urologists; these however are relatively new structures to colorectal surgeons. Bilateral injury of the bundles would undoubtedly render a male patient unable to achieve an erection. While performing surgical dissection close to these structures a surgeon would be warned about imminent danger of injury by bleeding. The pathway and location of the bundles can be usually identified by the experienced surgeon.
- Posterior dissection is the "easy" part of the operation, as the TME plane at this location remains the closest resemblance to what is known to the laparoscopic dissection appearance (2:51′ video).
- The circumferential bottom-up dissection can be completed either by a synchronous or a simultaneous approach. Regardless of the approach, once the rendezvous (2:40′, 3:12′ video) occurs, it requires traction and countertraction from both locations. Either both surgeons collaborate and work simultaneously or the assistant provides traction from the abdomen to facilitate the transanal detachment. Transillumination from above has been described as a useful technique to guide the transanal surgeon (2:46′ video).
- Once the rectal dissection has been completed (4:02″ video), we recommend performing a thorough pelvic washout with warm saline or sterile water, irrigated from both ends. This minimizes the risk of infection (4:36′ video).
- The decision to extract the rectum transanally versus transabdominally should not be taken lightly. In our practice we commonly lean toward using an abdominal incision since a transanal extraction can lead to disruption of the specimen of even devascularization of the conduit. The latter is only used when the specimen is thin or the patient's pelvis is wide enough that one can ascertain no extraction difficulties. In transanal specimen extraction the GelPOINT is removed, a small or medium size Alexis wound retractor® is inserted, and the entire rectosigmoid specimen is delivered via the anus (6:08′ video).
- Right at this point and before extraction if a stapled reconstruction is an option, placement of a purse string in the rectal stump is required. This itself has particular challenges and specific details have been described elsewhere [19].
- After the rectum is extracted, the bowel is divided at the selected point, either guided by Indocyanine green (ICG) or proximal to the inferior mesenteric artery (IMA) pedicle. The specimen is handled to be sent to the pathology lab (Fig. 9.5). The subsequent plan for bowel reconstruction includes placement of the anvil or mobile piece of the circular stapler in the proximal colonic stump. This is secured and placed either laterally or at the end of the bowel. There are different methods described to create an anastomosis when using a taTME approach [20].
- Bowel reconstruction (6:49′ video) is usually performed similarly to laparoscopic surgery with the use of a circular stapler to form a double purse string (8:24′ video) anastomosis (4:54′ video). The alternative is a handsewn anastomosis to the rectal cuff.

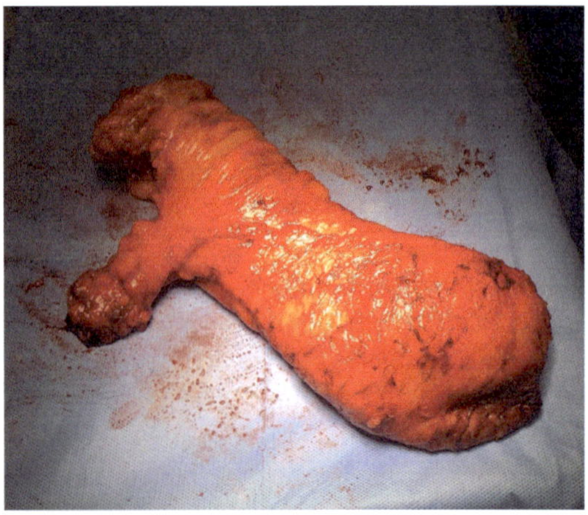

Fig. 9.5 taTME specimen

9.6 Postoperative Course and Management

The principles of postoperative management of patients who have undergone taTME remain similar to any surgical resection of the bowel. Indeed, the procedure is similar to a complex laparoscopic procedure as there are no additional wounds that require attention other than the conventional laparoscopic approach.

Postoperatively our patients are managed with enhanced recovery after surgery (ERAS) principles, which have benefit in both open and laparoscopic colorectal surgical patients [21]. The ERAS protocol includes early mobilization and feeding, minimizing opioid analgesia, early removal of Foley, and restricted use of IV fluids. Care is provided by a dedicated, well-trained multidisciplinary team. The stoma nurse sees the patient from postoperative day 1 and educates the patient on all aspects of stoma care.

The length of stay is similar to conventional laparoscopy and one would expect patients to remain in hospital for 3–5 days following surgery. It is not unusual to have 40% of patients discharged on day 2 or 3 after surgery. Inflammatory markers may be an important test to signify a pelvic collection or anastomotic leak (AL). Results from the recent PREDICT Study suggest a CRP above 150 or an increase of more than 50 between consecutive postoperative days may be indicative of a leak [22].

If there is a clinical suspicion for AL, then it is prudent for early and careful endoscopic assessment rather than waiting for radiological confirmation. In this situation a combination between a transanal and laparoscopic approach may salvage the anastomosis; this is more likely to be successful if identified early. Often radiology is not helpful in the immediate postoperative period.

Information on long-term postoperative bowel, sexual and urinary function should be sought. Continence scoring systems such as the Cleveland Clinic Incontinence Index [23] and the Low Anterior Resection Syndrome (LARS) score [24] are useful tools to assess and monitor postoperative function.

9.7 Complications

The international taTME registry reported overall morbidity of 30.4%, with visceral injuries during the transanal phase occurring in 1.8% [25]. The bottom-up approach to rectal dissection opens up anatomical planes in a different manner compared to the transabdominal approach. Recognition of these planes from below can be challenging, and inaccurate dissection can lead to injury to adjacent pelvic structures. During the posterior dissection there may be a breach of the mesorectum or rectal wall anteriorly, increasing the risk of recurrence and infection, or a breach of the presacral fascia posteriorly, which can lead to significant bleeding from the presacral venous plexus. Laterally structures of the pelvic side wall may be injured. In the anterior plane, injury to the vagina and urethra may occur. The international registry reported urethral injury in 0.8% of patients [25].

Surgeons embarking on this technique have described signs that can suggest dissection may have drifted into the incorrect plane. The correct plane can be indicated by the presence of "triangles" where the tethered point tents the fascia. If dissection proceeds and the fascial planes are disrupted, the pneumoperitoneum can take on the shape of a circle or "halo." Recognition of these signs can help guide dissection in the correct plane [26]. In the anterolateral aspect the appearance of skeletal muscle of the pelvic floor suggests the dissection is too anterior, and the prostate and urethra are at risk. Urethra identification can be aided with the use of ICG or lighted urethral stents [27, 28].

The position and quality of the purse string suture is vital to avoid the complication of a loose, broken or severed purse string, with resultant contamination with feces and tumor cells. Carbon dioxide embolism is a rare, severe complication that can occur when CO_2 insufflation gas is introduced into the low-pressure venous system during dissection [20].

As with all new techniques, implementation requires careful patient selection, detailed knowledge of the surgical anatomy, advanced technical skills, quality training, and detailed audit. To minimize the risks associated with learning curve, surgeons should access learning opportunities in the form of training courses, video-based learning, and conference tips and trick sessions. Having a proctor present for the first few cases is also advisable.

9.8 Personal Experience

One of the authors has acquired a large experience in the performance of the taTME procedure for both benign and malignant conditions. As experience and skills grow, one can expand the use and indications for the procedure, which includes extra-levator abdominoperineal resections, pelvic exenteration, or reexploration of the pelvis in cases of complications such as strictures, anastomotic dehiscence, or even local recurrences [25, 29]. Another potential use is the creation, redo, and excision of J-pouches [7]. Regardless, it is imperative to increase case complexity in a slow and progressive fashion. It is important to remain aware that the learning curve requires around 40–50 cases to master the technique [30–32] and the initial ten cases of a surgeon's experience bear a higher oncological risk (BMJ-Caycedo). It is only fair to question the applicability of a technique that can only be safely done by a group of few; nonetheless I personally think that it is rather a technique that can and should only be done at specialized and dedicated centers of excellence with concentrated expertise, this is not different than the performance of a Whipple procedure or a radical esophagectomy. Similar to those procedures, taTME requires skill, training, expertise, and consistent volumes. A surgeon who is looking to master this approach necessarily has to become abundantly familiar with the "inverted anatomy" and the potential variations one could encounter; this can only be developed by way of pattern recognition system, which in time allows the surgeon to successfully deal with both familiar and unfamiliar anatomical scenarios.

Many surgeons currently, and even myself during the early experience, are convinced that it is imperative to do all the TME dissection via taTME. This is far from being mandatory and it is important to understand that the real benefit of taTME lies on achieving distal margin control and allowing sound dissection of the lower third of the rectum. As such, one should do as much dissection it is safe and easy to do transabdominally before resorting to the taTME portion of the operation. In my current practice, it would not be unusual only do the perpendicular transection of the rectum followed by 1 or 2 cm of caudal to cephalic dissection before the rendezvous is achieved.

Performing a taTME procedure for a lesion located in the upper third of the rectum is essentially not indicated as it can be easily achieved by means of conventional laparoscopy. In my opinion and those of many, in order to consider taTME advisable, the lower edge of a rectal tumor should be below the peritoneal reflection. With that in mind it is still reasonable to say that every case needs to be individually analyzed. Similarly when considering any surgical approach for patients with rectal cancer, it is necessary to study and interpret the MRI images, it is not enough to have the radiologist report and the distance from the anal verge. The angulation of the sacrum, the distance between the tumor and the top of the sphincter, the size and configuration of the prostate, the exact circumferential location of the tumor and every other aspect usually considered in rectal cancer surgery needs to be thoroughly assessed by the surgeon; it is not unusual to have to look at those images while performing this, as one, for instance, needs to "project" the angulation of the sacrum to plan the posterior dissection or to assess the prostate/vagina configuration in order to avoid a devastating injury.

Performing cases with a proctor is strongly recommended as beneficial to reach technical proficiency; it also enables the novel surgeon to refine patient selection skills. There is a need to perform taTME from a well-equipped institution that not only has the surgeons willing and trained to take on this cases, it requires a center with enough volume where at least 25 extra-peritoneal rectal cancer cases per year are performed, in addition to the capabilities to deal with "complex" rectal cancer surgery as previously define elsewhere [30].

Just thinking and being convinced that one has good surgical and oncological results is not enough, this is particularly true when adopting novel and difficult techniques. Including taTME cases in a registry is an important method for quality assurance, similarly the performance of internal audits are valuable actions that help to monitor and enhance the procedure and technique-specific outcomes [33].

References

1. Sylla P, Rattner D, Delgado S, Lacy A. NOTES transanal rectal cancer resection using transanal endoscopic microsurgery and laparoscopic assistance. Surg Endosc. 2010;24(5):1205–10.
2. Buess G, Theiss R, Günther M, Hutterer F, Pichlmaier H. Endoscopic surgery in the rectum. Endoscopy. 1985;17(1):31–5.
3. Whiteford MH, Denk PM, Swanstrom LL. Feasibility of radical sigmoid colectomy performed as natural orifice translumenal endoscopic surgery (NOTES) using transanal endoscopic microsurgery. Surg Endosc. 2007;21(10):1870–4.
4. Marks JH, Salem JF. From TATA to NOTES, how taTME fits into the evolutionary surgical tree. Tech Coloproctol. 2016;20(8):513–5.
5. Heald B, Ryall RDH. Recurrence and survival after total mesorectal excision for rectal cancer. Lancet. 1986;1(8496):1479–82.
6. Burke JP, Martin-Perez B, Khan A, Nassif G, de Beche-Adams T, Larach SW, Albert MR, Atallah S. Transanal total mesorectal excision for rectal cancer: early outcomes in 50 consecutive patients. Colorectal Dis. 2016;18(6):570–7.
7. Caycedo-Marulanda A, Jiang HY, Kohtakangas EL. Outcomes of a single surgeon-based transanal-total mesorectal excision (TATME) for rectal cancer. J Gastrointest Cancer. 2018;49(4):455–62.
8. Lacy FB, van Laarhoven JJEM, Pena R, Arroyave MC, Bravo R, Cuatrecasas M, Lacy AM. Transanal total mesorectal excision: pathological results of 186 patients with mid and low rectal cancer. Surg Endosc. 2018;32(5):2442–7.
9. Mege D, Hain E, Lakkis Z, Maggiori L, Prost a la Denise J, Panis Y. Trans-anal total mesorectal excision: is it really safe and better than laparoscopic total mesorectal excision with perineal approach first in patients with low rectal cancer? A learning curve with case-matched study in 68 patients. Colorectal Dis. 2018;20(6):O143–51.
10. Atallah SB, DuBose AC, Burke JP, Nassif G, deBeche-Adams T, Frering T, Albert MR, Monson JRT. Uptake of transanal total mesorectal excision in North America: initial assessment of a structured training program and the experience of delegate surgeons. Dis Colon Rectum. 2017;60(10):1023–31.
11. Larsen SG, Pfeffer F, Korner H, On Behalf of the Norwegian Colorectal Cancer Group. Norwegian moratorium on transanal total mesorectal excision. Br J Surg. 2019;106(9):1120–1.
12. Wasmuth HH, Faerden AE, Myklebust TA, Pfeffer F, Norderval S, Riis R, Olsen OC, Lambrecht JR, Korner H, Larsen SG, Norwegian TaTME Collaborative Group on Behalf of the Norwegian Colorectal Cancer Group, Forsmo HM, Baekkelund O, Lavik S, Knapp JC, Sjo O, Rashid G. Transanal total mesorectal excision for rectal cancer has been suspended in Norway. Br J Surg. 2020;107(1):121–30.
13. Fearnhead NS, Acheson AG, Brown SR, Hancock L, Harikrishnan A, Kelly SB, Maxwell-Armstrong CA, Sagar PM, Siddiqi S, Walsh CJ, Wheeler JMD, Abercrombie JF, Association of Coloproctology of Great Britain, Ireland (ACPGBI) Executive, Getting It Right First Time (GIRFT). The ACPGBI recommends pause for reflection on transanal total mesorectal excision. Colorectal Dis. 2020;22(7):745–8.
14. Bonjer HJ, Deijen CL, Abis GA, Cuesta MA, van der Pas MH, de Lange-de Klerk ES, Lacy AM, Bemelman WA, Andersson J, Angenete E, Rosenberg J, Fuerst A, Haglind E, COLOR II Study Group. A randomized trial of laparoscopic versus open surgery for rectal cancer. N Engl J Med. 2015;372(14):1324–32.
15. Caycedo-Marulanda A, Brown CJ, Chadi SA, Ashamalla S, Lee L, Stotland P, Hameed U, Melich G, Ma G, Letarte F, Karimuddin A, Quereshy F, Phang T, Raval M, Vikis E, Liberman AS, Bouchard A, Bouchard P, Drolet S. Canadian taTME expert collaboration (CaTaCO) position statement. Surg Endosc. 2020;34(9):3748–53.
16. Hol JC, van Oostendorp SE, Tuynman JB, Sietses C. Long-term oncological results after transanal total mesorectal excision for rectal carcinoma. Tech Coloproctol. 2019;23(9):903–11.
17. Lacy AM, Tasende MM, Delgado S, Fernandez-Hevia M, Jimenez M, De Lacy B, Castells A, Bravo R, Wexner SD, Heald RJ. Transanal total mesorectal mesorectal excision for rectal cancer: outcomes after 140 patients. J Am Coll Surg. 2015;221(2):415–23.
18. Veltcamp Helbach M, Deijen CL, Velthuis S, Bonjer HJ, Tuynman JB, Sietses C. Transanal total mesorectal excision for rectal carcinoma: short-term outcomes and experience after 80 cases. Surg Endosc. 2016;30(2):464–70.
19. Wu R, Benedict R, Caycedo-Marulanda A. Distal purse-string suture technique for TaTME. Tech Coloproctol. 2019;23(1):67–68. https://doi.org/10.1007/s10151-018-1917-8. PubMed PMID: 30580385.

20. Atallah SB. Transanal minimally invasive surgery (TAMIS) and transanal total mesorectal excision (taTME). Cham: Springer; 2020.
21. Currie AC, Malietzis G, Jenkins JT, Yamada T, Ashrafian H, Athanasiou T, Okabayashi K, Kennedy RH. Network meta-analysis of protocol driven care and laparoscopic surgery for colorectal cancer. Br J Surg. 2016;103(13):1783–94.
22. Stephensen BD, Reid F, Shaikh S, Carroll R, Smith SR, Pockney P, On Behalf of the PREDICT Study Group Collaborators. C-reactive protein trajectory to predict colorectal anastomotic leak: PREDICT study. BJS. 2020;107(13):1832–7.
23. Jorge JM, Wexner SD. Etiology and management of fecal incontinence. Dis Colon Rectum. 1993;36(1):77–97.
24. Emmertsen KJ, Laurberg S. Low anterior resection syndrome score: development and validation of a symptom-based scoring system for bowel dysfunction after low anterior resection for rectal cancer. Ann Surg. 2012;255(5):922–8.
25. Penna M, et al. Transanal total mesorectal excision: international registry results of the first 720 cases. Ann Surg. 2017;266(1):111–7.
26. Bernardi MP, Bloemendaal AL, Albert M, Whiteford M, Stevenson AR, Hompes R. Transanal total mesorectal excision: dissection tips using 'O's and 'triangles'. Tech Coloproctol. 2016;20(11):775–8.
27. Atallah SB, Mabardy A, Volpato AP, Chin T, Sneider J, Monson JRT. Surgery beyond the visible light spectrum: theoretical and applied methods for localization of the male urethra during transanal total mesorectal excision. Tech Coloproctol. 2017;21(6):413–24.
28. Barnes TG, Volpi D, Cunningham C, Vojnovic B, Hompes R. Improved urethral fluorescence during low rectal surgery: a new dye and a new method. Tech Coloproctol. 2018;22(2):115–9.
29. Westerduin E, Bos K, Blok RD, Tanis PJ, Bemelman WA. Transanal minimal invasive surgical management for persisting pelvic sepsis or chronic sinus after low anterior resection. Dis Colon Rectum. 2019;62(12):1458–66.
30. Caycedo-Marulanda A, Verschoor CP. Experience beyond the learning curve of transanal total mesorectal excision (taTME) and its effect on the incidence of anastomotic leak. Tech Coloproctol. 2020;24(4):309–16.
31. Koedam TWA, Veltcamp Helbach M, van de Ven PM, Kruyt PM, van Heek NT, Bonjer HJ, Tuynman JB, Sietses C. Transanal total mesorectal excision for rectal cancer: evaluation of the learning curve. Tech Coloproctol. 2018;22(4):279–87.
32. Lee L, Kelly J, Nassif GJ, deBeche-Adams TC, Albert MR, Monson JRT. Defining the learning curve for transanal total mesorectal excision for rectal adenocarcinoma. Surg Endosc. 2020;34(4):1534–42.
33. Adamina M, Buchs NC, Penna M, Hompes R, On Behalf of the St.Gallen Colorectal Consensus Expert Group. St.Gallen consensus on safe implementation of transanal total mesorectal excision. Surg Endosc. 2018;32(3):1091–103.

Minimally Invasive Resection for Lung Cancer

10

G. Karimundackal, D. M. Niyogi, S. Nadkarni, and R. C. Mistry

Abstract

Surgery is the standard of care for early stage lung cancer. The traditional surgical approach for lung resection is through a posterolateral thoracotomy; this involves transecting muscles and retracting the ribs. This results in significant postoperative pain and compromised cough effort leading to high pulmonary morbidity. Researchers have been looking for alternatives to reduce trauma of access to thoracic cavity. Video-assisted thoracoscopic surgery (VATS) offers this alternative. While thoracoscopy dates back to 1910, it was after 1990, when modern telescopes, high definition camera, dedicated instruments, energy sources, and endoscopic staplers became available that complex thoracoscopic procedures were performed. First VATS lobectomy was reported in 1991; since then, more and more centers across the globe have adopted the technique for lung resection. The technique has been shown to reduce postoperative pain, pulmonary complications, hospital stay, and improved quality of life without compromising the oncological outcomes. Over the years, the technique of thoracoscopic surgery has evolved: from conventional "multi-port" approach to "uniportal" and "needle-scopic" approach. Also, complexity of surgery has increased: from simple lobectomy to bronchial and vascular sleeve resections. Advances in technology is improving the ease of performing VATS: introduction of telescope with three-dimensional vision, camera, and monitors with high resolution images. Introduction of robotic-assisted thoracoscopic surgery (RATS) has introduced a new dimension to minimal invasive thoracic surgery. Despite all the advances, it is imperative that the art of conventional thoracic surgery is imparted to all trainees as it will continue to be the backbone of lung surgery for years to come.

Keywords

MIS · VATS · Lung cancer

10.1 History

The history of minimally invasive lung surgery goes as far back as 1910, when Jacobaeus first used the thoracoscope for lysing adhesions in patients with tuberculosis. After a long period of

Supplementary Information The online version contains supplementary material available at https://doi.org/10.1007/978-981-97-7059-5_10.

G. Karimundackal · D. M. Niyogi · S. Nadkarni
Department of Thoracic Surgery, Tata Memorial Hospital, Mumbai, India

R. C. Mistry (✉)
Department of Thoracic Surgery, Kokilaben Dhirubhai Ambani Hospital, Mumbai, India
e-mail: RAJESH.MISTRY@kokilabenhospitals.com

M. Tewari (ed.), *Minimally Invasive Surgery in Cancer*,
https://doi.org/10.1007/978-981-97-7059-5_10

dormancy, thoracoscopy reemerged when Roviaro in Milan performed the first thoracoscopic lobectomy in 1991 [1]. This spurred worldwide interest in minimally invasive lung resection with the first international symposium being held in the USA in 1993. However, in 1994, a study by Landreneau et al. comparing minimally invasive and open approaches showed no significant difference in chronic pain scores and shoulder dysfunction between the two groups [2]. This, and a few more reports along similar lines, coupled with the technical challenges around major vascular structures, led to a decline in the original enthusiasm. The advent of better imaging technology and endo-stapling devices rekindled the interest, with a large number of reports in favor of minimally invasive lung cancer resection emerging world-over. The purported benefits included fewer in-hospital complications, shorter hospital stay, better pain scores, and quality of life, all while maintaining the oncological quality of surgery [3, 4]. Enough evidences of better perioperative outcomes and oncological equivalence made minimally invasive resection standard of care for early-stage lung cancer [5]. The constant criticism of lack of randomized evidence supporting minimally invasive lung resection ended recently with the publication of results from a number of multicenter randomized trials [3, 4]. The results uniformly favored video-assisted thoracoscopic surgery (VATS) in a few key short-term outcomes like operative time, intraoperative blood loss, postoperative pain, and quality of life (QOL). VATS was also shown to be non-inferior to open surgery in short-term oncological outcomes in the recently announced results of the VIOLET trial [6]. There is also emerging evidence for long-term oncological superiority in terms of overall and disease-free survival with minimally invasive resection for lung cancer [7, 8].

The simultaneous development of VATS lung surgery in different parts of the world has led to the evolution of the surgical technique in many directions. The earliest definition of VATS approach was by Swanson et al. in 2007 [9]. They recommended a 3-port approach with two 0.5 cm ports and one 4–8 cm access incision. The world has moved on from that early definition to a 2-port, needle-scopic and what is now the current favorite, the uniportal technique. The uniportal approach mimics open surgery with the camera and instruments being in the same line of vision, making the learning curve shorter and with no increase in complication rates [10]. Advances in surgical technology have made even complex resections like bronchial and vascular sleeves and non-intubated surgery a real-world possibility [11].

10.2 Introduction

The evolution of VATS lung resection in our institute has mirrored the practice patterns in most other parts of the world. We started off adopting the Japanese/East Asian style of operating with the surgeon standing to the right of the patient and soon moved on to the more Western, anterior approach to the hilum. This helped us in adopting the uniportal technique, which is easier with an anterior approach. In the following sections we will be delving in greater detail into the operative technique that we have developed with brief comments on anesthesia, equipment, and postoperative care.

10.3 Anesthesia Concerns, Patient Position, and Operating Room Setup

All patients are operated under general anesthesia with muscle relaxation and lung isolation. Although there have been reports of non-intubated lung surgery, even complex resections, we have not explored that avenue yet. Lung isolation is achieved with a double lumen tube introduced into the contralateral side where possible or a bronchial blocker in the ipsilateral side to allow for collapse of the lung on the side to be operated upon. Placement of the tube on the contralateral side aids in moving the bronchus around for lymph node dissection and reduces the chance of tube displacement. However, placing the tube on the right side optimally may be technically demanding. If a bronchial sleeve/bronchotomy is a possibility, it is mandatory to

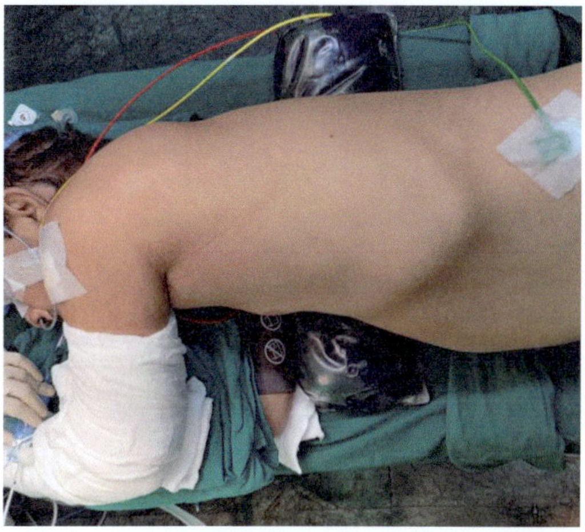

Fig. 10.1 Patient position

insert a double lumen tube into the contralateral side. In patients with a low likelihood of conversion and when no major blood loss is expected, arterial lines and epidural catheters may be avoided.

The patient is positioned in the lateral position, in the middle of the table with the side to be operated facing upward. The arms are kept folded together in front of the patient in their natural position. A bolster is placed under the patient at the level of the tip of the scapula or a table break performed at that level in order to open out the intercostal spaces. All pressure points are adequately padded and the patient is securely strapped to allow for tilting the table during the course of the surgery (Fig. 10.1).

The main operating screen is placed posterior to the patient. The surgeon stands anterior to the patient. The cameraperson may stand on the same side or opposite side as the surgeon depending on the surgeon's preference. The assisting surgeon stands on the opposite side. A slave monitor, if available may be used for the assistant. It is ergonomically important that the operating table is kept at an optimal height, preferably lower. This helps in keeping the surgeon's shoulders at a lower level while using longer instruments and helps in reducing shoulder fatigue and dysfunction. This is particularly important in prolonged surgeries (Fig. 10.2).

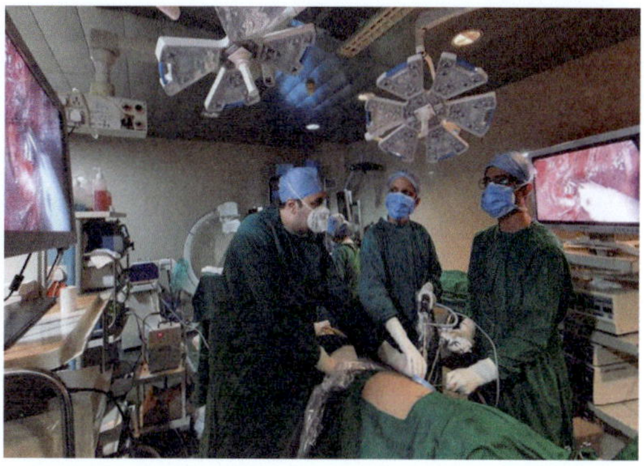

Fig. 10.2 Operating room setup

10.4 Equipment and Instrumentation

It is important to invest in good equipment when embarking on a thoracoscopic program. The bulk of the investment comes under three headings: imaging equipment, energy devices, and VATS instruments. The consumables that may be used during the course of the surgery are also an important consideration.

The imaging equipment should be of at least full HD resolution (1080p) and offer good illumination, contrast, and color gamut. While systems with 4 K resolution and 3D imaging are available and may help in complex resections, they are not mandatory. The preferred optics to go along with the imaging system is a 10 mm 30 degree rigid rod lens system. The angled view helps in better visualization of the thoracic cavity and the 10 mm lens provides better illumination than a 5 mm lens. However, some centers use a 5 mm lens to decrease the size of the port, but this may compromise vision. Advanced optical systems like the Endo Chameleon Telescope (Storz) or Endoeye system (Olympus) give more flexibility and help enhance visualization, particularly in uniportal surgery.

When it comes to energy sources, diathermy still plays a key role in thoracoscopic surgery. Both monopolar and bipolar diathermy instruments with suitable angulation are very useful. Energy sources like the Harmonic shears (Ethicon) and Ligasure (Medtronic) provide an additional advantage in terms of safety in dissection and reliable hemostasis. With multiple options available offering different advantages in terms of curvature, reliability, etc., it is safer to stay off recommending a particular device and leave it to the surgeon to choose.

There are a wide range of instruments designed for thoracoscopic lung resection varying in grip, length, and angulation. The surgeon may choose instruments depending on his technique, training, and skill. There are surgeons who use laparoscopic instruments too for lung resection. However, it is important to note that long angled instruments are preferable, for reasons of access and reducing fencing with the lens and other instruments (Figs. 10.3 and 10.4).

The consumables used for thoracoscopic surgery are a long list and form a considerable part of the expense of surgery. The use of surgical sleeves/ports for the access incision has been oft debated. The current consensus is to use surgical sleeves for reasons of wound protection and ease of passing instruments. The development of stapler technology has been a boon to thoracoscopic surgery and staplers are mandatory. The modern tip up cartridges and powered staplers developed by various companies have given us a tremendous advantage in negotiating tricky spaces and maintaining stability. It is important to maintain oncological principles including avoiding tumor spillage during the surgery and specimen bags, proprietary, or self-designed should be used when possible. While these items form the essentials for VATS, when considering complex resections,

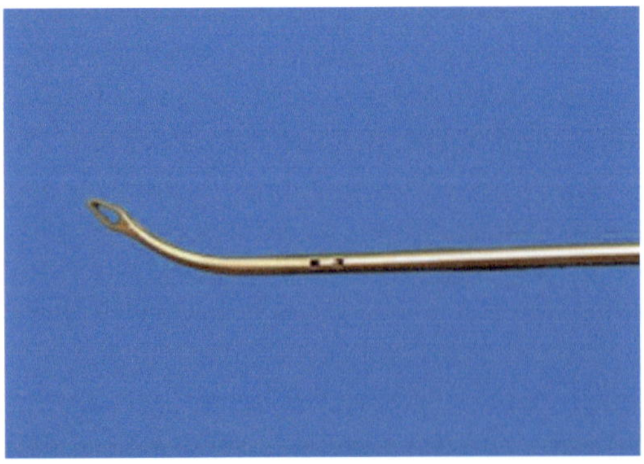

Fig. 10.3 Long, angled diamond forceps

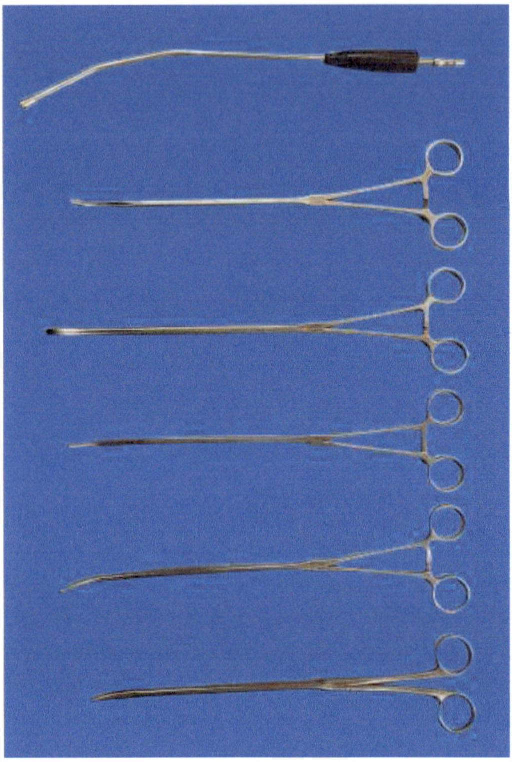

Fig. 10.4 Long, angled instruments developed for uniportal surgery

other devices like vessel tapes, snuggers, and minimal access needle holders should be kept in readiness.

10.5 Operative Technique

Coordinated teamwork is important in any thoracoscopic work and more so in uniportal surgery. The additional coordination required in this case is at the port, where the surgeon, cameraperson, and assistant have to utilize the limited space available to maneuver all the instruments. This can be partially resolved by assigning locations for each person at the port. For instance, the camera lens should occupy the top part of the port, while the surgeon and assistant use the remaining space as required. The exercise may start off with a lot of instrument fencing, with time and practice this reduces and the advantages in the hand -

eye coordination with the uniportal approach slowly kicking in.

An invasive mediastinal nodal staging is performed in all indicated patients prior to surgery. The port is placed in the 4th/ 5th intercostal space between the mid and posterior axillary lines, approximately 3–4 cm long. The port is placed slightly higher for right-sided resections taking into account the location of the hilum. The angle of scapula and nipple are taken as landmarks to mark the port (Fig. 10.5). The intention is to get the easiest and straightest access to the lung hilum, while still allowing reach to the apex and diaphragm.

While making the port, an energy source is avoided while dividing the intercostal muscles and entering the pleura to prevent lateral thermal damage to the intercostal nerve, which runs along the lower border of the rib. The surgical sleeve is then inserted to open out the port in keeping with the principle of "no rib spreading." All the instruments, including the lens are inserted through this single port (Fig. 10.6).

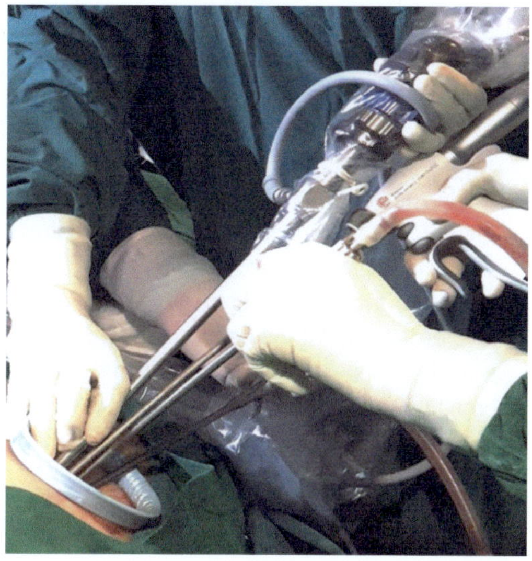

Fig. 10.6 All instruments, including the lens inserted through a single port

A staging thoracoscopy should be performed to rule out pleural deposits and assess the growth. Any pleural adhesions that may affect dissection should be taken down. Preemptive analgesia is an important consideration and we prefer to give intercostal nerve blocks in three intercostal spaces (space of the incision, one above, and below) as soon as we enter the thoracic cavity. We use a mixture of lignocaine and bupivacaine and prefer to inject as posteriorly as possible before the takeoff of the lateral branch of the intercostal nerve. This is particularly important since the use of epidural analgesia for VATS is on the decline. The first step in dissection is the division of the inferior pulmonary ligament. For lower lobectomies, this is to help isolate the inferior pulmonary vein. For upper lobectomies, it is for the lower lobe to expand and fill the cavity after surgery. We recommend this as an ideal first step for the beginner surgeon to get adapted to the system and her/his assistants.

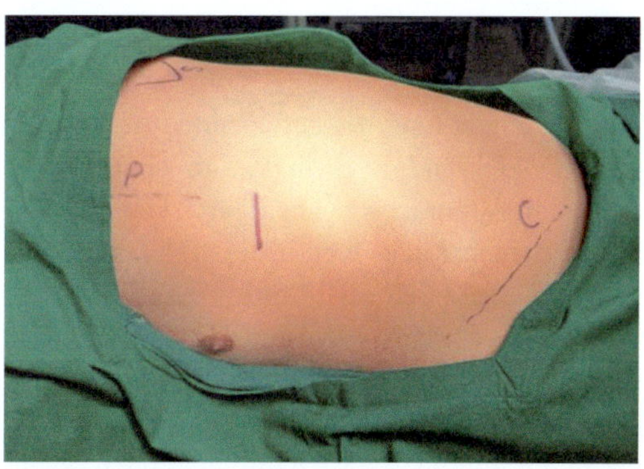

Fig. 10.5 Marking the port (S: Angle of the scapula, C: Costal margin, P: Posterior axillary line)

10.6 Lower Lobectomy

- The inferior pulmonary vein is dissected and isolated. Adequate space is made for passing a vascular stapler.
- The posterior pleural cut is taken, extending along the bronchus till the secondary carina.
- The fissure is dissected to locate the interlobar pulmonary artery and the segment 6 branch is identified.
- Anteriorly, the middle pulmonary vein is identified and the anterior fissure is created using a stapler/energy device depending on how well formed the fissure is.

- Similarly, the posterior fissure is divided between the interlobar pulmonary artery and secondary carina.
- The interlobar pulmonary artery is then dissected, isolated, and divided using a vascular stapler just proximal to the segment 6 branch.
- The inferior pulmonary vein is divided using a vascular stapler.
- Now, the lobe is attached only at the lower lobe bronchus. All the nodal tissue around the bronchus is swept onto the bronchus and the bronchus is clamped with a stapling device.
- The inflation of the upper and middle lobe is checked prior to firing the stapler.

10.7 Upper Lobectomy

- The anterior pleural cut is taken at the hilum, coursing superiorly around the hilum and posteriorly till the secondary carina along the bronchus.
- The superior pulmonary vein is identified, dissected, and isolated. The middle vein is identified and safeguarded.
- The truncus arteriosus/first branch is next identified, dissected, and isolated. It is then divided using a vascular stapler.
- The fissure is next dissected and the interlobar pulmonary artery identified within the fissure. The apicobasal and middle lobe branches are identified and safeguarded. Any further branches (2–5) to the upper lobe, including the recurrent branch (may arise from the interlobar artery or the apicobasal branch) are dissected and divided using staplers, clips, or ties.
- The anterior fissure between the interlobar artery and the space between the superior and middle pulmonary veins is divided using a stapler or energy device depending on how well the fissure is formed.
- Similarly, the posterior fissure is divided between the interlobar artery and the bronchial division.
- The upper lobe is now only attached at the bronchus. All the nodal tissue is swept off the bronchus onto the specimen side. The upper lobe bronchus is clamped with the stapling device. The stapler is only fired after ascertaining the expansion of the middle and lower lobes.
- The fissureless technique described by Decaluwe can be used in cases where the fissures are fused and difficult to dissect. In this technique, the superior pulmonary vein, the truncus arteriorus, and the upper lobe bronchus are taken early and individual arterial branches to the upper lobe are dissected and serially divided, with the fissure being divided last [12].

The specimen is extracted using a specimen retrieval bag. For slightly larger masses, it might help to first deliver the normal lung through the bag, making more space for extracting the specimen within the bag. A systematic mediastinal lymph node dissection (paratracheal, subcarinal, inferior pulmonary ligament, pre-vascular, AP window, and hilar stations) is performed. Hemostasis is confirmed. A wash is given; any air leak from the bronchial stump and parenchymal-stapled margins is identified and dealt with (sutures/fibrin sealants). A 24 Fr intercostal drain is inserted from the posterior part of the same incision. The muscle is closed with No 1 Vicryl, taking care to ensure that the closure is snug around the drain to avoid any subcutaneous emphysema. The skin is then closed with sutures/stapler. Local anesthesia is injected around the incision and ICD.

10.8 Multiportal VATS

Thoracoscopic lung resection started with multiportal VATS and it is the more conventional approach to thoracoscopic surgery. The lens and each instrument have their own port and one incision is enlarged to form the utility incision for staplers and specimen delivery (Fig. 10.7). The surgeon can choose to operate via the anterior or posterior approach to the hilum. Many surgeons prefer this approach since it mitigates the problem of instrument fencing and allows for finer dissection. However, the lack of triangulation of the

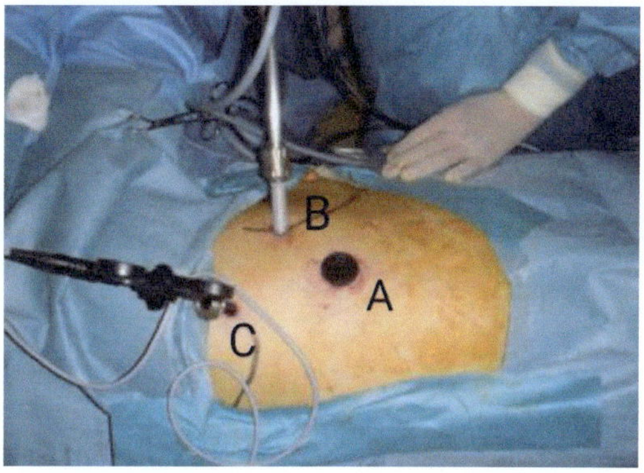

Fig. 10.7 Multiportal VATS: Port positions (A: camera port; B and C: Instrument ports)

camera affects depth perception and hence, coordination. The debate between which approach is better, multiportal or uniportal is unlikely to be resolved by any randomized trial since the differences are likely to be marginal. It would be best to leave the choice of the approach to the surgeon as long as it is minimally invasive.

10.9 Robotic Lung Resection

Robotic surgery was initially predicted to be a game changer in minimally invasive lung surgery and many centers adopted this technology to drive their minimally invasive programs [13].The impressive technology allows 3D imaging, better depth perception, better coordination, wristed instruments, and tremor filtration: all features favoring minimally invasive surgery. However, the master slave relationship, with the surgeon remaining away from the operating table and the need for a really competent surgical team proves a hindrance, particularly when one thinks that major bleeding requiring emergency conversion to open approach is a concern. This has not slowed the adoption and the rates of robotic lung resection consistently show an upswing across different databases. However, the adoption has not been uniform and this has brought about significant variations in practice patterns across hospitals and countries. While there have been a number of large single institution series and national database analyses showing impressive results as compared to open surgery there is no randomized evidence to support its routine use. Robotic surgery remains an important piece in the armamentarium in minimally invasive lung resection. While the technology favors those transitioning from open surgery to minimally invasive surgery, it provides no particular advantage to a surgeon already well versed in VATS. In our opinion, unless new technologies like haptic feedback, uniportal robotics, or robotic controlled staplers emerge; it will be difficult to recommend robotics over VATS especially considering the significant cost involved.

10.10 Alternate Approaches (Subxiphoid, Transcervical)

What we have discussed so far are variations that access the thorax through the intercostal spaces. Entry through the intercostal space and trauma to the intercostal nerve/spreading of the intercostal spaces is the primary cause of postoperative pain. A few groups have explored other options of accessing the thoracic cavity with reasonable success. Marcin Zielinski and his team in Poland have developed a transcervical, mediastinoscopic approach to lobectomy. A limited number of resections have been performed and the procedure appears feasible and results favorable [14]. Similarly, a few centers in South East Asia, majorly, Lei Jiang et al. at Shanghai Pulmonary Hospital have developed a subxiphoid uniportal technique for lobectomy. Their results of over 400 resections have been published and the results appear impressive [15]. However, both techniques appear to be technically demanding and require specially designed instruments for completion. Whether these techniques will be adopted into routine practice remain to be seen.

10.11 Postoperative Course and Management

Post an uneventful lung resection, the patient is generally extubated on table and shifted to the recovery room. As per Enhanced Recovery

After Surgery guidelines, the patient is given adequate analgesia. A Patient-Controlled Anesthesia (PCA) system is used when required [16]. Diet is initiated immediately after adequate recovery from anesthesia and after confirming vocal cord function (clinically). Once orals are initiated, intravenous fluids are stopped [16]. Chest physiotherapy and incentive spirometry are initiated as soon as the patient is wide awake and the patient is mobilized on the evening of surgery. This is made easier if a chest physiotherapist has trained the patient during the course of the preoperative workup. Lung expansion is monitored with the aid of a chest X-ray. If there is no air leak, the intercostal drain is removed once the output decreases to less than 5 ml/kg body weight, usually by postoperative day 2 or 3. The patient is discharged on oral analgesics and full diet by postoperative day 3 or 4.

10.12 Complications

10.12.1 Intraoperative Bleeding

The potential for torrential intraoperative hemorrhage is one of the major worries especially during complex pulmonary resections. The most important point in such a situation is not to panic. Most bleeding from the pulmonary vessels, although torrential, can be controlled with pressure. The first step should be to apply pressure with the adjacent lung or a sponge introduced through the utility incision. This arrests the bleeding in most cases, which gives the surgeon time to organize the team, including the anesthesiologist to manage potential blood loss. It is important to arrange good suction, clear the field of blood and get the optics ready before attempting further control. Any attempt at vascular control without these steps would be foolhardy. One cannot overemphasize the importance of keeping a thoracotomy set ready in the OR while performing minimally invasive surgery. There should be no hesitation in converting to open if the bleeding is massive. Having said that, most experienced minimal access surgeons develop the ability to manage most intraoperative bleeds thoracoscopically as they build on experience and expertise.

10.12.2 Postoperative Air Leak

Air leak should be carefully excluded prior to closure. A persistent air leak in the postoperative period manifests in the form of continuous bubbling in the intercostal drain. A digital drainage device with suction is extremely helpful in quantifying and mitigating the leak, enabling early chest drain removal and discharge from the hospital.

10.12.3 Subcutaneous Emphysema

It is one of the most common complications after uniportal VATS surgery. It can be easily avoided by ensuring that the muscle is closed snugly around the exit of the intercostal drain during closure. It only needs re-assurance and conservative management and usually settles spontaneously.

10.12.4 Bronchopleural Fistula

It manifests in the form of persistent, significant air leak in the intercostal drain, cough with expectoration. A bronchoscopy with a bronchogram is usually diagnostic. It can be managed endobronchially (gluin, spigot) or via a resurgery and buttressing of the bronchial stump depending on the severity.

10.13 Personal Experience

We started practicing minimally invasive lobectomy in our institute in 2009. We adopted the 3-port technique used by most South East Asian surgeons. A few surgeons also adopted the anterior approach advocated by McKenna et al. The cases were carefully selected early stage lesions with no lymphadenopathy or lung adhesions and we gradually progressed to more advanced lesions over a period of time. The initial difficulties we experienced due to lack of orientation and appropriate instrumentation resulted in a few conversions to open surgery. The major difficulties encountered were in dissecting off lung adhesions, adherent lymph nodes, and finding the appropriate angles for looping and dissecting pulmonary vessels. In fact, during our early practice we had a conversion rate of about 13%. A few of these conversions were emergent due to vascular injuries but we did not lose a single patient to any intraoperative event. One practice we have continued over the years is to keep a set of open thoracotomy instruments ready in the OR for any eventuality regardless of the simplicity of the procedure and experience of the surgeon. This has held us in good stead.

A few years ago, in 2015, we started using the uniportal technique as propagated by Rivas et al. for select cases. We soon found this technique easier to adopt, primarily because of the instruments being aimed in the line of sight of the camera. The problem of instruments fencing in the single port decreased over time. In the next 100 cases, our conversion rates dropped to 4%. It is difficult to determine whether the improved results are to be attributed to the new technique or to the accumulated experience of the past decade. Another pleasant surprise was the relatively easy adoption of the technique by trainee surgeons.

In our experience, minimally invasive lung resections significantly decreased postoperative pain and morbidity. The median hospital stay was also reduced by 1 day. We could not find any difference in these outcomes between the different techniques we used over this period: uniportal, multiportal, or robotic. The learning curve should be negotiated with care; progression from simpler to more complex cases should be planned over time with the whole team being part of the process. In terms of learning, the uniportal technique affords some advantages with trainees and younger colleagues finding it easier to adopt.

It is safe to say that minimally invasive surgery appears to be the future of lung resection with equivalent oncological outcomes and superior outcomes in terms of short-term morbidity and complications. Careful adoption of the technique is recommended.

References

1. Bertolaccini L, Rocco G. History and development of minimally invasive surgery: VATS surgery. Shanghai Chest. 2019;3:16.
2. Landreneau RJ, Mack MJ, Hazelrigg SR, et al. Prevalence of chronic pain after pulmonary resection by thoracotomy or video-assisted thoracic surgery. J ThoracCardiovascSurg. 1994;107:1079–85. discussion 1085-6
3. Bendixen M, Jørgensen OD, Kronborg C, et al. Postoperative pain and quality of life after lobectomy via video-assisted thoracoscopic surgery or anterolateral thoracotomy for early stage lung cancer: a randomized controlled trial. Lancet Oncol. 2016;17:836–44.
4. Long H, Tan Q, Luo Q, et al. Thoracoscopic surgery versus thoracotomy for lung cancer: short-term outcomes of a randomized trial. Ann ThoracSurg. 2018;105:386–92.
5. National Comprehensive Cancer Network. Non-small cell lung cancer. (Version4.2021). https://www.nccn.org/professionals/physician_gls/pdf/nscl_blocks.pdf. Accessed 3 Mar 2021.
6. Lim E, Batchelor T, Dunning J, et al. In hospital clinical efficacy, safety and oncological outcomes from VIOLET: a UK multi-center RCT of VATS versus open lobectomy for lung cancer. PLO206 J ThoracOncol. 2019;14:10S.
7. Whitson BA, Groth SS, Duval SJ, et al. Surgery for earlystage non-small cell lung cancer: a systematic review of the video-assisted thoracoscopic surgery versus thoracotomy approaches to lobectomy. Ann Thorac Surg. 2008;86:2008–16.
8. Ng CSH, MacDonald JK, et al. Optimal approach to lobectomy for non-small cell lung cancer: systemic review and meta-analysis. Innovations (Phila). 2019;14(2):90–116.
9. Swanson SJ, Herndon JE 2nd, D'Amico TA, Demmy TL, McKenna RJ Jr, Green MR, Sugarbaker DJ. Video-assisted thoracic surgery lobectomy: report of CALGB 39802--a prospective, multi-institution feasibility study. J ClinOncol. 2007;25(31):4993–7.
10. Gonzalez-Rivas D, Fieira E, Delgado M, et al. Uniportal video-assisted thoracoscopic sleeve lobectomy and other complex resections. J Thorac Dis. 2014;6(Suppl 6):S674–S68.
11. Hernandez-Arenas LA, Lin L, Purmessur RD, et al. Uniportal video-assisted thoracoscopic early learning curve for major lung resections in a high-volume training center. J Thorac Dis. 2018;10(Suppl 31):S3670–7.
12. Decaluwe H, Sokolow Y, Deryck F, et al. Thoracoscopic tunnel technique for anatomical lung resections: a 'fissure first, hilum last' approach with staplers in the fissureless patient. Interact Cardiovasc Thorac Surg. 2015;21(1):2–7.
13. Wei B, Eldaif SM, Cerfolio RJ. Robotic lung resection for non-small cell lung cancer. SurgOncolClin N Am. 2016;25(3):515–31.

14. Zielinski M, Nabialek T, Pankowski J, et al. Transcervicaluniportal pulmonary lobectomy. J Vis Surg. 2018;4:42.
15. Abdellateef A, Ali JM, Aresu G, et al. Tips and tricks for success in subxiphoid video-assisted thoracic surgery. J Thorac Dis. 2019;11(1):292–301.
16. Haro GJ, Sheu B, Marcus SG, et al. Perioperative lung resection outcomes after implementation of a multidisciplinary, evidence-based thoracic ERAS program. Ann Surg. 2019.

Minimal Access Breast Cancer Surgery

11

Chi Wei Mok, Hung-Wen Lai,
Jun Xian Jeffrey Hing, and Su-Ming Tan

Abstract

Minimally invasive or minimal access breast surgery techniques were developed over the past two decades with the aim to achieve the same oncological safe surgical margins as conventional surgery but with smaller and/or fewer incisions. Specialized surgical instruments were utilized to give better visualization of the operative field while keeping the incision small and hidden in inconspicuous areas. There are a few broad categories of minimally invasive breast surgery (MIBS) techniques, which are but not limited to minimally invasive surgery techniques using moving window, retraction with light handle retractors; endoscopic MIBS using laparoscopic system, with or without insufflation, single or multiple ports and 3-dimensional (3D) or 4 K resolution system, depending on the location and size of the breast lesion; robotic breast surgery using robotic surgical system. With smaller and well-hidden incisions, postoperative recovery has been reported to be shorter with improved patients' and surgeons' satisfactions. In this chapter, commonly used minimally invasive breast surgery techniques in the surgical manage-

Supplementary Information The online version contains supplementary material available at https://doi.org/10.1007/978-981-97-7059-5_11.

C. W. Mok (✉) · J. X. J. Hing · S.-M. Tan
Division of Breast Surgery, Department of Surgery, Changi General Hospital, Singapore, Singapore

Singhealth Duke-NUS Breast Centre, Singapore, Singapore
e-mail: mok.chi.wei@singhealth.com.sg

H.-W. Lai
Endoscopic and Oncoplastic Breast Surgery Center, Department of Surgery, Changhua Christian Hospital, Changhua, Taiwan

Division of General Surgery, Department of Surgery, Changhua Christian Hospital, Changhua, Taiwan

Comprehensive Breast Cancer Center, Department of Surgery, Changhua Christian Hospital, Changhua, Taiwan

Minimal Invasive Surgery Research Center, Department of Surgery, Changhua Christian Hospital, Changhua, Taiwan

Department of Surgery, Kaohsiung Medical University, Kaohsiung, Taiwan

Division of Breast Surgery, Department of Surgery, Yuanlin Christian Hospital, Yuanlin, Taiwan

Department of Surgery, School of Medicine, National Yang Ming University, Taipei, Taiwan

Department of Surgery, School of Medicine, Chung Shan Medical University, Taichung, Taiwan

Department of Surgery, Chang Gung University College of Medicine, Taoyuan City, Taiwan

Division of General Surgery, Department of Surgery, Kaohsiung Chang Gung Memorial Hospital, Kaohsiung, Taiwan

M. Tewari (ed.), *Minimally Invasive Surgery in Cancer*,
https://doi.org/10.1007/978-981-97-7059-5_11

ment of breast cancer will be discussed along with pictorial and video illustrations.

Keywords
Minimally invasive breast surgery · Minimal access breast surgery · Keyhole breast surgery · Endoscopic assisted · Robotic assisted · Single-port

11.1 Introduction

Minimal access breast surgery, a term used interchangeably with minimally invasive breast surgery (MIBS) refers to surgical techniques performed with the assistance of endoscopic instruments and over the last 4–5 years, with robotic surgical system. MIBS techniques emphasized on adequate yet small incision(s) placed in hidden areas such as the axilla or anterior axillary line, thereby leading to better cosmetic outcomes, while at the same time offering comparable safety and allowing for breast reconstruction to be performed through the same incision(s) [1, 2]. All these are made possible with improved optics and visualization accorded by the endoscopic instruments or robotic surgical platforms. Endoscopic-assisted breast surgery was first popularized in a few Asian countries [3–6], where superior cosmetic outcomes were achieved in women with small breasts and in whom a breast conserving surgery would have resulted in either poor aesthetic outcomes as well as the risk of inadequate resection margins. Multiple studies reporting on the technical feasibility, aesthetic and safety outcomes of the technique have been published over the years but MIBS has yet to become the mainstream or standard treatment [7–10]. The lack of long-term follow-up data to establish oncologic safety in terms of locoregional and distant recurrence as well as disease survival outcomes data could have been postulated to be one of the main reasons for the lack of uptake of MIBS techniques. In this chapter, the authors will strive to discuss the use of minimal access breast surgery techniques in the management of breast cancer from the following aspects or perspectives: oncological resection, axillary staging, reconstruction, and future prospects/advancements.

11.2 Minimal Access/Minimally Invasive Techniques in Different Aspects of Breast Cancer Surgery

11.2.1 Oncological Resection

Minimal access breast surgery techniques can be employed in both mastectomy as well breast conserving surgery/wide excision. In the initial stage of development, most surgeons used dual-incision technique [9, 11], which commonly referred to an axillary incision that was used for axillary staging as well as dissection of the posterior breast parenchyma. The second incision was a peri-areolar incision, which was important for raising the skin flap as well as dissection of breast parenchyma off the peripheral margins. Advancement over the last 5–6 years have witnessed the conduct of the surgery through a single incision [4, 12, 13]. Depending on the tumor location as well as the need for axillary staging, single incision was commonly either in the anterior axillary line or in the axilla. The authors believe that single incision surgery is the future of minimal access breast surgery, especially single incision endoscopic mastectomy.

11.2.1.1 Description of Technique

(i) *Endoscopic Nipple-Sparing/Skin-Sparing Mastectomy (E-NSM/E-SSM)* (Fig. 11.1 [14] and Video 11.1)

Preoperative Positioning and Marking

As per conventional breast surgery, patient was marked in standing and supine position. Under general anesthesia, patient was then placed in supine position with the ipsilateral arm abducted to 90°. This was done to avoid collision of the ipsilateral arm with the instruments. Endoscopic systems were set up on both sides of the patient's head so as to allow both the surgeon and first assistant to view the monitors with ease. An oblique-ended 30° rigid endoscope measuring 5 mm in diameter was used.

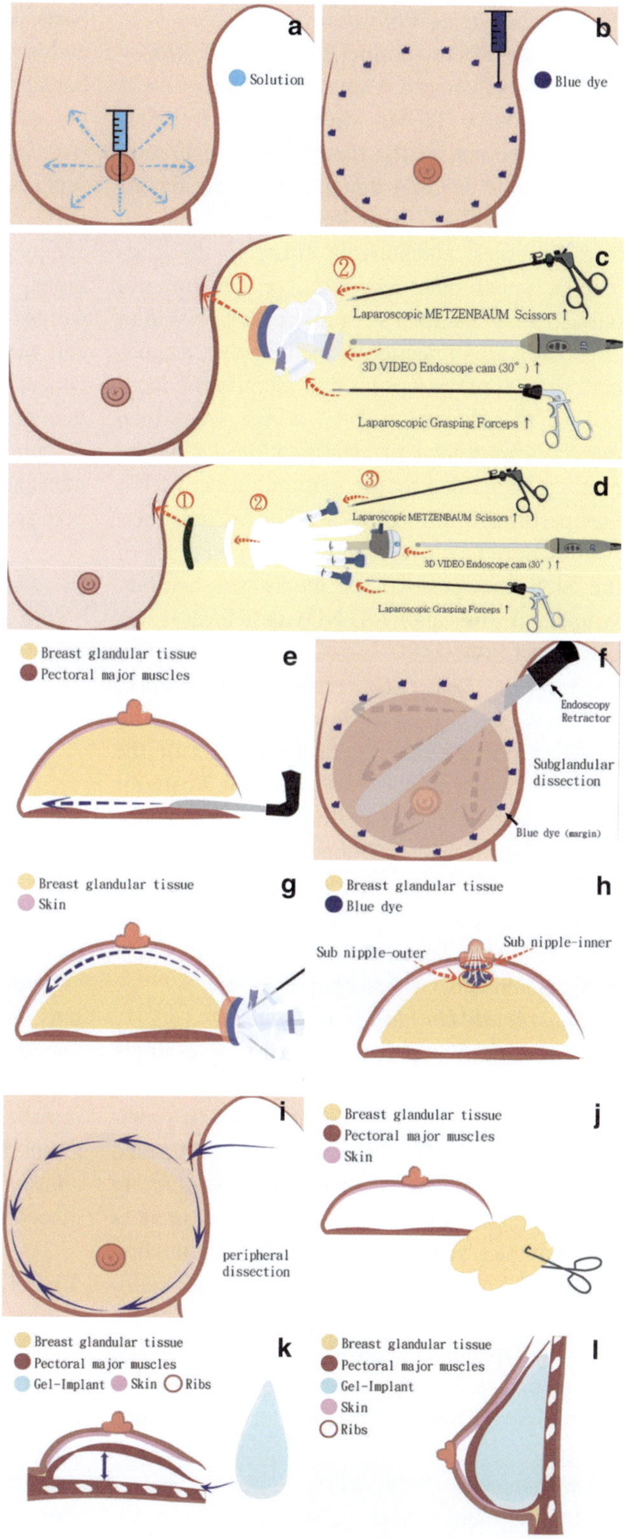

Fig. 11.1 (**a**) A physiological saline solution containing lidocaine 0.05% and epinephrine 1: 1,000,000 was injected subcutaneously into the whole breast to minimize bleeding. (**b**) Injection of jelly containing methylene blue as a guide to mark the boundaries of resection. (**c, d**) Illustration of insertion of single port (commercial—**c** or DIY—**d**) and placement of instruments in endoscopic mastectomy (video camera, monopolar scissors, and forceps or grasper). (**e, f**) Posterior dissection of breast parenchyma off pectoralis major fascia with endoscopic vein harvester all around breast boundaries marked with blue dye. (**g**) Dissection was commenced from the superficial skin flaps in all quadrants. (**h**) Intraoperative sub-nipple biopsies were performed and sent for frozen section analysis. (**i**) Peripheral and posterior dissection was performed with the guidance of the blue dye markings. (**j**) Mastectomy specimen removed intact and in entirety from single incision and oriented. (**k**) Breast reconstruction was performed with dissection of subpectoral muscular pocket. (**l**) Implant was placed via the single incision in the submuscular pocket

Axillary Staging Procedure

In cases where sentinel lymph node biopsy (SLNB) was indicated, a small amount (2–3 mCi) of radioisotope Tc99m was injected intradermally at the site of the tumor before operation (either on the day or 1 day prior). On the day of surgery, 5 ml of 1% methylene blue was injected into the breast parenchyma either in the peri-areolar, upper outer quadrant, or peri-tumoral based on surgeon's preferences. Within 20–30 min after injection of the blue dye, a hand-held gamma probe was used to identify the location of the "hottest nodes," which were then marked for subsequent identification. Using the marking as guided by the gamma probe, SLNB was performed through a 2–3 cm axillary incision. If intraoperative frozen section analysis of the SLN was positive for metastases, axillary lymph node dissection (ALND) up to level II was performed.

Posterior Breast Dissection (dissection of breast parenchyma off pectoralis major fascia)

After axillary staging, lateral border of the pectoralis major muscle was identified. Posterior breast dissection can be performed with an endoscopic Ultra Retractor (Johnson & Johnson KK or Karl Storz) vein harvester with or without the use of CO_2 insufflation. The use of bipolar scissors in securing hematostasis of penetrating vessels ensured better visual clarity.

Superficial Skin Flap Development

A semicircular peri-areolar skin or a single axillary incision was made (depending on surgeon's preference and tumor location) as previously described. Hydrodissection was performed using a physiological saline solution containing lidocaine and epinephrine. An approximately 3–5 mm thick skin flap was created via tunneling method using Metzenbaum scissors under endoscopic guidance. Subsequently, the septa between the skin flap and parenchyma were dissected and taken off under endoscopic guidance using endoscissors, bipolar scissors, or a harmonic scalpel.

Mastectomy

Both retraction (gasless) or insufflation methods can be employed for the mastectomy. The authors used both techniques on a case-to-case basis. Retraction technique involved the use of endoscopic Ultra Retractor in dissection of septa between skin flap and breast parenchyma. After placement of a single port and CO_2 insufflation (for insufflation technique), dissection of the septa between the skin flap and parenchyma was performed under endoscopic guidance. Following adequate skin flap development, a sub-nipple biopsy and frozen section analysis can be performed in a nipple sparing mastectomy. If cancer cell was found, the entire NAC was removed and conversion to a skin sparing mastectomy was then performed. After detaching the breast off the pectoralis major fascia, the entire breast specimen can be removed in entirety via the axillary or peri-areolar incisions.

(ii) *Endoscopic Breast Conserving Surgery (E-BCS)* (Video 11.2)

The following aspects of E-BCS were similar to that of E-NSM/SSM and will not be discussed under this section: preoperative marking and positioning; axillary staging; axillary staging procedure; dissection of breast parenchyma off pectoralis major fascia; tunneling and development of skin flap.

Performing Wide Excision and Repair of Resection Cavity

In order to guide resection with adequate margins, the authors recommended the use of intraoperative ultrasound and marking of resection margin with blue dye injection. Specimen was retrieved thereafter and hemostasis secured. Level I oncoplastic techniques were used to approximate breast parenchyma and drain was placed on a case-to-case basis.

11.2.1.2 Pearls and Tricks

Patient positioning: In the conduct of endoscopic-assisted mastectomy, placement of incision will determine the ipsilateral arm position. This is to avoid conflict between patient's arm and instruments. For example, the ideal ipsilateral arm position if an axillary or anterior axillary line incision is used would be above the head.

Skin Incision for E-NSM: Skin incision can be either dual or single incision. If dual incisions are used, it would normally be the peri-areolar as well as the axillary incision. Axillary incision is commonly used for axillary staging procedure as well as posterior parenchyma dissection. Peri-areolar incision is then used for skin flap dissection and tumor resection. Beginners might find dual incisions technique easier in the initial learning curve.

Carbon Dioxide (CO_2) Insufflation: CO_2 insufflation is useful in the conduct of E-NSM as it helps in tissue/plane dissection as well as hemostasis due to positive pressure provided by the insufflation.

Sub-Nipple Biopsy: When performing sub-nipple biopsy in E-NSM, care has to be taken not to de-vascularize the NAC complex. Avoidance of coagulation when performing sub-nipple biopsy could reduce the risk of NAC ischemia or necrosis.

11.2.2 Axillary Staging

Axillary staging procedures refers to both sentinel lymph node biopsy as well as axillary dissection/clearance. There were a few small case series reporting on institutional experiences in endoscopic axillary dissection but this technique has not taken a firm footing as the mainstay technique for axillary staging. Possible reasons include technical difficulties such as the lack of triangulation and adequate space. The authors developed a novel hybrid technique where an optical trocar was used to guide the sentinel lymph node biopsy. This technique is as described below.

11.2.2.1 Endoscopic-Assisted ICG (EASI) Technique for Sentinel Lymph Node Biopsy in Breast Cancer [15] (Video 11.3)

Detailed description of the technique along with video illustrations and pictorial guide was described by the authors in a previous publication [15].

Indocyanine Green (ICG) Preparation and Injection

Indocyanine green (ICG) VERDYE (Diagnostic Green, Bavaria) powder 1.25 mg/0.5 ml (Vial of 25 mg diluted with 10 ml of water for injection) was prepared and injected intradermally at the peri-areolar region after general anesthesia (Fig. 11.1). In order to avoid contamination of the surgical field with ICG, which may subsequently reduce artifacts under fluorescence imaging, massage of the dye was not recommended. Instead, 5 min of waiting time was advised to allow adequate lymphatic flow to the axilla. Lymphatic flow could then be visualized under fluorescence imaging to aid in optimal placement of the axillary incision. Alternatively, a direct axilla incision could be made within the axillary skin crease without prior identification of lymphatic flow.

Endoscopic-Assisted ICG (EASI) Technique and Identification of SLN

This technique involved the use of an optical trocar (Endopath Xcel® Bladeless Trocar, Johnson & Johnson, USA), a 5- or 10-mm 30 degrees endoscope and ICG system in performing sentinel lymph node biopsy. A 5 mm or 10 mm stab incision was placed along the axillary skin crease. In the authors' institution, methylene or patent blue dye was used as a second modality. Direct optical entry was then performed with slow and controlled movement while observing for lymphatic flow, either blue or green (under fluorescence imaging). Direction of entry was then guided by the lymphatic flow till the first sentinel lymph node was identified.

Retrieval of Sentinel Lymph Node

Once the first sentinel lymph node was identified, camera was then removed. With the optical trocar still in place, minimal extension of the skin incision was then performed to allow retrieval of sentinel lymph node (SLN). A focused and directed dissection toward the SLN as guided by the optical trocar resulted in minimal tissue/lymphatic disruption or damage. After retrieval of the first SLN, fluorescence imaging was then used to trace the lymphatic flow beyond the first SLN and detect further SLN, if any. Nodes were sent for intraoperative frozen section analysis and axillary dissection performed as deemed necessary based on current evidence should the frozen section analysis return positive for metastatic carcinoma.

11.2.2.2 Pearls and Tricks

Planning the Incision for SLNB: When using ICG, the optimal incision can be placed at the point where the lymphatic channels enter into the axilla.

Using ICG: When dealing with ICG, extra care has to be taken not to massage the injection site but instead use gentle tapping with an instrument to encourage lymphatic flow. This is to avoid contamination of the breast or surgical field with fluorescence, which can affect the visualization of sentinel lymph nodes.

11.2.3 Reconstruction

Minimally invasive techniques are also used in breast reconstruction after breast cancer surgery. It can be used either in autologous tissue or implant-based reconstruction. These techniques were mostly performed with the use of endoscopic instruments with a few small studies reporting on initial experience in free autologous tissue harvest using robotic system. In this chapter, the authors will discuss endoscopic-assisted latissimus dorsi (LD) flap harvest. The authors' experience and detailed technique descriptions for implant-based reconstruction as well as pedicled omental flap reconstruction can be accessed from the following articles/resources [6, 12, 16, 17].

11.2.3.1 Endoscopic-Assisted Latissimus Dorsi Flap Reconstruction [18] (Video 11.4)

Positioning

The thoracodorsal pedicle can be identified and marked with a vessel loop to prevent injury during the flap harvest before positioning into the lateral decubitus position.

Flap Dissection

Posterior dissection along the under surface of the latissimus dorsi muscle can be performed with an endoscopic ultra-retractor (Johnson & Johnson KK or Karl Storz) vein harvester and harmonic scalpel. Thereafter, further dissection over the superficial surface of the muscle ensued and it was then disconnected from the infero-posterior and scapular border. Afterward, the pedicled LD flap was exteriorized from the axilla wound.

Flap Inset

Reconstruction of the excision defect was performed with the patient turned back to a supine position. Flap inset was performed with assistance from a handle light retractor to ensure full coverage of the defect. Care must be taken to ensure the correct axis of the vascular pedicle in order to prevent torsion of the blood supply. Drains were then placed both in the donor site as well as resection cavity.

11.2.3.2 Pearls and Tricks

Patient Selection: In this technique, the volume/size of flap harvested is greatly variable and it is important to take this into consideration when offering this technique for immediate reconstruction especially after mastectomy. It is most suitable in ladies with small to moderate breasts.

Use in Combination with Other Techniques: In centers where the use of acellular dermal matrix or synthetic meshes are not routine, LD flap harvested can serve as a sling to be used in combination with implant as a reconstructive option.

11.2.4 The Future Is Here: Advancements and Progress of Minimally Invasive Breast Surgery Techniques

11.2.4.1 Robotic Breast Surgery

Robotic breast surgery has gained much traction as the possible next step in the evolution of minimally invasive breast surgery over the past few years. So far, there have been a number of studies reporting on the technical feasibility, safety, early oncologic outcomes as well as aesthetic outcomes of robotic-assisted mastectomy in a few centers worldwide [19–24]. The results were promising and encouraging, however there is still a need for further evaluation of this technique to ensure oncological safety are not compromised in breast cancer patients.

11.2.5 Special Instruments Used and Settings

It has to be noted that there are no special instruments, and minimally invasive breast surgery are performed using standard laparoscopic instruments. However, in the early days of technique development, an endoscopic vein harvester was used for the dissection of pectoral muscle fascia off posterior portion of breast parenchyma. This has been replaced with CO_2 insufflation in recent years.

11.2.6 Postoperative Management and Complications

Postoperative management of patients who underwent minimal access/minimally invasive breast surgery did not differ from conventional surgery. In fact, studies had reported earlier recovery owing to smaller incision and lesser pain [3–6]. In terms of complications, there were no significant differences if compared to conventional surgery but a significant advantage of endoscopic nipple sparing mastectomy performed through an axillary or anterior axillary line incision had been showed to reduce the incidence of nipple areolar complex (NAC) necrosis [4, 12, 13] owing to the avoidance of peri-areolar incision. Sparing of peri-areolar incision and thereby preserving blood flow to the nipple areolar complex has been postulated to be the cause of the lower incidence of NAC necrosis.

11.2.7 Personal Experience in the Last 5 Years or So

The authors had a combined experience of approximately 15–20 years in the field of minimal access/minimally invasive breast surgery. This field is ever evolving and the last 5–10 years have witnessed what would be considered a tsunami of change and newfound interest in this field with new technique modifications/developments. It is heartening to witness this change as more and more breast surgeons understand the advantages of minimally invasive breast surgery and embark on it. The limitations to widespread adoption would be access to quality training and education as well as accreditation.

References

1. Mok CW, Lai H-W. Endoscopic-assisted surgery in the management of breast cancer: 20 years review of trend, techniques and outcomes. Breast. 2019;46:144.
2. Mok CW, Lai H-W. Evolution of minimal access breast surgery. Gland Surg. 2019;8(6).
3. Hung CS, Chang SW, Liao LM, Huang CC, Tu SH, Chen ST, et al. The learning curve of endoscopic total mastectomy in Taiwan: a multi-center study. PLoS One. 2017.
4. Lai H-W, Chen S-T, Mok CW, Lin S-L, Tai C-M, Chen D-R, et al. Single-port 3-dimensional Videoscope-assisted endoscopic nipple-sparing mastectomy in the management of breast cancer. Plast Reconstr Surg - Glob Open. 2019;7(8)
5. MokCW LHW. Endoscopic-assisted surgery in the management of breast cancer: 20 years review of trend, techniques and outcomes. Breast. 2019;
6. Hung-Wen L, Shou-Tung C, Dar-Ren C, Shu-Ling C, Tsai-Wang C, Kuo S-J, et al. Current trends in and indications for endoscopy-assisted breast surgery for breast cancer: results from a six-year study conducted by the Taiwan endoscopic breast surgery cooperative group. PLoS One. 2016.
7. Saimura M, Mitsuyama S, Anan K, Koga K, Watanabe M, Ono M, et al. Endoscopy-assisted breast-conserving surgery for early breast cancer. Asian J Endosc Surg. 2013;6(3):203–8.
8. Tamaki Y, SakitaI, Miyoshi Y, Sekimoto M, Takiguchi S, Monden M, et al. Transareolar endoscopy-assisted partial mastectomy: a preliminary report of six cases. Surg Laparosc Endosc Percutaneous Tech. 2001;11:356.
9. Owaki T, Yoshinaka H, Ehi K, Kijima Y, Uenosono Y, Shirao K, et al. Endoscopic quadrantectomy for breast cancer with sentinel lymph node navigation via a small axillary incision. Breast. 2005;14(1):57–60.
10. HN, KS, NM, TH, SO, KS. Section 5. Breast: video-assisted total glandectomy and immediate reconstruction for breast cancer. Biomed Pharmacother [Internet]. 2002;56(SUPPL. 1):205s–208s. http://www.embase.com/search/results?subaction=viewrecord&from=export&id=L35448047, http://sfx.library.uu.nl/utrecht?sid=EMBASE&issn=07533322&id=do

i:&atitle=Section+5.+Breast%3A+Video-assisted+total+glandectomy+and+immediate+reconstruction+for+breast+ca
11. Tamaki Y, Noguchi S. Endoscopy-assisted breast cancer surgery - long-term results from a single institute. Eur J Surg Oncol [Internet]. 2010;36(9):849. Available from: http://www.embase.com/search/results?subaction=viewrecord&from=export&id=L70272391, https://doi.org/10.1016/S0748-7983(10)00156-3, http://sfx.library.uu.nl/utrecht?sid=EMBASE&issn=07487983&id=doi:10.1016%2FS0748-7983%2810%2900156-3&atitle=Endoscopy-
12. Lai HW, Lin SL, Chen ST, Kuok KM, Chen SL, Lin YL, et al. Single-axillary-incision endoscopic-assisted hybrid technique for nipple-sparing mastectomy: technique, preliminary results, and patient-reported cosmetic outcome from preliminary 50 procedures. Ann Surg Oncol [Internet]. 2018;25(5):1340–9. https://doi.org/10.1245/s10434-018-6383-z.
13. Tukenmez M, Ozden BC, Agcaoglu O, Kecer M, Ozmen V, Muslumanoglu M, et al. Videoendoscopic single-port nipple-sparing mastectomy and immediate reconstruction. J Laparoendosc Adv Surg Tech [Internet]. 2014;24(2):77–82. https://doi.org/10.1089/lap.2013.0172.
14. Lai HW, Mok CW. Endoscopic-assisted nipple and skin sparing mastectomy. In: Vidya R, Becker H, editors. Prepectoral breast reconstruction. Cham: Springer; 2023. https://doi.org/10.1007/978-3-031-15590-1_23.
15. Mok C, Hing JX, Tan S-M. Endoscopic-assisted ICG (EASI) technique for sentinel lymph node biopsy in breast cancer. Mini-Invasive Surg [Internet]. 2020;4(26). Available from: https://misjournal.net/article/view/3452
16. Lai HW, Lin SL, Chen ST, Chen SL, Lin YL, Chen DR, et al. Robotic nipple-sparing mastectomy and immediate breast reconstruction with gel implant. Plast Reconstr Surg - Glob Open. 2018.
17. Lai HW, Chen ST, Lin SL, Lin YL, Wu HK, Pai SH, et al. Technique for single axillary incision robotic assisted quadrantectomy and immediate partial breast reconstruction with robotic latissimus dorsi flap harvest for breast cancer. Med (United States). 2018.
18. Mok CW, Hing JXJ, Tan S-M. Latissimus Dorsi flap: safe, reliable and versatile workhorse flap in the era of minimally invasive breast surgery—a case series. Ann Breast Surg. 2020;20(62)
19. Sarfati B, Honart JF, Leymarie N, Rimareix F, AlKhashnam H, Kolb F. Robotic da Vinci Xi-assisted nipple-sparing mastectomy: first clinical report. Breast J. 2018.
20. Toesca A, Peradze N, Galimberti V, Manconi A, Intra M, Gentilini O, et al. Robotic nipple-sparing mastectomy and immediate breast reconstruction with implant: first report of surgical technique. Ann Surg. 2017;266:e28.
21. Park HS, Lee J, Lee DW, Song SY, Lew DH, Kim SII, et al. Robot-assisted nipple-sparing mastectomy with immediate breast reconstruction: an initial experience. Sci Rep [Internet]. 2019;9(1):15669. https://doi.org/10.1038/s41598-019-51744-2.
22. Lai H-W, Chen S-T, Mok CW. Robotic nipple-sparing mastectomy: a preliminary report of a single institute and joint collective analysis of current reported series. Formos J Surg [Internet]. 2019.; Available from: http://www.e-fjs.org/text.asp?2019/52/5/175/269922
23. Lai H-W, Chen S-T, Mok CW, Lin Y-J, Wu H-K, Lin S-L, et al. Robotic versus conventional nipple sparing mastectomy and immediate gel implant breast reconstruction in the management of breast cancer- a case control comparison study with analysis of clinical outcome, medical cost, and patient-reported cosmetic result. J Plast Reconstr Aesthetic Surg. 2020;73:1514.
24. Lai HW, Chen ST, Tai CM, Lin SL, Lin YJ, Huang RH, et al. Robotic- versus endoscopic-assisted nipple-sparing mastectomy with immediate prosthesis breast reconstruction in the management of breast cancer: a case–control comparison study with analysis of clinical outcomes, learning curve, patient-reported aestheti. Ann Surg Oncol. 2020;27:2255.

Laparoscopic Radical Hysterectomy

12

Shailesh Puntambekar, Madhavi Patil, Seema Puntambekar, Ravindra Sathe, Suyog Bharambe, Nikesh Gandhi, Aishwarya Puntambekar, and Mohm. Azharuddin Azim Attar

Abstract

The gold standard treatment of uterine cancer is radical hysterectomy. With technological advances, radical hysterectomy can now be performed with minimally invasive techniques, such as laparoscopy and robotics. Laparoscopic procedure offers less postoperative pain, an early recovery of the patient, allowing the patient to take up adjuvant treatment as early as possible and overall a good quality of life of the patient. In this chapter, the "*Pune technique*" of laparoscopic radical hysterectomy is described by the authors with operative steps that are standardized. It makes this technique universally acceptable as it is easily duplicable. Knowledge of avascular spaces of pelvis and understanding of anterior parametrium makes this technique unique with lesser recurrence rate. Laparoscopic radical hysterectomy is onco-logically comparable to open surgery in terms of margins, lymph node clearance, and parametric resection, resulting in a successful type III radical hysterectomy. It is technically feasible and economically viable, and it has less postoperative complications and lower morbidity than the abdominal approach. We can replicate the traditional steps of multiport laparoscopic radical hysterectomy using alternative minimally invasive techniques such as LESS (Laparoendoscopic Single-Site Surgery), OASIS (One-Access Surgery), and Robotic surgery.

Keywords

Laparoscopic radical hysterectomy · Pune technique · Gynecological onco-surgery

12.1 Introduction

Uterine corpus cancer ranked as the sixth most frequently identified cancer in women, witnessing 417,000 new cases and 97,000 fatalities in 2020 [1]. Notably, birth cohort effects were prominently observed in several countries, including Japan, the Philippines, Belarus, Singapore, India, Lithuania, Costa Rica, and New Zealand. This trend may be attributed, at least in part, to the growing prevalence of risk factors such as excess body weight and physical inactivity in more recent generations [2]. The reported

Supplementary Information The online version contains supplementary material available at https://doi.org/10.1007/978-981-97-7059-5_12.

S. Puntambekar (✉) · M. Patil · S. Puntambekar · R. Sathe · S. Bharambe · N. Gandhi · A. Puntambekar · M. A. A. Attar
Department of Gynaecology, Galaxy care hospital, Pune, India

M. Tewari (ed.), *Minimally Invasive Surgery in Cancer*,
https://doi.org/10.1007/978-981-97-7059-5_12

increase in incidence in recent years is likely due to heightened awareness and improved screening practices [3].

Cervical cancer ranks as the fourth most commonly identified cancer and the fourth primary contributor to cancer-related fatalities among women. In 2020, there were approximately 604,000 new cases and 342,000 deaths globally associated with this disease [4]. It stands out as the most prevalent cancer in 23 nations and holds the position of the primary cause of cancer-related deaths in 36 countries [5]. Due to inadequate screening initiatives and a lack of awareness, a significant majority—70% or more—of patients are diagnosed at stage III or beyond when seeking medical attention [6]. The treatment options available to these patients are limited because they present with advanced diseases [7].

The primary and most widely accepted method for treating uterine cancer is a radical hysterectomy. Since the first radical hysterectomy performed by Clark in 1895 and the advent of Wertheim's technique of radical hysterectomy in 1898, radical hysterectomy has evolved into a simpler procedure and the surgical approach has also transformed over a period of time into a highly specialized and minimally invasive modality [8]. With technological advances, we can now perform the radical hysterectomy with minimally invasive techniques, such as laparoscopy and robotics [9]. The mainstay of these procedures is less postoperative pain, an early recovery of the patient due to smaller incisions, allowing the patient to take up adjuvant treatment as early as possible and overall, a good quality of life of the patient [10]. Thus, the acceptance of minimally access surgeries in recent years has increased [11].

In this chapter, the "*Pune technique*" of laparoscopic radical hysterectomy is described by the authors with operative steps that are standardized. This method becomes widely embraced due to its ease of replication. Its application in robotic radical hysterectomy, pelvic exenterations, and single-port surgeries are also covered.

12.1.1 Laparoscopic Radical Hysterectomy

12.1.1.1 Indications

1. Cervical cancer ranging from stage 1A2 to stage 2A is encompassed in this category. Additionally, instances of stage 1A1 exhibiting a heightened risk of lymph node dissemination are also considered within this group.
2. Laparoscopic surgery is not contraindicated for endometrial cancer up to stage 2, even in cases where preoperative irradiation has been administered.

12.1.1.2 Contraindications

1. Tumor size of more than 4 cm at the largest diameter.
2. Evidence of peritoneal carcinomatosis or distant metastatic disease.
3. Evidence of grossly involved lymph nodes.

12.1.1.3 Preoperative

Liquid diet 1 day prior to surgery. Polyethylene glycol the night before the operation to clear the bowels so as to keep them away from the operative field. Enema and bowel wash should be avoided as this leads to dilatation of sigmoid colon.

12.1.1.4 Anesthesia

A combined regional and general anesthesia is administered. Regional anesthesia—blocking the sympathetic activity, contracts the small bowel and keeps it away from the operative field.

12.1.1.5 Patient Position

Patient is placed in a "Modified Lloyd Davis position." A bolster is placed at the level of the anterior superior iliac spine, which causes elevation of the pelvis and results in a drop of the intestines cephalad. A gauze piece is kept in the vagina to prevent loss of peritoneum after colpotomy.

A total of *five ports* are used. (Fig. 12.1)

Camera port (10 mm) at infraumbilical.

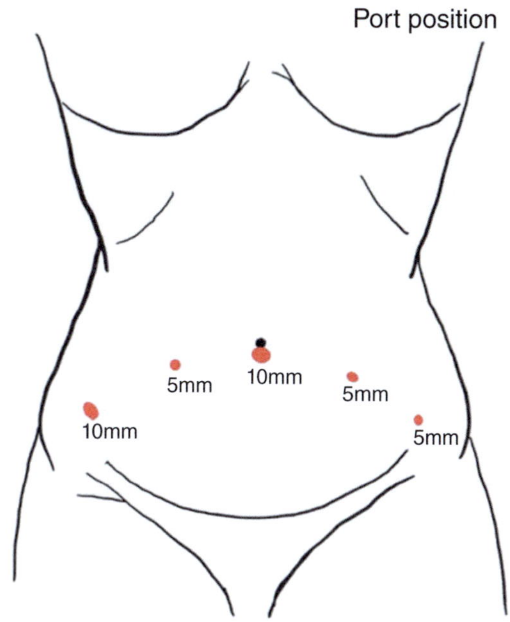

Fig. 12.1 Port positions

Working port (10 mm) at McBurney's point on right side.

Port para (5 mm)-rectally at midclavicular line at the level of umbilicus.

A set of two 5 mm ports are inserted as mirror image on left side.

Procedure

The uterus is hitched regarding endometrial cancer and cervical cancer for uterine manipulation. Monofilament polyamide suture on needle is used for hitching the uterus. The suture is passed through the uterine fundus anteroposteriorly and brought out to the exterior through the anterior abdominal wall (Fig. 12.2) In cases of cervical malignancies for uterine manipulation, tenaculum forceps may be used.

Step 1: Posterior U Cut (Fig. 12.3)

Uterus is anteverted. The right ureter is identified underneath the peritoneum at the level of sacral promontory. The peritoneum excised medial to ureter with the help of harmonic shears to expose the ureter. This cut is extended down up to the pouch of Douglas keeping the ureters laterally

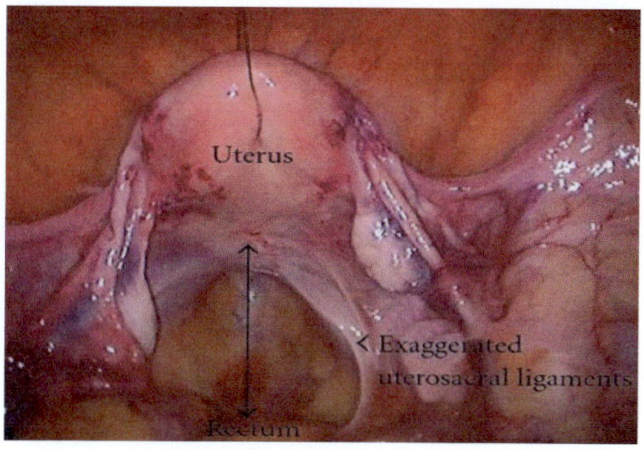

Fig. 12.2 Uterine hitched

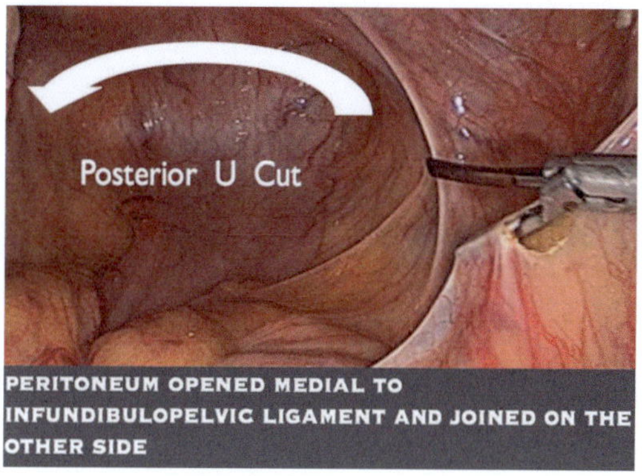

Fig. 12.3 Posterior "U cut"

and constantly under vision. The same steps are repeated on the left side and both the peritoneal cuts joined in the POD forming the posterior U cut (Figs. 12.3 and 12.4).

Step 2: Examination of Rectovaginal Space (Figs. 12.5 and 12.6)

The aide repositioned the rectum in a cranial direction to extend the peritoneum within the Douglas pouch. Subsequently, the Harmonic Shears were used to make an incision in this peritoneum. The insufflation of CO_2 gas opens the loose areolar planes between the two layers of Denonvilliers' fascia. The dissection is carried out between the two layers of Denonvilliers' fascia (Fig. 12.5). The plane between the fat and the posterior vaginal wall is dissected keeping in mind the dictum "*fat belongs to the rectum*" (Fig. 12.5). The rectum was dissected off the posterior vaginal wall up to the levator ani muscle.

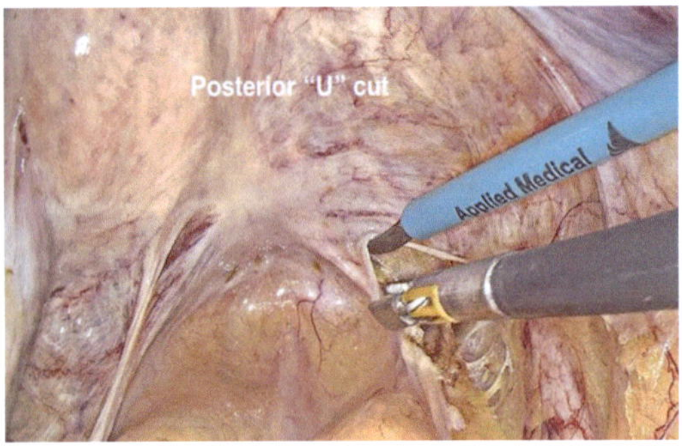

Fig. 12.4 Posterior U cut extended toward the pouch of Douglas

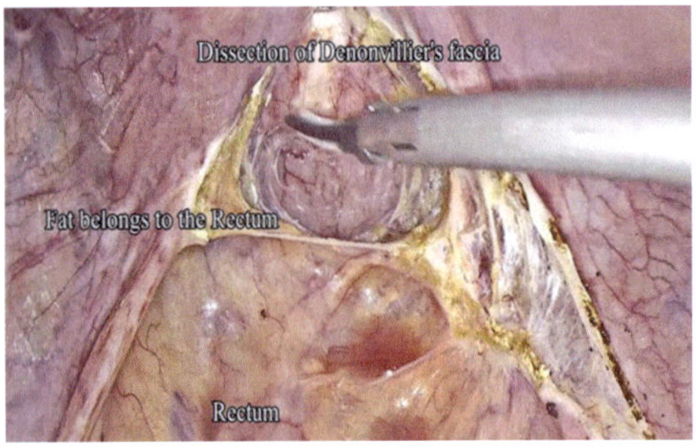

Fig. 12.5 Two layers of Denon-Villiers fascia

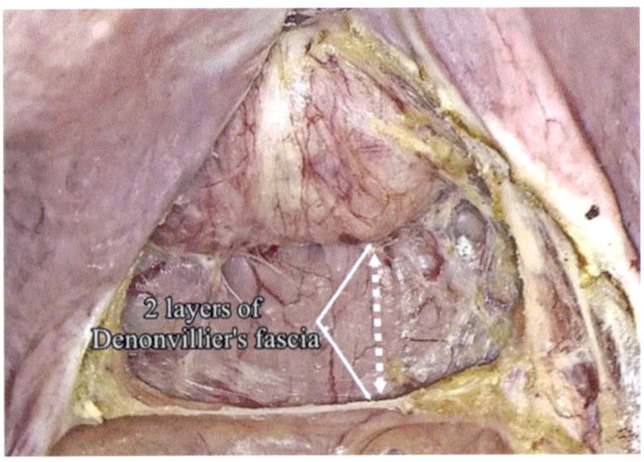

Fig. 12.6 Dissection in POD Fats belongs to the rectum

Step 3: Dissection of the Pararectal Space (Fig. 12.7)

The left ureter is retracted medially and the posterior leaf of broad ligament above the ureter is cut. The incision was prolonged downward, reaching the bladder and resulting in the formation of a window in the broad ligament. The ureter was once more moved medially, and the

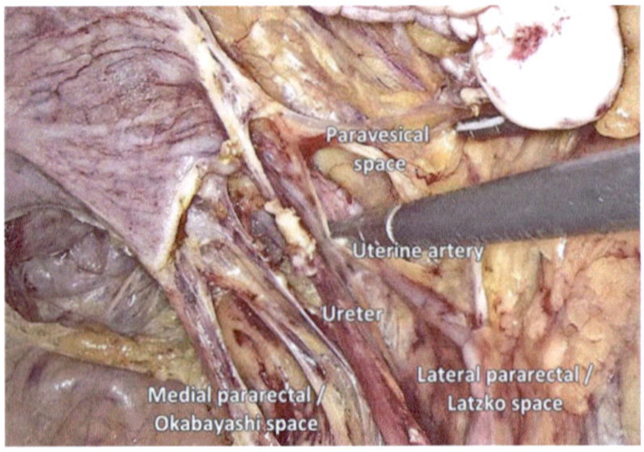

Fig. 12.7 Para-rectal space dissection

Harmonic Shear was used in a parallel and lateral motion to the ureter, thereby exposing the pararectal space. The internal iliac artery, serving as the lateral boundary of this space, became immediately visible.

The sole anatomical formation traversing the pararectal space horizontally is the uterine artery. Subsequently, the uterine artery underwent either clipping or ligation, followed by cutting, a process executed using Harmonic Shears. Within the pararectal space, the ureter demarcates both medial, also referred to as "Okabayashi Space," and lateral sections, commonly known as "Latzko Space." The ureter is pulled inward, and the dissection is carried out alongside it to expose the pararectal space. The medial pararectal space houses the hypogastric nerves, crucial for nerve-sparing radical hysterectomy. On the other hand, the lateral pararectal space accommodates the pelvic splanchnic nerves and the uterine artery. This location is optimal for clamping the uterine artery, a necessary step in any hysterectomy procedure. The uterine artery traverses the pararectal space in a horizontal direction. The area located in front of the uterine artery and toward the inner side of the obliterated hypogastric artery is explored and referred to as the paravesical space (refer to Fig. 12.8). This exploration extends through the paravesical space until reaching the levator ani. Within the paravesical space, one finds the umbilical artery, superior vesical artery, the neurovascular bundle of the obturator, lymphatic tissue, and accessory obturator vessels.

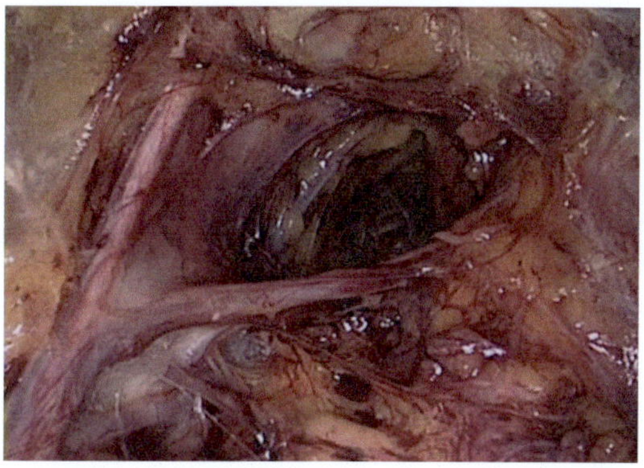

Fig. 12.8 Left para-vesical space

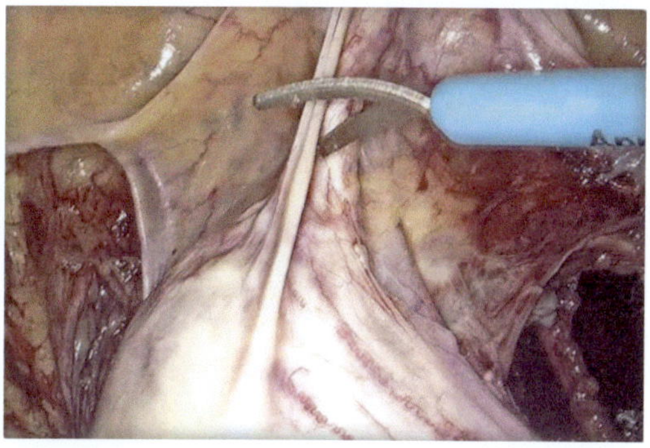

Fig. 12.10 Anterior U cut

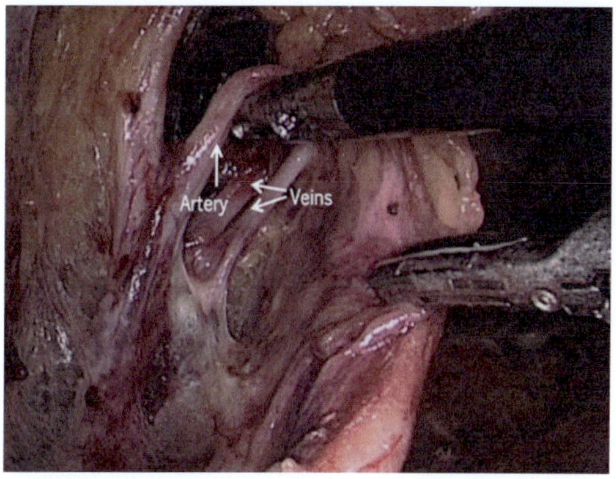

Fig. 12.9 Uterine artery–vein–ureter complex

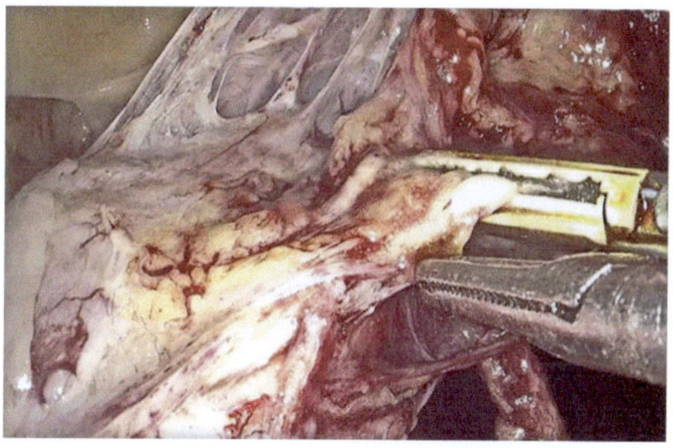

Fig. 12.11 Dissection of BladdePiller

This dissection helps to best access to lateral pelvic wall for optimal oncological clearance and lymph node dissection. The uterine vein is seen below the artery. Both the artery and the vein are individually clipped or ligated and then cut. The ureter is retracted medially to expose the utero-sacral's and Mackenrodt's ligaments, which are seen as a single fan-shaped structure. They are then cut with the harmonic shears in the downward direction toward the levator ani. The identical procedures are replicated on the right-hand side, as depicted in Fig. 12.8.

Step 4: Anterior U-cut (Figs. 12.9 and 12.10)
The uterus exhibits a retroverted position. Utilizing harmonic shears, an incision is made in the peritoneum over the utero-vesical fold, commencing from one round ligament and extending across to the other, creating a U-shaped cut in the anterior region. The fascial layer separating the bladder and the uterus was carefully established with consideration for the principle that emphasizes the association of fat with the bladder, as illustrated in Fig. 12.11. The dissection process was aided by the use of CO_2 insufflation. The peritoneal cut is further extended up to the infundibulopelvic ligaments. An incision is created in the wide ligament, revealing the ureter visible through this opening in the broad ligament.

Step 5: Ureteric Tunnel Dissection (Figs. 12.12 and 12.13)
The uterus is pulled upward and toward the right, while the entire length of the left ureter is carefully followed toward the bladder. The peritoneum covering the bladder is grasped, and the bladder is lifted upward by the assisting surgeon.

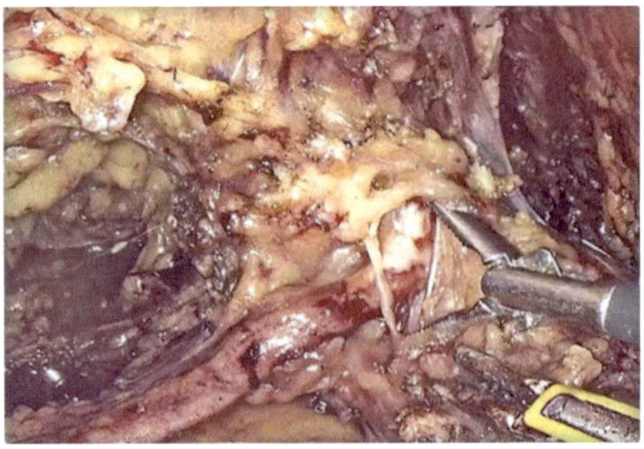

Fig. 12.12 Dissection of the tunnel

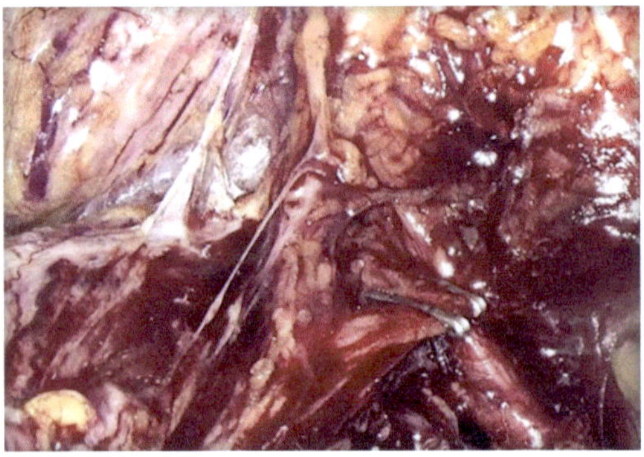

Fig. 12.13 Right ureteric tunnel dissection on the left ureter

This maneuver allows for clear visualization of the uretic tunnel, revealing small veins. The tunnel is dissected using Maryland's forceps, and within its roof, two veins are identified, clipped, and subsequently cut (refer to Figs. 12.12 and 12.13). This process facilitates the lateral movement of the ureter. The point where the ureter enters the bladder at the utero-vesical junction becomes visible. To achieve a well-formed vaginal cuff below the growth, the bladder is further pushed downward. Understanding of Anterior Parametrectomy, Ans To "LACC TRAIL" as complete parametrium dissection, help in prevention of local or pelvic recurrence of cervical cancers (Fig. 12.14). The paracolpos is then cut as laterally as possible. These procedures guarantee the attainment of the maximum paracolpos and visibility of the vaginal margin. The identical steps are iterated on the right side to expose the trigonal area. Purse-string suturing is taken above colpotomy to prevent spillage. A colpotomy is performed beyond this point using harmonic shears (Figs. 12.15, 12.16, and 12.17).The infundibulopelvic ligaments are subsequently incised, and the complete specimen is then isolated and placed inside an endobag (see Fig. 12.18).

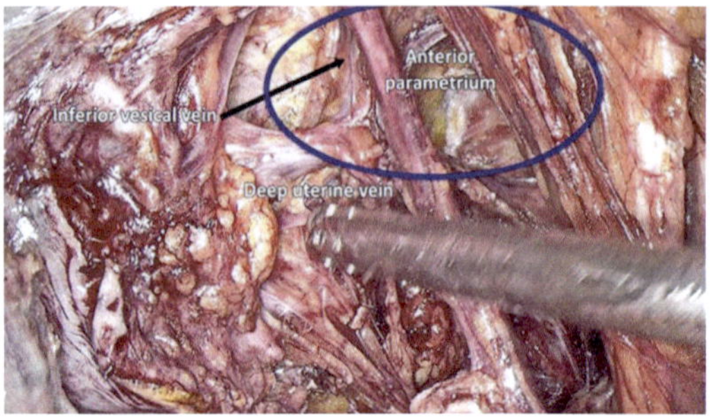

Fig. 12.14 Dissection of anterior parametrium

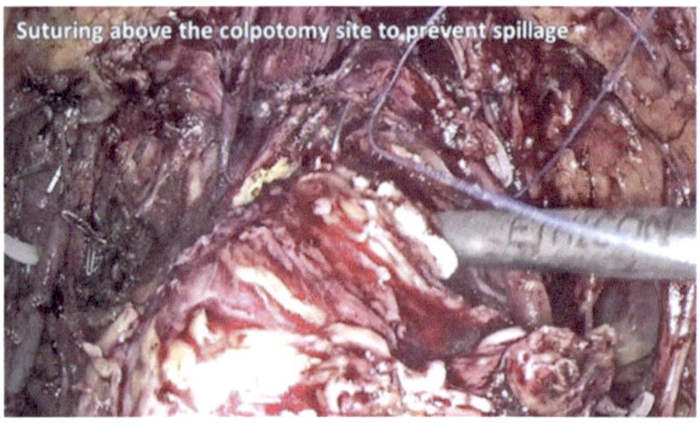

Fig. 12.15 Purse string suturing above colpotomy to prevent spillage

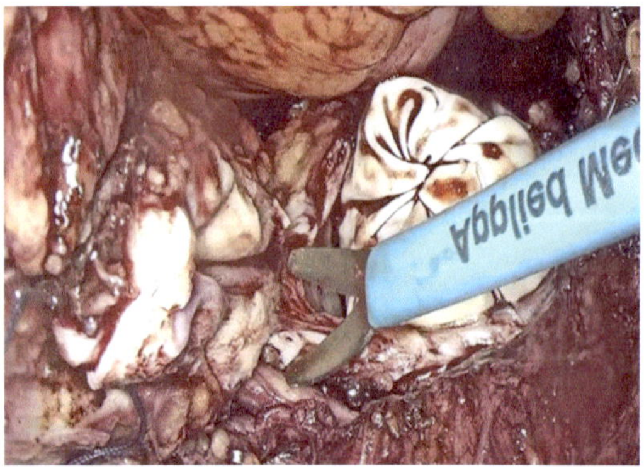

Fig. 12.16 Completed colpotomy

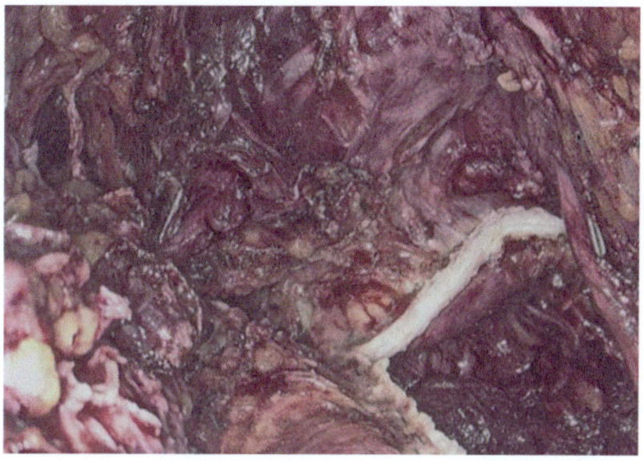

Fig. 12.17 Use of stapler for colpotomy

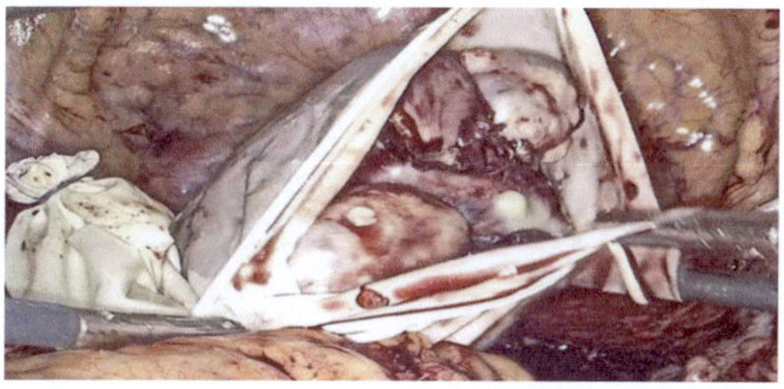

Fig. 12.18 Specimen put in an endobag

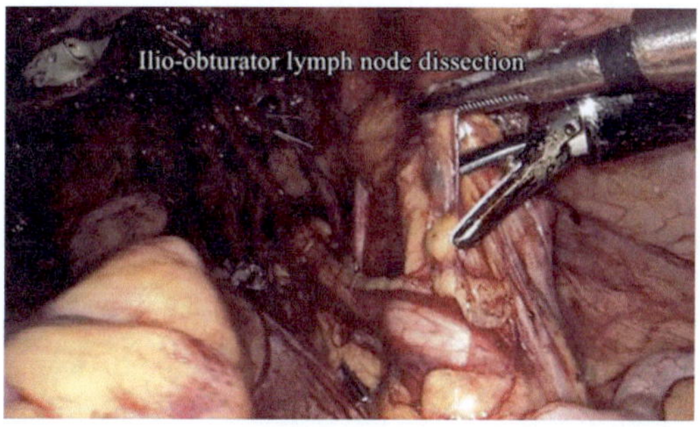

Fig. 12.19 Dissection of the lymph nodes in the right ilio-obturator region

Step 6: Lymph Node Excision (Fig. 12.19)

The dissection of lymph nodes commences at the bifurcation of the common iliac artery. This procedure utilizes a suction cannula for its relatively gentle approach, making it the preferred tool for dissection. No energy source is employed in this process. The fibro-fatty tissue along the external iliac vein is meticulously dissected using the suction cannula, moving in a direction parallel to the vessels and extending up to the iliac bone, which

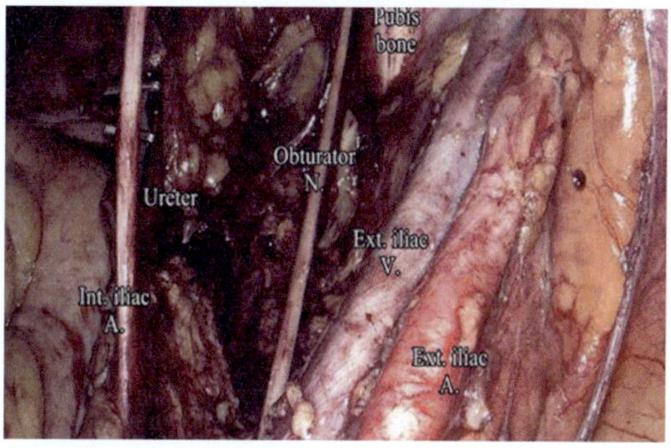

Fig. 12.20 Ilio-obturator lymph node dissection has been successfully performed

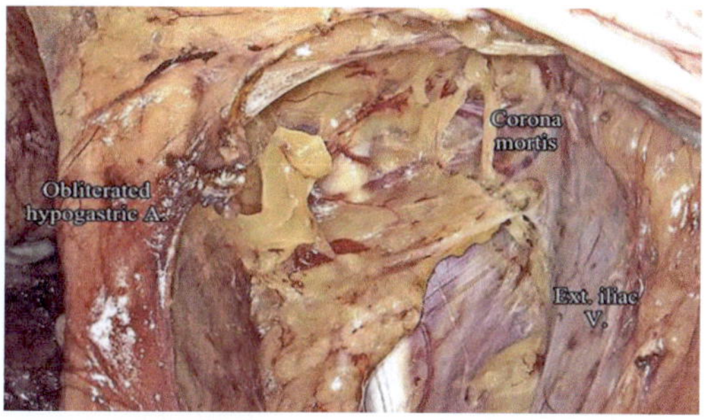

Fig. 12.21 Corona mortis

serves as the lateral boundary of the dissection. To visualize nodes in the obturator fossa, the peritoneum is stretched by the assistant, and the nodes are systematically cleared from the pubic bone in a cranial direction. Exposure of the obturator nerve occurs, and all nodes situated above the nerve are meticulously removed. The medial limit is defined by the internal iliac artery, while the lower limit is determined by the obturator nerve (refer to Fig. 12.20). Be aware of "*corona mortis*" an anastomosis between the obturator and external iliac vein (Fig. 12.21). A comparable analysis is conducted on both sides, as illustrated in Fig. 12.19. The complete nodal tissue extracted is placed inside the endobag. The endobag is removed vaginally. Hemostasis is achieved. The wound is irrigated with normal saline. The enclosure is securely shut by employing a consistent internal stitching technique using Vicryl 2–0, threaded through the 10 mm operational opening. The utilization of intra-abdominal drainage is deemed unnecessary. The removal of ports is conducted under visual guidance, followed by the closure of the port sites.

The sample: This method accomplishes a Pivers type III radical hysterectomy (Type C2 Querlow and Moore) with a paracervical clearance exceeding 3 cm. It also ensures a distal vaginal margin of over 2.5–3 cm and a retrieval of at least 18–20 nodes, as illustrated in Fig. 12.17.

Complications

1. Hemorrhage
2. Bladder injury
3. Ureteric injury
4. Bowel injury
5. Fistulas

12.2 Laparoscopic Nerve-Sparing Radical Hysterectomy (Figs. 12.22 and 12.23)

The main disadvantage of laparoscopic radical hysterectomy is the bladder dysfunction. This arises from a disturbance in the autonomic nerves, leading to a lack of support for the anatomical bladder neck and the overexpansion of the bladder. A nerve-preserving radical hysterectomy aims to protect the superior and inferior hypogastric nerves, as well as the pelvic splanchnic plexus. This approach successfully addresses the issue of bladder dysfunction. The process closely resembles laparoscopic radical hysterectomy. The hypogastric plexus is positioned on the side of the uterosacral ligaments (Fig. 12.22). Therefore, the dissection at the uterosacral level is performed with great care. The nerves are located to the side of the uterosacrals and toward the inner side of the ureter. The branches of the hypogastric nerve that extend to the uterus are found in the connective tissue just behind and to the side of the vagina. These branches are carefully severed, and the nerve plane is shifted to the posterior side. The preservation of the bladder branch of the inferior hypogastric plexus is achieved by lateralizing both the nerve plane and the ureter. Within the posterior leaf of the vesicouterine ligament, there are vesical veins that flow into the deep uterine veins. These veins are carefully identified and individually clipped and ligated on the medial side of the ureter. Additionally, the bladder branch, situated just beneath the inferior vesical vein, is also safeguarded. The inferior hypogastric plexus is selectively severed in the front section, including its uterine and cervical branches. As the colpotomy is performed, the nerve is situated laterally to the ureter, whereas in the initial dissection stages, the hypogastric nerve and inferior hypogastric plexus were anatomically positioned posteromedially to the ureter. The remainder of the procedure follows the same steps as outlined in the previously described laparoscopic radical hysterectomy.

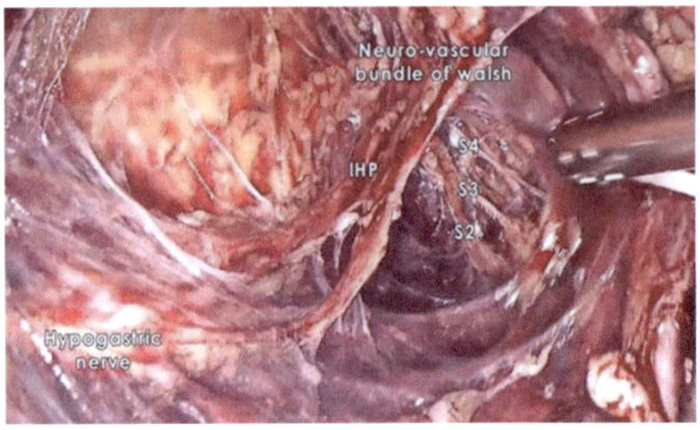

Fig. 12.22 Hyogastric nerve preservation

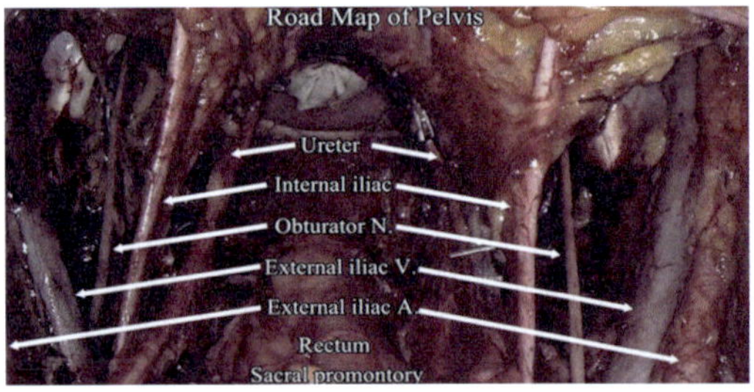

Fig. 12.23 Post dissection, there is a plan or a course of action laid out to guide the subsequent steps or directions

12.2.1 After Surgery

Foley catheter is removed after 48 h. If urinary retention occurs, Foley Catheterization is done again and patient is reassessed every 7 days.

12.2.2 Conclusion

In summary, we want to emphasize that laparoscopic radical hysterectomy demonstrates comparable oncological outcomes to open surgery regarding margins, lymph node clearance, and parametric resection, achieving successful type III radical hysterectomy. This approach is both technically feasible and economically advantageous, exhibiting fewer postoperative complications and lower morbidity compared to the abdominal method. Additionally, patients experience less postoperative pain, earlier ambulation, and a quicker return to work. Moreover, this approach allows for the initiation of adjuvant therapy at an earlier stage. We can perform duplication of conventional multiport laparoscopic radical hysterectomy steps with other minimal access modalities (LESS, OASIS, Robotic) [12].

Video Link

Video describing nerve sparing radical hysterectomy

https://drive.google.com/file/d/1HKdBBAoNvQaFtTghdzoqn5J1bZyqwLku/view?usp=share_link

References

1. Global Cancer Statistics 2020: GLOBOCAN Estimates of Incidence and Mortality Worldwide for 36 Cancers in 185 Countrieshttps://acsjournals.onlinelibrary.wiley.com/doi/full/10.3322/caac.21660
2. Bray F, Laversanne M, Weiderpass E, Soerjomataram I. The ever-increasing importance of cancer as a leading cause of premature death worldwide. Cancer (In press).
3. World Health Organization (WHO). Global Health Estimates 2020: Deaths by Cause, Age, Sex, by Country and by Region, 2000–2019. WHO; 2020. Accessed December 11, 2020. who.int/data/gho/data/themes/mortality-and-global-health-estimates/ghe-leading-causes-of-death
4. Omran AR. The epidemiologic transition. A theory of the epidemiology of population change. Milbank Mem Fund Q. 1971;49:509–38.
5. Piver MS, Rutledge F, Smith JP. Five classes of extended hysterectomy for women with cervical cancer. Obstet Gynecol. 1974;44:265–72.
6. Nandakumar A, Anantha N, Venugopal TC. Incidence, mortality and survival in cancer of the cervix in Bangalore, India. Br J Cancer. 1995;71:1348–52.
7. Morrow CP, Curtin J. Gynecologic cancer surgery. Philadelphia, PA: Churchill Livingstone; 1996.
8. Canis M, Mage G, Wattiez A, Ponly JL, Manhes H, Bruhat MA. Does endoscopic surgery have a role in radical surgery of cancer of the cervix uteri? [in French]. J Gynecol Obstet Biol Reprod (Paris). 1990;19:921.
9. Shoup M, Brennan MF, Karpeh MS, Gillern SM, McMahon RL, Conlon KC. Port site metastasis after diagnostic laparoscopy for upper gastrointestinal tract malignancies: an uncommon entity. Ann Surg Oncol. 2002;9:632–6.
10. Abu-Rustum NR, Rhee E, Chi DS, Sonoda Y, Sonoda Y, Gemignani M, Barakat RR. Subcutaneous tumor implantation after laparoscopic procedures in women with malignant disease. Obstet Gynecol. 2004;103:480–7.
11. Abu-Rustum NR, Gemignani ML, Moore K, et al. Total laparoscopic radical hysterectomy with pelvic lymphadenectomy using the argon- beam coagulator: pilot data and comparison to laparotomy. Gynecol Oncol. 2003;91:402–409. Erratum in Gynecol Oncol 2004;93:275.
12. Duplication of Conventional Multiport Laparoscopic Radical Hysterectomy Steps with Other Minimal Access Modalities (LESS, OASIS, Robotic) Shailesh P. Puntambekar, MS*, S. Katakdhond, MS, S. Galgali, MS, A. Iche, MS, S. Barik, MS, and A. S. Puntambekar, MS From the Galaxy Care Laparoscopy Institute, Pune, India (all authors). https://www.researchgate.net/publication/272028069_Duplication_of_Conventional_Multiport_Laparoscopic_Radical_Hysterectomy_Steps_with_Other_Minimal_Access_Modalities_LESS_OASIS_Robotic

13 Minimally Invasive Inguinal Lymph Node Dissection

James W. Jakub and Nicolas Contreras-Peraza

Abstract

Minimally invasive inguinal lymph node dissection (MILND) is a three-trocar technique that respects the same anatomic boundaries and oncologic principles of its open predecessor. As with any oncologic procedure, judgment is essential in patient selection and multidisciplinary input is critical for optimal management. MILND has significantly decreased the incidence of wound complications, surgical site infections, and all but eliminated wound dehiscence, which are problematic in the groin. Prolonged drain days and seroma remain an unresolved issue. This chapter provides the reader a step-by-step outline of the how to perform the procedure in text form as well as pictorial and a video accompaniment.

Keywords

Minimally invasive · Videoscopic · Laparoscopic · Inguinal · Groin · Melanoma · Lymphadenectomy · Dissection

J. W. Jakub (✉)
Mayo Clinic, Jacksonville, FL, USA
e-mail: Jakub.James@mayo.edu

N. Contreras-Peraza
Mayo Clinic, Rochester, MN, USA

13.1 History of the Procedure

13.1.1 Inguinal Lymphadenectomy

Cutaneous malignancies and malignancies of the perineum commonly metastasize to the inguinal lymph nodes. Inguinal lymphadenectomy has historically been the standard of care for inguinal lymph node metastases. In 1912, Besset first described the open Inguinal lymphadenectomy in detail, even though the procedure had been performed nearly three decades earlier by Sir William Mac Cormac in 1885 for penile carcinoma [1, 2]. Cabanas later described sentinel lymph node (SLN) biopsy and its utility in determining the necessity for inguinal lymph node dissection in penile carcinoma in 1977 [3]. Unfortunately, the wound complication rate for open inguinal lymphadenectomy from three prospective high-volume single institution studies was found to be significant with the incidence of infection, wound dehiscence, seroma formation, lymphocele, and chronic lymphedema approaching 70% [4–6]. Due to the high complication rate and failure of interventions to reduce these complications [7], a minimally invasive inguinal lymph node dissection (MILND) has gained popularity over the last decade [8–11]. This procedure has also been termed video endoscopic inguinal lymphadenectomy (VEIL) and videoscopic inguinal lymphadenectomy (VIL). MILND is defined as an inguinal lymph node dis-

M. Tewari (ed.), *Minimally Invasive Surgery in Cancer*,
https://doi.org/10.1007/978-981-97-7059-5_13

section performed through trocar ports. MILND has shown to have decreased rates of wound infection, wound dehiscence, hospital length of stay, and readmission rates when compared to the open technique [9, 12]. Lymph node yield is a surrogate marker for the oncologic completeness of the procedure and has also been shown to be comparable to the open technique [8, 12, 13]. Similar recurrence rates have also been demonstrated in two single institution retrospective reviews of 88 total MILND procedures [8, 13]. A recently published retrospective series of 228 MILNDs performed at 14 institutions demonstrated similar oncologic outcomes compared with a contemporary cohort of 288 open ILNDs performed in MSLT-II [14].

13.2 Anatomy

Understanding the anatomy of the inguinal nodes is imperative to performing inguinal lymph node dissections. Inguinal nodes can be subdivided into ilioinguinal and inguinalofemoral nodes. The ilioinguinal nodes extend from the bifurcation of the common iliac artery proximally, to the undersurface of the inguinal ligament distally, the pelvic sidewall laterally, and the bladder medially. These are part of the pelvic nodes and removed with the obturator nodes during a standard pelvic/ilioinguinal lymph node dissection for melanoma.

The inguinalofemoral nodes are located within the confines of the femoral triangle, which is bound superiorly by the inguinal ligament, laterally by the sartorius muscle, and medially by the adductor longus muscle (Fig. 13.1). The apex of the triangle occurs at the location where the sartorius muscle crosses over the femoral vessels and the adductor longus muscle. The femoral nerve, artery, and vein are located within the femoral triangle, and at the level of the inguinal ligament are aligned in the same plane from lateral to medial, respectively. The empty space and Cloquet's Lymph node are located medially (acronym NAVEL). It should be noted that the empty space medial to the femoral vein can be enlarged after MILND leading to femoral hernia.

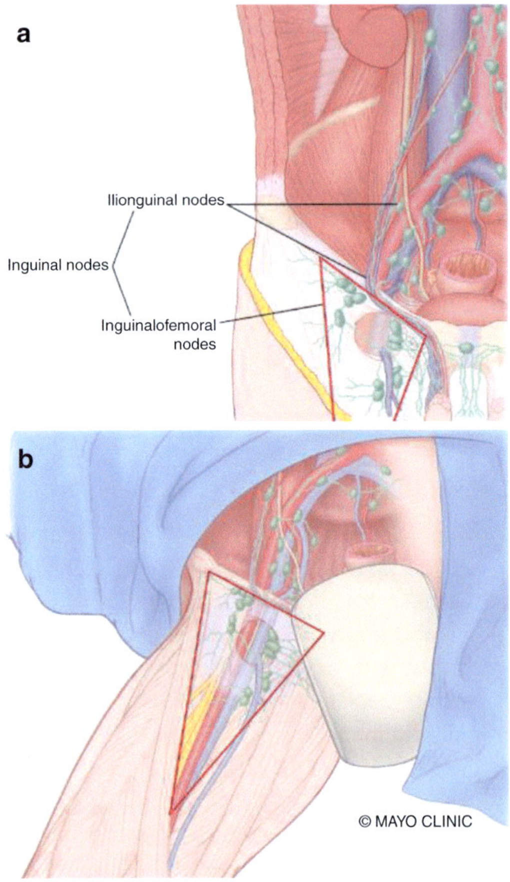

Fig. 13.1 Anatomy of the inguinal lymph nodes. (**a**) The inguinal nodes are composed of both the ilioinguinal nodes and the inguinalofemoral nodes. The inguinalofemoral nodes are those lymph nodes contained within the boundaries of the femoral triangle. This chapter focuses on minimally invasive dissection of the inguinalofemoral nodes referred in this chapter as the inguinal lymph nodes. (**b**) Superficial depiction of the femoral triangle bounded by the inguinal ligament superiorly, the sartorius muscle laterally, and the adductor longus muscle medially. The femoral triangle contains the femoral nerve, artery, and vein as well as the great saphenous vein as it courses proximally to join the femoral vein at the saphenofemoral junction after traversing the fossa ovalis. *Image used with permission of Mayo Clinic*

This is especially true if combined with an ilioinguinal dissection. The contents of the femoral triangle can be divided into superficial and deep compartments, which are separated by the cribriform fascia (Fig. 13.2). The cribriform fascia is an extension of the fascia lata and is violated at the fossa ovalis (saphenous opening) by the great

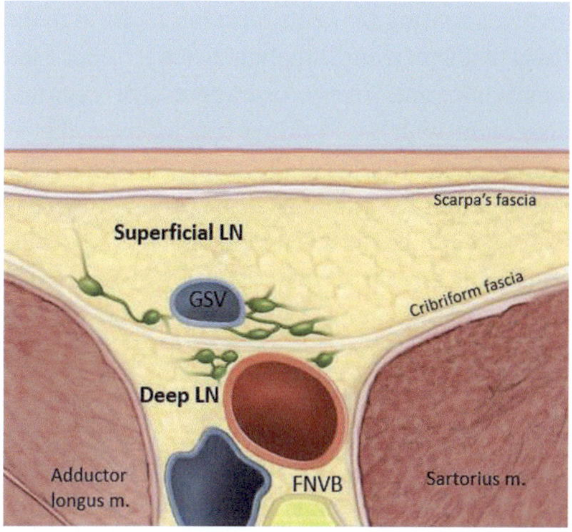

Fig. 13.2 The cross-sectional anatomy of the femoral triangle of a left lower extremity. The femoral triangle is confined by the sartorius muscle laterally and the adductor longus muscle medially. The femoral neurovascular bundle (FNVB) is contained within the boundaries of the triangle, as well as the proximal greater saphenous vein (GSV). The femoral triangle is divided into deep and superficial compartments by the cribriform fascia, which is an extension of the fascia lata. This fascia separates the superficial and deep inguinal lymph nodes (LN) in our dissections. *Image used with permission of Mayo Clinic*

saphenous vein (GSV) as it dives deep to the fascia to join the femoral vein at the saphenofemoral junction (SFJ). There are approximately ten lymph nodes in the femoral triangle superficial to the cribriform fascia and five lymph nodes deep to the fascia. The bulk of the lymph nodes are superficial and medial to the femoral vein. The most proximal lymph node, Cloquet's node, lies just medial to the common femoral vein, posterior to the inguinal ligament. Cloquet's node has been thought to be the "sentinel lymph node" of the pelvis for lower extremity malignancies; however, in practice the utility of Cloquet's node as a marker for disease spread into the pelvis has been unreliable [15].

It is important to note that there are additional nodes continuous with those in the inguinalofemoral region extending cephalad to the inguinal ligament superficial to the external oblique musculature. These supra-inguinal nodes extend to the level of the umbilicus superiorly, the pubic tubercle medially, the anterior superior iliac spine (ASIS) laterally, and the external oblique musculature posteriorly.

The nomenclature of the inguinal lymph node basins can be confusing because it varies among surgical subspecialties. By convention some melanoma specialists define the "deep" inguinal nodes as the ilioinguinal (pelvic) nodes and the "superficial" inguinal nodes as those contained within the confines of the femoral triangle. In this chapter, however, we refer to the inguinal nodes exclusively as the lymph node contents of the femoral triangle. Our distinction between superficial and deep inguinal nodes is in reference to the contents of the femoral triangle and those nodes that lie above and below the cribriform fascia, respectively. The inguinalofemoral nodes, the nodes within the confines of the femoral triangle, are the focus of this chapter.

13.3 Operative Indications and Preoperative Planning

A MILND is indicated for essentially the same reasons as an open inguinal lymph node dissection. These indications include metastatic spread to the regional basin from cutaneous malignancies (melanoma and squamous cell carcinomas (SCC) most commonly), urologic malignancies such as penile cancer and vulvar cancers, distal rectal and anal adeno and squamous cancers. Familiarity with cancer society guidelines and multidisciplinary management of gross or microscope disease and the role of surgery, systemic therapy, and radiation for inguinal lymph node disease is of the essence, as indications for lymphadenectomy continue to evolve. For example, in the melanoma literature, completion lymphadenectomy is much less common and is no longer the only accepted standard of care following a positive SLN biopsy. The practice changing Multicenter Selective Lymphadenectomy-2 (MSLT-2) trial demonstrated decreased disease-specific survival but no improvement in melanoma-specific survival with lymphadenectomy compared to active surveillance for microscopic nodal disease, i.e., a positive SLN [16]. As such, inguinal lymph node dissections are decreasing as a result of the MSLT-2 data in melanoma as well as the increasing efficacy of systemic therapy for melanoma. The role of neoadjuvant systemic therapy is becoming the new standard for clinical nodal disease in melanoma and the role of systemic therapy alone in exceptional responders is still being defined [17, 18].

The value of a thorough physical examination cannot be overstated for preoperative planning prior to any lymph node dissection. A detailed inspection of the regional nodal basins draining from the primary, including bilateral inguinal regions, as well as the popliteal fossa for primaries distal to the knee, and inspection for in-transit disease is essential for cutaneous malignancies of the lower extremity and lower trunk. Examination cephalad to the inguinal ligament (including the axilla) and superficial to the external oblique is also important as this may be a site of in-transit disease, especially for truncal malignancies. Detailed heat maps showing regional lymph node drainage from greater than 5000 SLN biopsies has been performed by the Sydney Melanoma Unit and is a great reference for this information [19]. A pelvic and genital examination should also be performed for perineal malignancies and metastatic inguinal nodal disease from an unknown primary.

In my personal practice, the location of the primary tumor and the route of lymph node metastasis impacts the extent of my dissection in MILND and helps me focus on which areas to be more or less aggressive. For example, in lower extremity melanoma with limited metastasis to the inguinal lymph node basin, both a superficial and deep inguinal lymph node dissection is required throughout the femoral triangle, including a more aggressive dissection at the apex of the femoral triangle as the route of metastasis traverses this region. In contrast, the dissection for truncal malignancies and anogenital malignancies can likely spare some of the dissection at the apex of the triangle and focus the majority of lymphadenectomy at the middle and proximal part of the femoral triangle, as most of the disease burden will be in this region. My practice now involves sparing the cribriform fascia distal to the fossa ovalis in truncal malignancies to reduce the magnitude and likely overaggressive regional dissection with these primaries, whereas this is removed en bloc in dissections performed for lower extremity malignancies. Although there is an inherent logic to this approach there is no outcome data to support this focused dissection; it has been an evolving shift in our practice in an effort to minimize the morbidity of MILND, namely, seroma formation and prolonged drain days (discussed below).

Finally, knowing the main complications and pitfalls of any operative procedure prior to proceeding to the operating room can assist with operative planning, patient counseling, and expectation management. Although MILND offers multiple benefits when compared to the open technique, seroma formation and prolonged drain days remain the major source of morbidity for the minimally invasive approach, as postoperative seroma can be observed in up to 50% of patients [20]. The cause of seroma/lymphocele and lymphedema is thought to occur secondarily to a combination of lymphatic injury, tissue trauma, and dead space formation. As such, when choosing to pursue MILND and the extent of dissection, one must be aware of the pros and cons between an adequate lymph node dissection and risk of recurrence while attempting to minimize the factors that may lead to lymphedema and seroma formation. Careful examination of a patient's bilateral lower extremities with baseline limb volume measurements is often undertaken preoperatively. We typically refer our patients to a lymphedema specialist prior to proceeding to surgery. Postoperatively, patients will leave with an operative drain and are monitored clinically for seroma formation. Management of postoperative complications is discussed later in the chapter.

Hypercarbia is to be expected during MILND. As opposed to most laparoscopic operations that occur within the peritoneal cavity, MILND dissection and CO_2 insufflation in the subcutaneous tissue results in much higher levels of systemically absorbed CO_2. The anesthesia team must be aware of this expected physiologic change and make ventilator adjustments to account for this increased systemic absorbance of CO_2. Failure to manage this expected change may lead to patient intolerance of the procedure requiring conversion to an open technique.

13.4 Surgical Management

13.4.1 Technique of MILND

A detailed step-by-step video can be seen at:

https://medprofvideos.mayoclinic.org/videos/minimally-invasive-inguinal-lymph-node-dissection-milnd

Positioning and OR Setup

- After induction of general endotracheal anesthesia, the patient is positioned supine in the split-leg position. The operative leg is abducted and flexed at the knee, exposing the femoral triangle (Fig. 13.3).
- Sequential compression devices are placed for DVT prophylaxis and prophylactic subcutaneous heparin is administered. A Foley catheter is placed in a sterile fashion after the field has been prepped. Preoperative antibiotics are administered. Expected physiologic changes of intraoperative hypercarbia are discussed with the anesthesia team.
- The operative leg is prepped circumferentially and draped into the surgical field, as well as the genitals and the contralateral anterior thigh and abdomen up to the umbilicus. The genitals and operative site are sealed over with a blue towel and Ioban™ (3M™, Minneapolis, Minnesota)
- The surgeon alternates with the assistant as necessary, standing in between the legs of the patient and standing lateral to the surgical leg. Monitors are placed at the head of the table, one over each shoulder of the patient.
- Minimal instrumentation is needed on the Mayo Stand; however, appropriate instruments for an open operation should be immediately available in case there is an operative emergency or vascular injury.

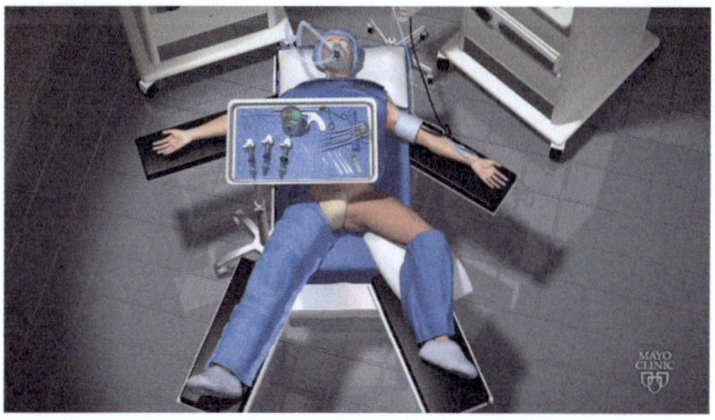

Fig. 13.3 Operating room setup for MILND. The patient is positioned in the split-leg position with flexion of the knee and external rotation of the hip of the operative leg. This position is critical to bring the femoral triangle anterior. The surgeon alternates between standing between the patient's legs and lateral to the operative leg. Video monitors are placed above each shoulder of the patient. *Image used with permission of Mayo Clinic*

Trocar Placement

- Using palpation, the landmarks of the femoral triangle are identified and outlined with a marking pen—the medial border of the Sartorius muscle, the lateral boarder of the adductor longus muscle, and the inguinal ligament. The proximal dissection will be carried 2–5 cm proximal to the inguinal ligament when removing the supra-inguinal lymph nodes overlying the external oblique aponeurosis. This is also marked. Next, the location for the three 10 mm/12 mm trocars are marked (Fig. 13.4). The distal most trocar is placed 3 cm distal to the apex of the triangle, while the other two trocars are placed 5 cm proximal to this, one on the medial edge and the other on the lateral edge of the triangle. Both the medial and lateral trocars are placed two fingerbreadths from the triangle edge.
- Incisions are made and kept as small as possible to minimize a CO_2 leak through the incisions, which can be a major nuisance throughout the case. We mark the length of the incision by pushing and indenting the skin with the blunt end of the open trocar. Classically, blunt dissection with an index finger being swept from side-to-side through the trocar site along the subcutaneous tissue plane has been described. This separates a

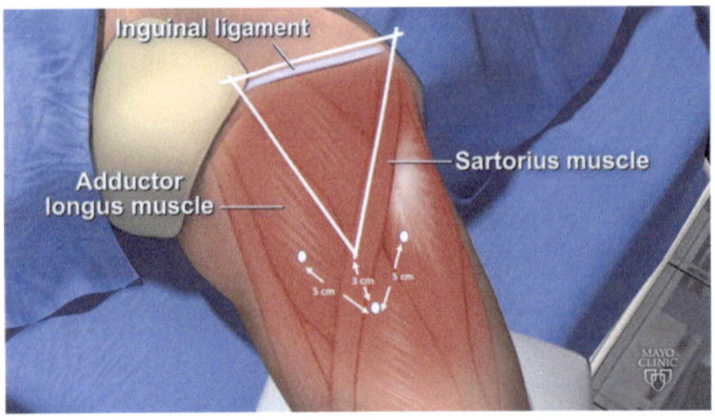

Fig. 13.4 Surface anatomy of the lower extremity. The boundaries of the femoral triangle are marked on the lower extremity. The 10 mm/12 mm trocar sites are also marked. The apical trocar site should be marked 3 cm distal to the apex of the triangle. The other two trocar sites are marked 5 cm proximal to this on each side of the triangle. They should be two finger breadths from the triangle edge. The inguinal ligament is located approximately 2 cm proximal to the inguinal crease. *Image used with permission of Mayo Clinic*

space for the trocar to be placed along the natural avascular plane between the subcutaneous fat and the underlying soft tissue. This will typically require one incision to be extended slightly. If utilizing this approach, I place a figure-of-eight silk suture through one side of the incision and tie this down after the trocar is placed to prevent an air leak. Most frequently, I now introduce a fine curved instrument and use bunt dissection to create the initial working space. I advance the tip of the instrument into all three skin entry sites in a natural superficial plane for the full length of the instrument and spread. The 10 mm/12 mm trocars are then placed (Fig. 13.5). Carbon dioxide insufflation is initially set at a pressure of 25 mmHg with a flow of 20 L/min for 10 min to further dissect the working space and then turned down to 15 mmHg.

Dissection

- Our approach is broken down into a series of steps. We have found implementing a stepwise approach to our minimally invasive procedure has complemented our open approach, organically leading us to more formally structure our open approach into a series of steps as well. These steps consist of a superficial dissection of the anterior skin flap, followed by a Sartorius dissection, adductor longus dissection, exposure and identification of the distal great saphenous vein (GSV), apical and deep dissection, and finally proximal dissection with management of the proximal GSV.

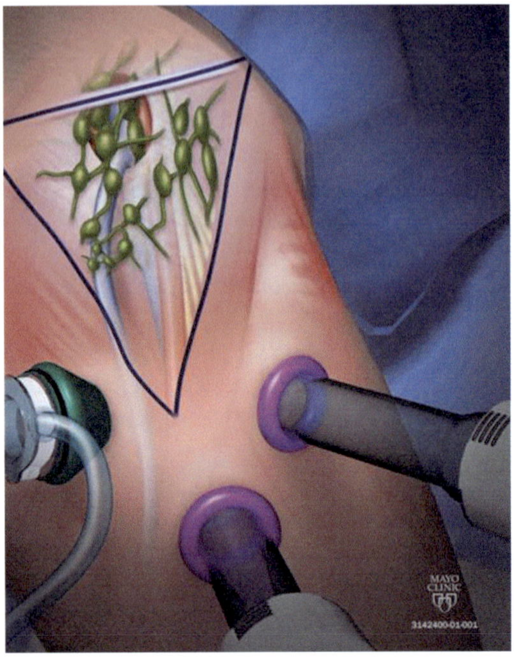

Fig. 13.5 Depiction of the femoral triangle with trocar placement. The 10 mm/12 mm trocars are placed at the apex and to the sides of the femoral triangle. *Image used with permission of Mayo Clinic*

Superficial Dissection of the Anterior Skin Flap

- We perform the entire dissection with a harmonic scalpel. A 30-degree laparoscopic camera is placed in the apical port, and an atraumatic grasper and an energy devise are placed in the lateral and medial ports. The superficial dissection consists of creating a thin tissue flap within the confines of the previously outlined femoral triangle from the apex of the triangle to the eternal oblique aponeurosis more proximally. The dissection plane occurs just superficial to Scarpa's fascia, effectively separating the subcutaneous fat from the underlying regional contents (Fig. 13.6). A thin layer of fat is left on the skin flap, which will vary in thickness depending on body habitus. The flap is fairly thin and

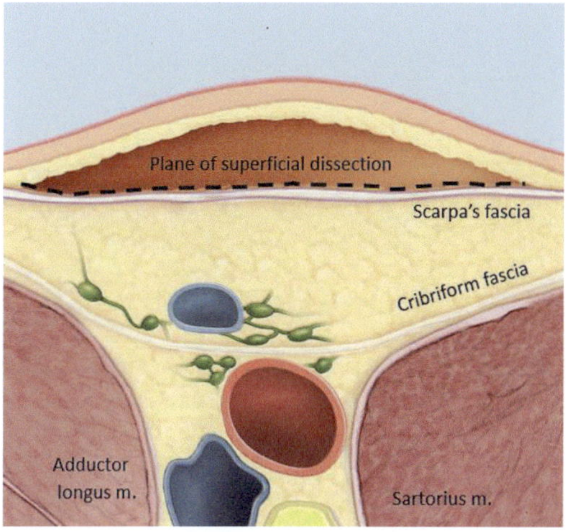

Fig. 13.6 Superficial dissection of MILND. The superficial dissection plane should occur beneath Camper's fascia but superficial to Scarpa's fascia separating the soft tissue flap from the underlying regional contents of the groin. The dissection should take place within the marked outline of the femoral triangle and extend 2–5 cm above the inguinal ligament, over the external oblique aponeurosis to encompass the supra-inguinal nodes. *Image used with permission of Mayo Clinic*

can be appreciated by the transillumination of the light source through the tissue flap (Fig. 13.7). The light emanating from the camera should appear as a red hue through the skin. If it appears white, the flap is too thin and the dermis is likely being exposed. The dissection is aided by palpating over the previously marked boundaries of the femoral triangle externally and viewing this internally with the camera to define the extent of dissection. As the dissection approaches the proximal base of the triangle, the loose areolar tissue overlying the external oblique aponeurosis can be appreciated and can be divided with hook cautery. Note, proximally Scarpa's fascia can be quite thick and be confused with the external oblique aponeurosis. This dissection extends 2–5 cm proximal to the inguinal ligament. The entire superficial dissection over the externally marked triangle should be completed in this step.

Sartorius Dissection

- The subsequent portion of the operation focuses on the lateral dissection. The subcutaneous tissues are divided distally and laterally to identify the sartorius fascia. Once the fascia is identified, it is divided to expose the underlying fibers of the sartorius muscle (Fig. 13.8). The dissection is initially preformed distally and then marched proximally, scoring and

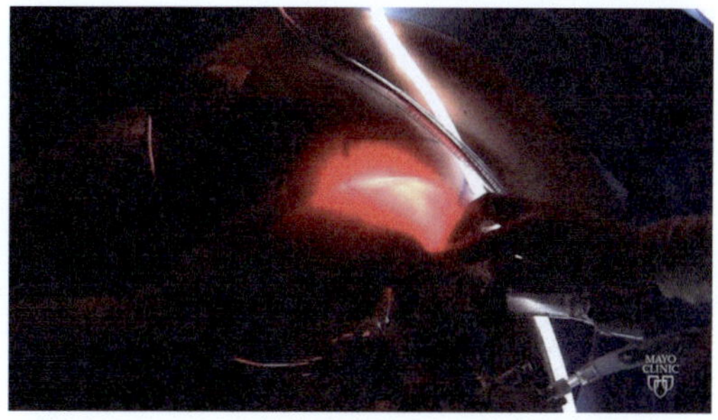

Fig. 13.7 External view of superficial dissection. Once initial CO_2 insufflation has been achieved, external pressure on the marked skin outline of the femoral triangle can be viewed intracorporeally to help define the boundaries for the superficial dissection. The thin tissue flap should appear to have a red hue with transillumination of the flap. If a white hue is present, the flap is too thin. *Image used with permission of Mayo Clinic*

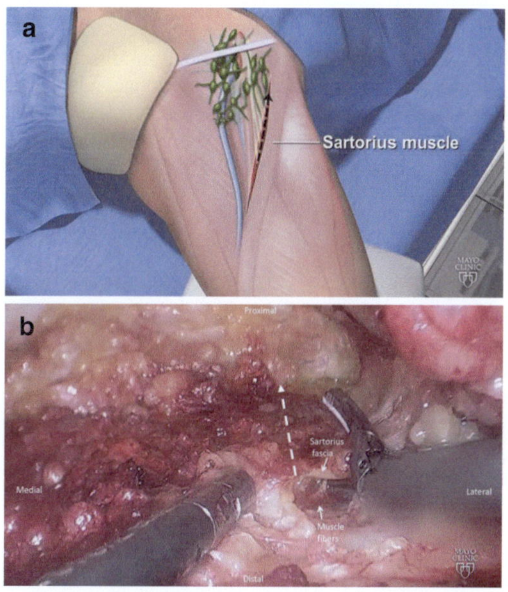

Fig. 13.8 The lateral border of the deep dissection on the sartorius muscle. Diagram (**a**) and intraoperative picture (**b**) of the lateral dissection. Once the sartorius fascia is exposed distally, it is divided exposing the underlying muscle fibers. The specimen is retracted medially and anteriorly while the sartorius fascia is divided until reaching the inguinal ligament proximally (arrow). *Image used with permission of Mayo Clinic*

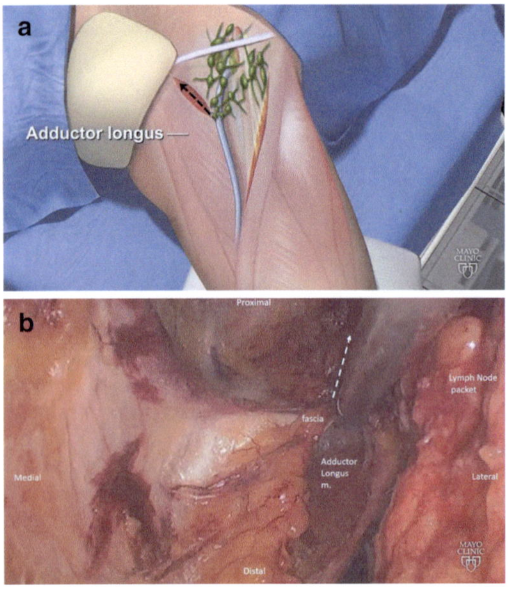

Fig. 13.9 The medial border of the deep dissection on the adductor longus muscle. Diagram (**a**) and intraoperative picture (**b**) of medial border of deep dissection. The adductor longus fascia is divided from distal to proximal to expose the underlying muscle fibers. This is started just proximal to the crossing GSV and carried until reaching the inguinal ligament. *Image used with permission of Mayo Clinic*

dividing the sartorius fascia until the inguinal ligament is reached. The entire medial boarder of the sartorius muscle should be exposed.

Adductor Longus Dissection

- In a similar fashion to the lateral dissection, the medial dissection is performed identifying the adductor longus muscle. The fascia is scored and divided exposing the underlying muscle fibers. Because of the crossing GSV, this dissection is started more proximally on the thigh than the lateral dissection but is also carried until reaching the inguinal ligament (Fig. 13.9).
- The specimen is progressively rolled laterally as this dissection is continued proximally. The underlying pectineus muscle will be exposed more proximally and medially as the inguinal ligament is approached (Fig. 13.10).
- It is not uncommon for the surgeon to feel that the knee is "in the way" during this medial dissection and can be accommodated by flipping the instrument handles "upside-down."

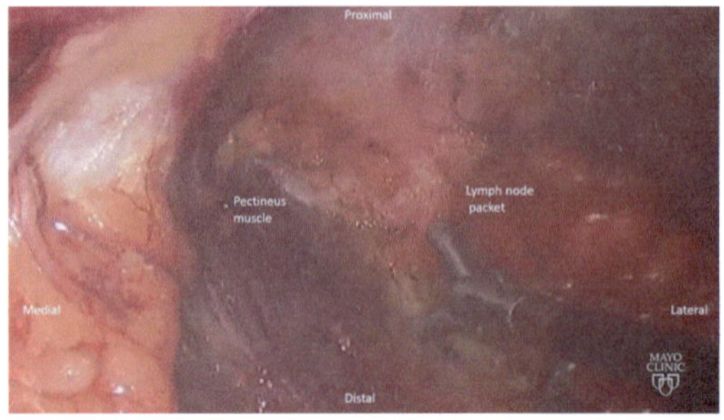

Fig. 13.10 Exposure of the pectineus muscle during the deep medial dissection. The pectineus muscle will be exposed during the proximal portion of the deep medial dissection as the specimen is rolled laterally. *Image used with permission of Mayo Clinic*

Exposure and Identification of Distal Great Saphenous Vein

- The GSV crosses the adductor longus muscle at approximately two-thirds of the distance from the inguinal ligament to the apex of the femoral triangle.
- In order to identify the GSV distally, the dissection is started at the apex of the triangle and carefully dissected proximally until the vein is encountered (Fig. 13.11). Once circumferentially dissected, the vein can be clipped or divided with either an energy device or with an endoscopic stapler, depending on the preference of the surgeon and the quality and size of the vessel. If the vein is entered, there will likely be minimal bleeding secondary to the low venous pressure and CO_2 insufflation. The distal end must be identified and controlled to prevent postoperative bleeding. Division of the GSV is not mandatory in the dissection and we attempt to preserve the GSV when it is not grossly involved with disease.

Apical Dissection and Deep Dissection

- Next, the apical contents of the femoral triangle are dissected free. This is the soft tissue between the sartorius and the adductor longus muscles at the most distal aspect of the opera-

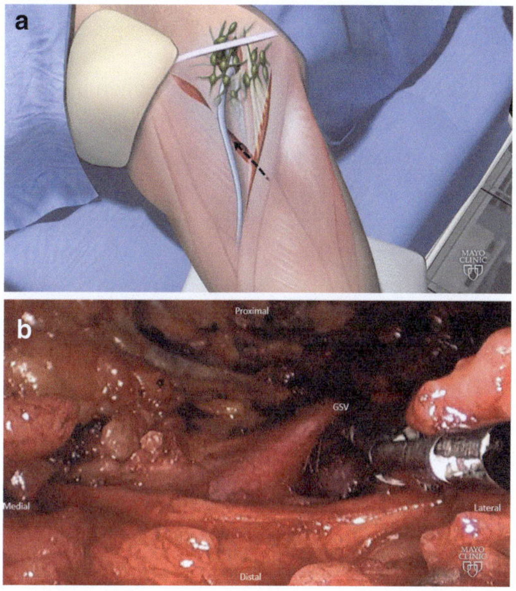

Fig. 13.11 Exposure and division of the distal great saphenous (GSV). Diagram (**a**) and intraoperative picture (**b**) of the deep medial dissection where the GSV is exposed and circumferentially dissected as it crosses the adductor longus muscle. The GSV crosses at two thirds of the distance from the inguinal ligament to the apex of the femoral triangle. Division of the GSV is not mandatory and can be preserved when possible. *Image used with permission of Mayo Clinic*

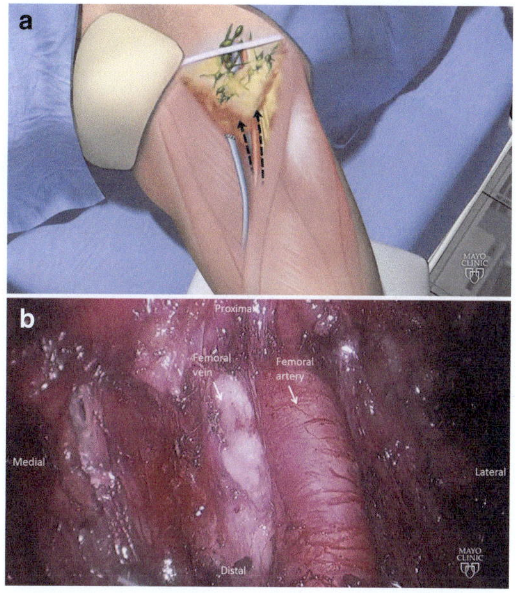

Fig. 13.12 The apical dissection. Diagram (**a**) and intraoperative picture (**b**) of the apical dissection. As the apical dissection and deep dissection proceeds from distal to proximal, the femoral vessels will be encountered. The dissection plane should be carried on the adventitia of the vessels. Dissection should not extend beyond 180 degrees of the femoral vessels. This is most critical laterally to avoid injury to the femoral nerve. Trendelenburg position often aids in the dissection as the contents fall cephalad. *Image used with permission of Mayo Clinic*

tive field. The soft tissue is grasped, elevated, and retracted cephalad while the dissecting hand frees the tissue from any remaining attachments. This is best done with the patient placed in Trendelenburg position. I initially start dividing the distal attachment by making an imaginary line between the medial and distal trocars, joining my distal most, previously created dissection of the adductor and sartorius muscles. As long as the dissection is distal enough, the vessel will be protected and deep to the musculature that forms Hunter's canal. If the dissection is too proximal in this maneuver, the femoral neurovascular bundle may be directly encountered and potentially injured. Identifying the deep border of the dissection distally will allow the dissection to proceed safely proximally and the femoral vessels will gradually come into view (Fig. 13.12).

- It should be noted that because the lower extremity is abducted and flexed at the knee, the femoral artery lies anterior and slightly lateral to the femoral vein within the femoral triangle distally. More proximally, however, the vessels spiral and transition to a more parallel relationship with each other, where the femoral vein lies directly medial to the femoral artery (Fig. 13.13).
- Knowing the relationship of the vessels in the femoral triangle is of paramount importance. Dissection should stay on the peri-adventitial plane. A laparoscopic Kittner blunt dissector can be used to aid in the dissection along with an energy device. The anterior 180 degrees of the vessels should be fully exposed, but there is no need for the vessels to be circumferentially dissected and should be avoided.
- The dissection is then continued by dividing the tissue on the medial aspect of the sartorius muscle and rotating the inguinal contents medially. The femoral nerve lies in this loca-

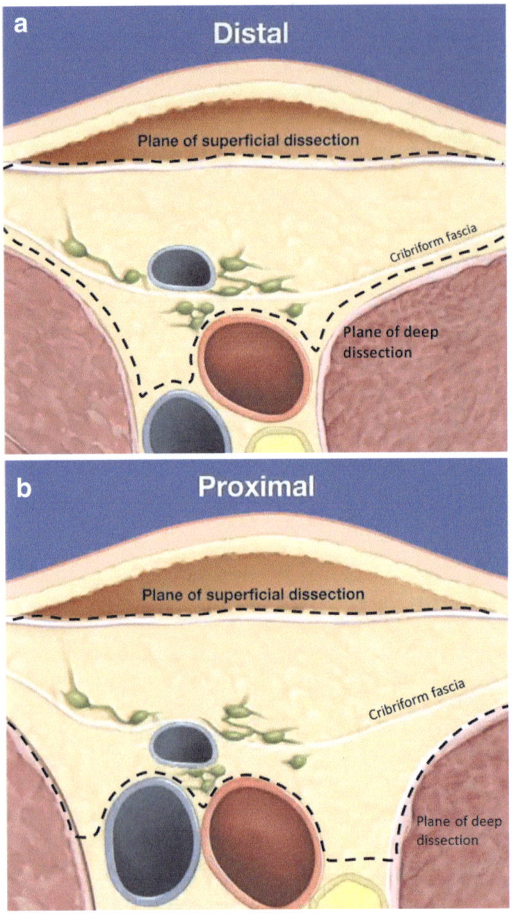

Fig. 13.13 Cross-sectional depictions of the proximal and distal superficial and deep dissection planes. (**a**) The distal dissection starts at the apex of the femoral triangle. The femoral artery here lies anterior and slightly lateral to the femoral vein. The femoral vein will be quite collapsed secondary to the CO_2 insufflation and even more so if Trendelenburg position is utilized. (**b**) The proximal deep dissection extends to the inguinal ligament. The superficial proximal dissection exposes 2–5 cm of the external oblique aponeurosis. The femoral vessels at this location have rotated to reach a parallel configuration with the femoral vein being medial to the femoral artery and nerve. *Image used with permission of Mayo Clinic*

tion, so a thin layer of fat is left on the nerve. The nerve does not need to be exposed and should be at a level about midway the circumference of the artery. Attention to detail here is necessary to avoid a femoral nerve injury.

- This process is repeated sequentially and continued, beginning at the apex and dissecting proximally. The floor of the central dissection will become the adventitia of the femoral vessels.
- During this deep dissection, the deep inguinal nodes, posterior to the cribriform fascia, are elevated and removed en bloc with the specimen. The specimen is continually rotated from distal to proximal, medially off the sartorius and laterally off the adductor, mobilizing all contents centrally onto the femoral vessels. The dissection directly over the vessels is performed last. The femoral vein will be collapsed because of the positive pressure exerted by the CO_2 insufflation and the Trendelenburg position. The caliber of the vein will also fluctuate with respirations. Continued "upward" or anterior tension with the nondominant hand will aid in the dissection over the vessels.

Proximal Dissection

- The medial and anterior surface of the femoral vein should be completely skeletonized. The dissection should be carried proximally with the pectineus muscle becoming the posterior border of the medial dissection. Thorough dissection medial to the common femoral vein is critical as this is where a bulk of the regional lymph nodes resides. The dissection is carried beneath the inguinal ligament (Fig. 13.14). Cloquet's lymph node will be encountered here and can be teased out and removed en bloc with the specimen. Be conscious of a crossing artery and vein that can be spared. A suture can be used to mark the location of Cloquet's node on the specimen if desired. The anterior dissection off the artery should be completed as well. An aggressive dissection lateral to the femoral artery does not need to be performed as there are fewer lymph nodes in this location and the femoral nerve resides there.
- Dissection of the soft tissue off the external oblique is performed with a hook cautery from proximal to distal in the avascular plane directly on the musculature fascia. The cautery is run with the tip parallel to the muscle fibers. The specimen should peel off easily. Positioning the patient into reverse

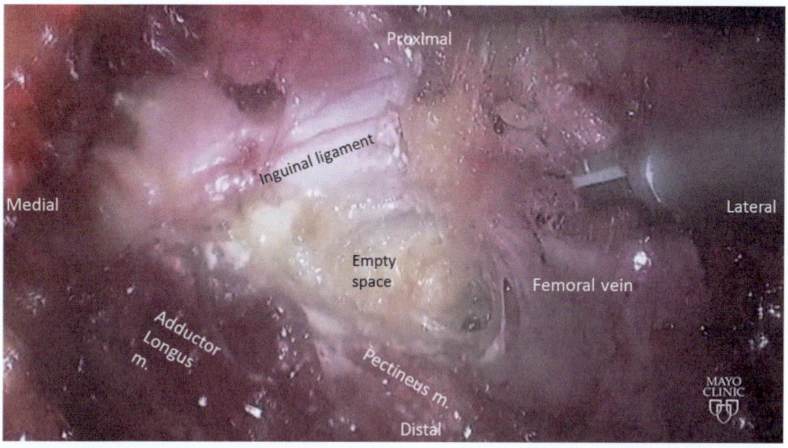

Fig. 13.14 The completed medial dissection. Dissection medial along the femoral vein, including proximally under the inguinal ligament is critical as this is where nodal disease is frequently encountered. After completion of the medial dissection, the inguinal ligament should be exposed proximally, the adductor longus and pectineus muscles distally, and the empty space previously containing Cloquet's node medially, and the media surface of the common femoral vein laterally. *Image used with permission of Mayo Clinic*

Trendelenburg can assist with the proximal dissection.

- As the inferior edge of the inguinal ligament is encountered, the soft tissue should be superficially scored. This will allow entry back into the femoral triangle. Proceeding with caution here is paramount as the femoral vessels are quite superficial with only a thin layer of fat overlying them. As the soft tissue plane at the inferior edge of the inguinal ligament is scored, only the tip of the hook cautery should be used with a lifting motion during cauterization to avoid underlying thermal injury.
- Note that during the most proximal part of the dissection, the surgical instruments will be essentially running parallel to one another making the dissection challenging and frustrating. Patience will be needed as instrument triangulation is not possible. Placement of an additional trocar here may be needed to complete the dissection, especially early in one's experience. We have not had to do this except once in an extremely obese patient, although if struggling a fourth 10mm trocar site will be of no added consequence to the patient.

Proximal Dissection of the Great Saphenous Vein at the Fossa Ovalis

- At this point, the SFJ will be encountered as the GSV enters the femoral vein. After piercing the cribriform fascia at the fossa ovalis, the GSV drains directly into the anterior surface of the femoral vein, approximately 3 cm distal to the inguinal ligament. If a SFV preserving procedure is not possible, the SFJ should be cleared of any soft tissue and divided with a linear endovascular stapler (Fig. 13.15). A generous dissection around the SFJ will need to be undertaken, including proximal on the common femoral vein in order to have an adequate working space for the stapler. The stapler tips must be seen prior to firing and the superficial and common femoral vein visualized continuously posterior to the stapler. Slight rotation of the stapler and changing the camera angles is helpful. After dividing the GSV at the SFJ, the remaining tissue is then removed as necessary from the proximal vessels.
- Any additional medial and lateral attachments should be divided so that the specimen is com-

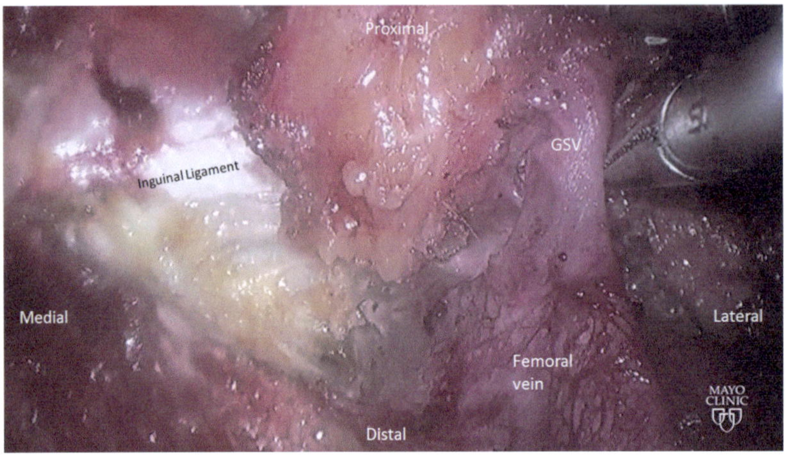

Fig. 13.15 Division of the GSV at the saphenofemoral junction. The GSV pierces the cribriform fascia and enters the femoral vein anteriorly, approximately 3 cm distal to the inguinal ligament. The soft tissue surrounding the saphenofemoral junction should be cleared, and the GSV can be divided with a linear stapler. *Image used with permission of Mayo Clinic*

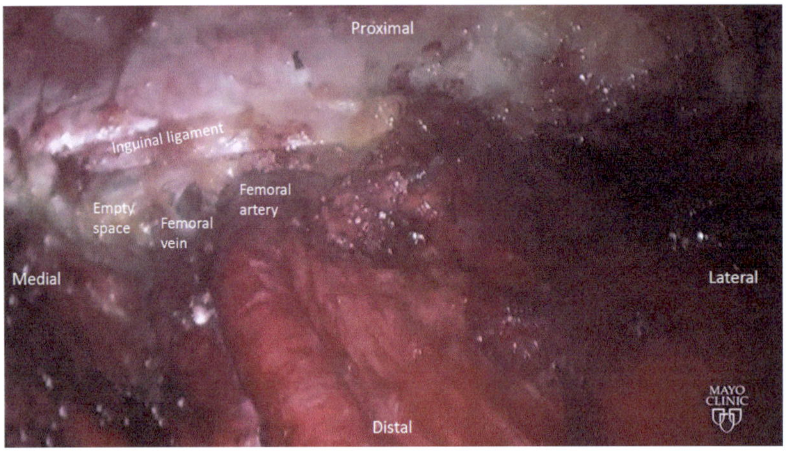

Fig. 13.16 The completed MILND. Intraoperative picture of the completed dissection field with removal of the inguinal lymph node contents. Note the femoral vessels exposed at the deep margin of the dissection plane and the inguinal ligament and external oblique aponeurosis at the most proximal border of the dissection field. *Image used with permission of Mayo Clinic*

pletely free. The dissection should now be complete (Fig. 13.16).

Preservation of the Great Saphenous Vein

- As previously discussed, the GSV can be preserved and division is not mandatory. It is generally our preference to do so if the vein is not involved by metastatic disease. For GSV preservation, dissection from distal to proximal on the GSV should be performed. As the dissection is carried proximal and the SFJ is approached, additional branches entering the vein will need to be divided with harmonic scalpel or other energy devise. On the posterior aspect of the proximal GSV, a small portion of the soft tissue specimen will need to be divided to allow 360-degree exposure of the GSV as it enters the femoral vein and allow the specimen to be freed from the GSV.

Specimen Removal

- The specimen is placed in an endobag. The surgical field is carefully inspected, and hemostasis is ensured. Topical TXA can be applied to the wound bed. A trocar site incision is extended as minimal as possible to allow extraction. Backward, forward, and circular rotation of the bag while applying a steady pull will allow the specimen to slowly creep out of the defect. Spreading with a Wiley retractor can assist in this maneuver. A 15 French round Jackson-Pratt drain is introduced through the medial trocar site and brought out through the lateral trocar site. The drain is secured with a nylon suture (Fig. 13.17). All incisions are closed with interrupted 3-0 Vicryl® (Ethicon, Inc, Bridgewater, NJ) in the deep dermis. A running 4-0 Monocryl® (Ethicon, Inc., Bridgewater, NJ) subcuticular stitch is used to close this skin. The deep dermal sutures around the drain must be placed as secure and abutting the drain as possible to avoid an air leak. The nylon stitch securing the drain is placed abutting the drain as well to eliminate the possibility of air leak and the drain not holding suction. Sterile dressings are applied. The lower extremity can be wrapped in Ace compression bandages or the patient can be seen by a lymphedema specialist on postoperative day 1 for leg compression. Similarly, compression shorts are placed intraoperatively or on postoperative day 1. It is common for the scrotum to be edematous from CO_2 insufflation. This typically resolves by the morning after surgery. Crepitance up to the level of the chest strap can at times be observed from the CO_2 insufflation and is not uncommon. This is of no clinical significance and will resolve without intervention. A low placed chest strap can be used during the operative procedure to avoid subcutaneous air dissecting into the neck, which is also of no consequences but can cause the anesthesia team angst.

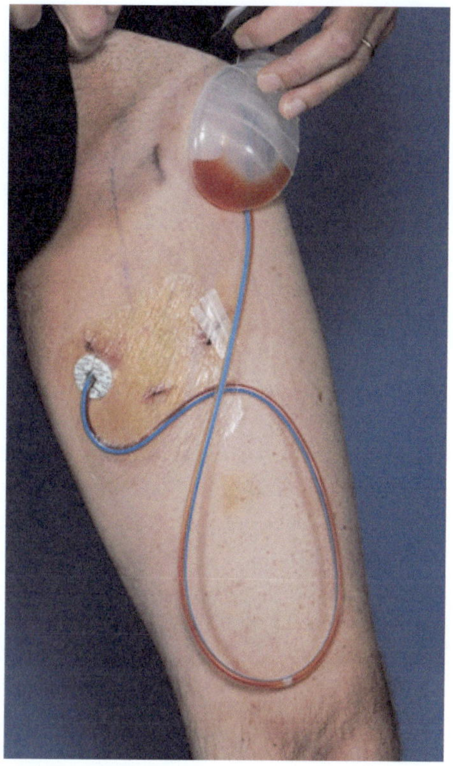

Fig. 13.17 Picture of the postoperative leg. A Jackson-Pratt drain is brought out through the incision and secured with a nylon stitch. Our practice has evolved into placing the drain through the lateral trocar site as it results in better ergonomics for the patient. It is placed through the medial trocar site in this picture. Note that the most proximal incision adjacent to the inguinal ligament is from a previous sentinel lymph node biopsy. *Image used with permission of Mayo Clinic*

13.5 Intraoperative Techniques to Reduce Seroma Formation

- Seroma formation and prolonged drain days remains the major morbidity associated with MILND. Our practice has evolved throughout the years employing different techniques intended to reduce the incidence of seroma based on literature from open inguinal lymphadenectomy and breast surgery. We have attempted using different tissue sealing devises (LigaSureTM vs Harmonic Scalpel), performing a more superficial deep dissection when oncologically appropriate and reducing the bulk of the lymphadenectomy by preserving the cribriform fascia distal to the fossa ovalis, quilting the tissue flaps at the end of the operation to reduce the postoperative dead space, and preserving the saphenous vein, all with no significant changes in the seroma rate. In general, there is no need to dissect the soft tissue and muscular fascia off the anterior surface of the sartorius and adductor muscles except what is needed centrally to expose the femoral triangle. We also have attempted lymphatic channel mapping with blue dye injections at the end of surgery to identify any leaking lymphatic channel; however, this too has shown little promise in reducing our postoperative seroma rate. We have used postoperative external compression as standard. Asking patients to minimize mobilization and at the extreme bedrest can have some efficacy; however, this must be balanced with the risk of venous thromboembolic events. At this time, we have not yet attempted immediate lymphatic reconstruction via a prophylactic lympho-venous bypass at the completion of the procedure.

13.6 Postoperative Care

- Patients are scheduled as outpatient overnight procedures and can be considered for same day discharge as long as all drain instructions, education, and wound care instructions have been provided in advance and are able to be followed.
- As previously mentioned, postoperative care is aimed at reducing drain days, reducing the risk of lymphedema and seroma formation. Our patients undergo baseline preoperative limb volume measurements and lymphedema education.
- Patients are seen prior to discharge by the physical medicine and lymphedema therapists. Compression dressings are applied to the thigh and operative sites.
- Our practice continues to evolve. Initially, patients were recommended to have limited activity until the drains were removed. This later changed to no activity with bed rest at home and now has changed back to limited activity as the "no activity" regimen did not seem to reduce the incidence of seroma or drain days in our patients. In patients with high prolonged drain output we have seen a dramatic impact with strict bedrest. Unfortunately, this is not practical for a prolonged period and has its own set of consequences.
- Postoperative antibiotics are not indicated. Redness of the flap is common and seen on the first postoperative day and on the first postoperative visit a week later. This represents mild ischemia and bruising. Cellulitis and surgical site infection are very rare, and antibiotics are not indicated for this expected postoperative finding.
- Patients are educated on drain care prior to discharge and are appropriately counseled to expect surgical drains for a prolonged period of time. Our practice has taken two approaches to determining when drains can be removed:
    1. Leave the drain until the output is 30–40 mL for 2 consecutive days. This can mean keeping the drain in for as long as 7 weeks before outputs decrease enough to meet criteria.
    2. Remove the drain in 4 weeks and accept an increased risk of seroma. If seromas do occur, observing asymptomatic seromas is reasonable. They can also be managed with serial ultrasound-guided drainage and not infrequently placement of a new drain through a new cutaneous entry site. This is probably preferred secondary to increased risk of infection with prolonged drain days.
- Drain care consists of placement of a Biopatch® (Wolf Medical Supply Inc, Sunrise, FL) at the drain skin exit site, which is covered with a Tegaderm™ (3M, Minneapolis, MN) dressing and changed every 3 days.
- Patients can shower on postoperative day 1. They should not submerge the drain or incisions under water while the drain remains in place.

13.7 Potential Complications

- Seroma
- Hematoma
- Flap necrosis
- Major vascular injury
- Deep venous thrombosis
- Femoral nerve injury
- Lymphedema
- Infection
- Anesthesia risks
- Hypercarbia intraoperatively leading to conversion to open technique
- Recent incisions in the dissection field, such as a SLN biopsy site, can dehisce postoperatively.

13.8 Our Tips

- If performing MILND for positive SLN biopsy, we typically wait a minimum of 6 weeks to allow the acute inflammation to subside.
- Schedule a light day for your first few cases, especially if bilateral, until you gain more experience. Consider making this your only scheduled case for the day while starting out.
- Communicate with anesthesia to adjust minute ventilation and avoid hypercarbia. Failing to do so can require unnecessary conversion to an open procedure.
- Consider a chest strap to prevent crepitance up the chest/neck from insufflation. This is not a medical issue, even though it can be unsettling to the anesthesia team.
- If the operative leg is not abducted and the knee not flexed, the femoral triangle will not be brought anterior. This may result in misidentification of the dissection field and starting the dissection too laterally.
- Creating the initial working plane without marking the trocar sites can make the incisions too large and create a CO_2 leak. If there is not sufficient attention to detail during these steps, unnecessary frustration throughout most of the case can follow.
- The initial working space will have limited view and exposure. It takes some patience to create this working space. In the first few cases, it may be unsettling to have such a limited working space. With experience, creating the anterior flap through this initial limited exposure can be done very quickly and safely.
- Bring the drain out through the lateral trocar site. This will result in better patient comfort.
- Be very conscious to seal the skin and soft tissue around the drain. Unlike in other locations, there is only skin separating the dissection cavity from the outside world with essentially no additional soft tissue to internally buttress. Failing to seal around the drain can lead to air leak and inability to hold suction, which may necessitate additional drain placement to decompress the dissection cavity.

References

1. MacCormac W. Five cases of amputation of the penis for epithelioma. Br J Med. 1886;1:343.
2. Basset A. L'epithelioma primitif du clitoris; son retenissement ganglionaire et son traiement operatoire. Paris: G Steinheil; 1912.
3. Cabanas RM. An approach for the treatment of penile carcinoma. Cancer. 1977 Feb;39(2):456–66. https://doi.org/10.1002/1097-0142(197702)39:2<456::aid-cncr2820390214>3.0.co;2-i.
4. Chang SB, Askew RL, Xing Y, et al. Prospective assessment of postoperative complications and associated costs following inguinal lymph node dissection (ILND) in melanoma patients. Ann Surg Oncol. 2010;17(10):2764–72.
5. Serpell JW, Carne PW, Bailey M. Radical lymph node dissection for melanoma. ANZ J Surg. 2003;73(5):294–9.
6. Coit DG, Peters M, Brennan MF. A prospective randomized trial of perioperative cefazolin treatment in axillary and groin dissection. Arch Surg. 1991;126:1366–71.
7. Sarnaik AA, Puleo CA, Zager JS, Sondak VK. Limiting the morbidity of inguinal lymphadenectomy for metastatic melanoma. Cancer Control. 2009;16(3):240–7.
8. Martin BM, Etra JW, Russell MC, et al. Oncologic outcomes of patients undergoing videoscopic ingui-

nal lymphadenectomy for metastatic melanoma. J Am Coll Surg. 2014;218(4):620–6.
9. Abbott AM, Grotz TE, Rueth NM, et al. Minimally invasive inguinal lymph node dissection (MILND) for melanoma: experience from two academic centers. Ann Surg Oncol. 2013;20(1):340–5.
10. Sommariva A, Pasquali S, Cona C, et al. Videoscopic ilioinguinal lymphadenectomy for groin lymph node metastases from melanoma. Br J Surg. 2016;103(8):1026–32.
11. Jakub JW, Terando AM, Sarnaik A, et al. Training high-volume melanoma surgeons to perform a novel minimally invasive inguinal lymphadenectomy: report of a prospective multi-institutional trial. J Am Coll Surg. 2016;222(3):253–60.
12. Jakub JW, Terando AM, Sarnaik A, et al. Safety and feasibility of minimally invasive inguinal lymph node dissection in patients with melanoma (SAFE-MILND): report of a prospective multi-institutional trial. Ann Surg. 2017;265(1):192–6.
13. Sommarivia A, Cona C, Tonello M, et al. Oncological outcome of videoscopic groin dissection for lymph node metastasis from melanoma. Surg Endoscopy. 2020. https://doi.org/10.1007/s00464-020-07675-5
14. Jakub JW, Lowe M, Howard JH, et al. Oncologic outcomes of multi-institutional minimally invasive inguinal lymph node dissection for melanoma compared with open inguinal dissection in the second multicenter selective lymphadenectomy trial (MSLT-II). Ann Surg Onc. published on line May 2, 2022. https://doi.org/10.1245/s10434-022-11758-z
15. Teramoto Y, Nakamura Y, Sato S, Yamazaki N, Yamamoto A. Low probability of lymphatic drainage to Cloquet's node is of limited value as indicator for pelvic lymph node dissection in patients with lower limb melanoma. Lymphat Res Biol. 2016;14(2):109–14. https://doi.org/10.1089/lrb.2015.0007.
16. Faries MB, Thompson JF, Cochran AJ, Andtbacka RH, Mozzillo N, Zager JS, Jahkola T, Bowles TL, Testori A, Beitsch PD, Hoekstra HJ, et al. Completion dissection or observation for sentinel-node metastasis in melanoma. N Eng J Med. 376: 2211–222
17. Blank CU, Lucas MW, Scolyer RA, van de Wiel BA, Menzies AM, Lopez-Yurda M, Hoeijmakers LL, Saw RPM, Lijnsvelt JM, Maher NG, Pulleman SM, Gonzalez M, Torres Acosta A, van Houdt WJ, Lo SN, Kuijpers AMJ, Spillane A, Klop WMC, Pennington TE, Zuur CL, Shannon KF, Seinstra BA, Rawson RV, Haanen JBAG, Ch'ng S, Naipal KAT, Stretch J, van Thienen JV, Rtshiladze MA, Wilgenhof S, Kapoor R, Meerveld-Eggink A, Grijpink-Ongering LG, van Akkooi ACJ, Reijers ILM, Gyorki DE, 2 Grünhagen DJ, Speetjens FM, Vliek SB, Placzke J, Spain L, Stassen RC, Amini-Adle M, Lebbé C, Faries MB, Robert C, Ascierto PA, van Rijn R, van den Berkmortel FWPJ, Piersma D, van der Westhuizen A, Vreugdenhil G, Aarts MJB, Stevense-den Boer MAM, Atkinson V, Khattak M, Andrews MC, van den Eertwegh AJM, Boers-Sonderen MJ, Hospers GAP, Carlino MS, de Groot JB, Kapiteijn E, Suijkerbuijk KPM, Rutkowski P, Sandhu S, van der Veldt AAM, Long GV. Neoadjuvant Nivolumab and Ipilimumab in Resectable Stage III Melanoma. N Engl J Med. 2024;391(18):1696–1708. https://doi.org/10.1056/NEJMoa2402604. Epub 2024 Jun 2. PMID: 38828984.
18. Reijers ILM, Menzies AM, van Akkooi ACJ, Versluis JM, van den Heuvel NMJ, Saw RPM, Pennington TE, Kapiteijn E, van der Veldt AAM, Suijkerbuijk KPM, Hospers GAP, Rozeman EA, Klop WMC, van Houdt WJ, Sikorska K, van der Hage JA, Grünhagen DJ, Wouters MW, Witkamp AJ, Zuur CL, Lijnsvelt JM, Torres Acosta A, Grijpink-Ongering LG, Gonzalez M, Jóźwiak K, Bierman C, Shannon KF, Ch'ng S, Colebatch AJ, Spillane AJ, Haanen JBAG, Rawson RV, van de Wiel BA, van de Poll-Franse LV, Scolyer RA, Boekhout AH, Long GV, Blank CU. Personalized response-directed surgery and adjuvant therapy after neoadjuvant ipilimumab and nivolumab in high-risk stage III melanoma: the PRADO trial. Nat Med. 2022;28(6):1178–1188. https://doi.org/10.1038/s41591-022-01851-x. Epub 2022 Jun 5. PMID: 35661157.
19. Reynolds HM, Dunbar PR, Uren RF, Blackett SA, Thompson JF, Smith NP. Three-dimensional visualization of lymphatic drainage patterns in patients with cutaneous melanoma. Lancet Oncol. 2007;8:801–12.
20. Contreras N, Jakub JW. The Achilles heel of minimally invasive inguinal lymph node dissection: Seroma formation. Am J Surg. 2020;219(4):696–700.

14 Transoral Robotic Surgery for Head and Neck Cancer

Albert Y. Han and Abie H. Mendelsohn

Abstract

Transoral robotic surgery (TORS) has rapidly changed the field of head and neck surgery since its initial FDA approval in 2009. By combining excellent visualization and multiple degrees of freedom, robotic surgical systems allow precision surgery in areas that were previously only accessible through open approaches associated with high morbidity. In this chapter, we will review the history of TORS and its expanding application for minimally invasive surgical resection of the upper aerodigestive tract. The use of the robotic system requires specialized training for the surgeon as well as trained staff to maintain efficiency throughout the case. This includes availability of consistent room setup, ergonomic interior layout, wide range of available retractors and instruments, and personnel such as a surgical assistant and operating room staff. Operative techniques used in common TORS surgeries are introduced in this chapter. We conclude the chapter by illustrating the postoperative course, complications, and a clinical case example.

Keywords

Transoral robotic surgery · Da Vinci surgical robot · Oropharyngeal cancer · Throat cancer

14.1 Introduction

The development of robotic instrumentation for surgery of the head and neck grew out of advancements in camera and robotic technology. Transoral robotic surgery (TORS) has gained popularity especially due to the increasing incidence of human papillomavirus-related oropharyngeal cancers that often present as surgical resectable lesions in the throat [1]. The clearance of gross disease by robotic surgery has gained favor in the interest of deintensifying postoperative chemoradiation after excision [2]. The advancement of sophisticated robotic systems from multiport to single port, and the

Supplementary Information The online version contains supplementary material available at https://doi.org/10.1007/978-981-97-7059-5_14.

A. Y. Han
Department of Otolaryngology—Head and Neck Surgery, Keck School of Medicine of USC, University of Southern California, Los Angeles, CA, USA

A. H. Mendelsohn (✉)
Department of Head and Neck Surgery, David Geffen School of Medicine at University of California, Los Angeles (UCLA), Los Angeles, CA, USA

UCLA Head and Neck Cancer Program, UCLA Medical Center, Los Angeles, CA, USA
e-mail: AMendelsohn@mednet.ucla.edu

M. Tewari (ed.), *Minimally Invasive Surgery in Cancer*,
https://doi.org/10.1007/978-981-97-7059-5_14

development of wireless capabilities and miniaturization allow the use of robotic systems in head and neck surgery to expand dramatically the diversity of surgical options available for the patient.

14.2 History of Transoral Robotic Surgery

The use of robotic arms initially began with image-guided precision biopsies of the brain. In 1985, Unimation PUMA 560 was designed to assist with accurate CT-guided brain biopsies [3]. Innovations in robotic surgery continued with miniaturization and high-definition 3D cameras [4]. The first robotic surgical system approved by the United States Food and Drug Administration (FDA) was the ROBODOC developed in 1992, which was designed for use during total hip arthroplasty [5]. With the advent of high-definition endoscopes, robotic surgical systems evolved to include three-dimensional views of the operative field. Following the success of ZEUS, where the surgical console is physically distant from the robotic instrumentation, Intuitive Systems (Sunnyvale, CA) designed the da Vinci robotic systems [6].

The feasibility of TORS was initially confirmed in animal and cadaver models. Early studies were based on multiport systems. The first documented use of a robot for head and neck surgery was the robot-assisted salivary gland resection and neck dissection in Yorkshire pigs [7]. McLeod et al. performed the first pharyngeal surgery (excision of vallecular cyst) in a patient [8]. Subsequently, Hockstein and O'Malley demonstrated TORS in patients with base of tongue cancers in 2006 [9]. Since this time, the indications of TORS have rapidly expanded to the larynx, hypopharynx, and parapharyngeal space. The FDA approved the use of da Vinci robots to perform TORS for oropharyngeal squamous cell carcinomas in 2009. It continues to provide an effective, minimally invasive approach for optimal patient outcomes. Most recently, a novel single-port flexible robot was developed and was successfully tested in Phase I and II clinical trials [10, 11]. The SP system utilizes three 6-mm instruments attached via flexible joints that are deployed into the surgical target.

14.3 Patient Positioning and Operating Room Setup

Optimal layout of equipment and instrumentation is key for efficient flow of robotic surgeries. The patient is generally intubated by a seasoned anesthesiologist to avoid avulsing the tumor. A shoulder roll and mouth guard are placed. The patient is positioned supine and turned 180-degrees away from the anesthesiologist. The operating room setup is outlined in Fig. 14.1. The da Vinci robotic system consists of the surgeon console (Fig. 14.2a) and patient-side cart (Fig. 14.2b, c). The patient side cart is introduced from the patient's right side after the patient has been turned. The assistant is positioned at the head of the patient to provide retraction and suction. The surgeon console is ideally positioned close to the assistant, nursing staff, and the anesthesiologist to ensure close communication.

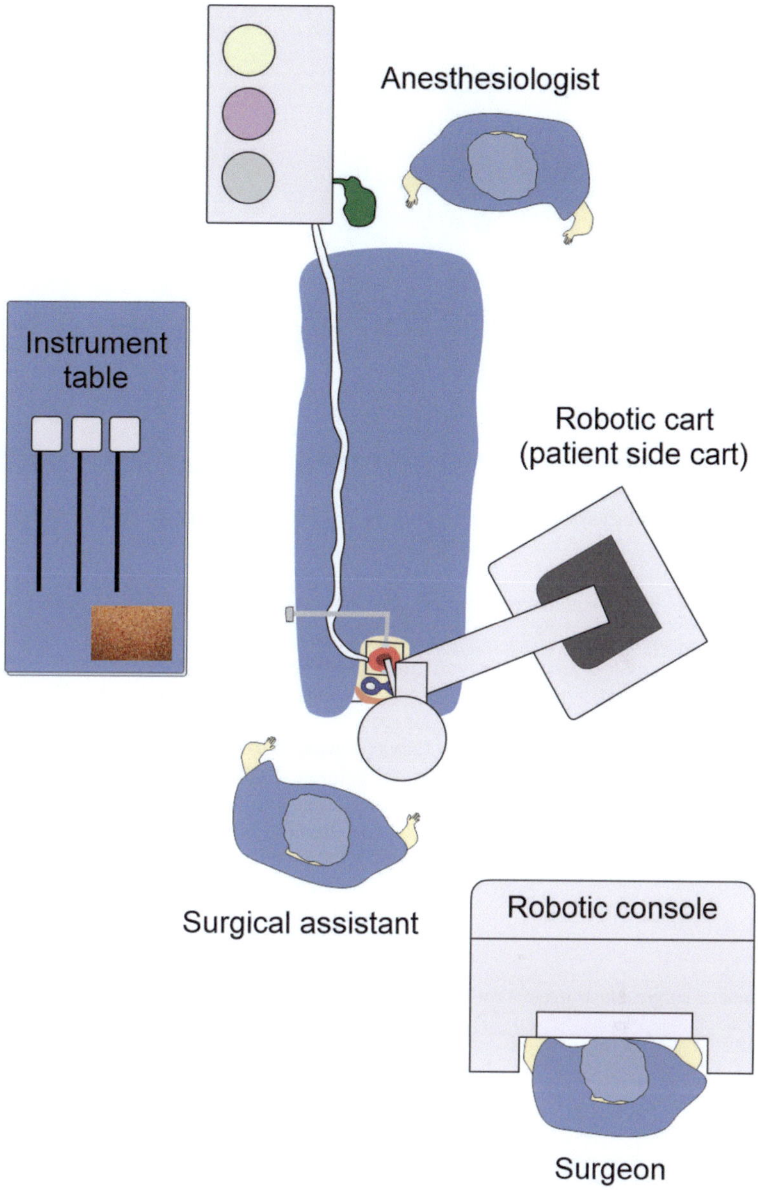

Fig. 14.1 Transoral robotic surgery room layout. For optimal communication, the anesthesiologist, surgical assistant, and the surgeon should all be in close proximity from one another

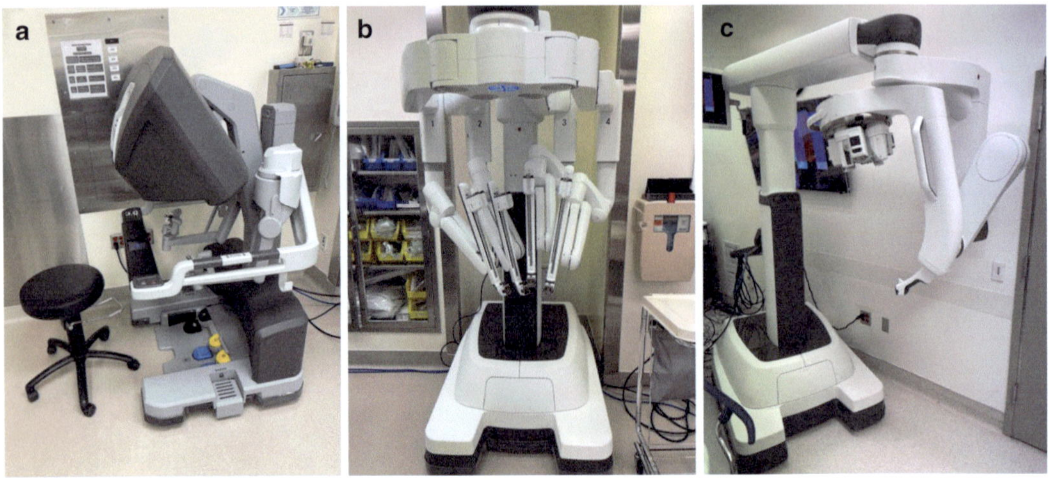

Fig. 14.2 Da Vinci system surgeon console (**a**), Xi patient side cart (**b**), and SP patient side cart (**c**)

Table 14.1 Equipment, instruments and consumables frequently used for transoral robotic surgeries

Mouth gags/retractors	Dingman mouth gag: oral cavity Crowe-Davis retractor: oropharynx (tonsils, base of tongue) Feyh-Kastenbauer (FK) retractor: larynx, hypopharynx, and select base of tongue Larynx Advanced Retractor System (LARS)
Equipment specific to robot arms	Intuitive Surgical high-magnification camera head (45 FOV) Intuitive Surgical wide-angle camera head (60 FOV) 30-degree Intuitive Surgical endoscope 0-degree Intuitive Surgical endoscope Chairs with adjustable height using a foot pedal 5 mm Endowrist Instrumentation – Monopolar cautery with spatula tip – Maryland dissector
General surgical instrumentation	Electrocautery unit Bipolar electrocautery Headlamps Kelly clamps Needle driver 2–0 Silk sutures (for specimen orientation); 3–0 Vicryl for parapharyngeal space tumors Surgical clips for ligation of vessels by assistant
Consumables	Tooth guard Shoulder roll Eye protection goggles Flexible suction to be placed in the nose Mini Yankauer suction Specimen Cork Board with 25G needles for fixation

14.4 List of Specific Equipment and Instruments Used

An array of equipment and instruments must be prepared for both initial setup and surgical manipulation. This includes standard mouth retractors for optimal exposure of the surgical site and instruments for suctioning secretions and smoke in addition to the robot-specific instrumentation. The recommended list of equipment and consumables can be found in Table 14.1.

14.5 Operative Techniques Used in Common TORS Procedures

TORS can be applied to disease localized in all parts of the upper aerodigestive tract, including the oral cavity, oropharynx, larynx, and hypopharynx. The operative techniques used in common surgeries are illustrated in this text.

14.6 TORS for Base of Tongue Resection

After informed consent is obtained, the patient is brought to the operating room where general endotracheal anesthesia is administered after which the patient is rotated 180 degrees away from anesthesia, and a shoulder roll and tooth guard are placed. The patient is intubated with oral or nasal intubation using a laser-safe endotracheal tube [12]. The authors usually begin with a careful assessment for visualization and palpation of the tumor for operative planning. A Dedo laryngoscope is then placed intraorally and advanced to the glottis, the pyriform sinuses bilaterally, the vallecula, and bilateral tonsillar fossa. Each of these areas is closely inspected with the use of operative telescope. The pharyngoepiglottic fold is carefully inspected to determine whether it is involved in any detected mucosal region. The procedure proceeds with selective neck dissection with ipsilateral arterial branch ligation.

Once the selective neck dissection is completed, the procedure continues with the transoral robotic portion. The TORS portion may be performed prior to open neck surgery per surgeon preference. A Crowe-Davis, Feyh-Kastenbauer (FK) or LARS retractor is introduced into the mouth, advanced to the base of tongue. It is held in open retraction and placed in suspension.

The choice of retractor depends on the location of the tumor. Feyh-Kastenbauer (FK) retractors are most widely used with the tongue apex retracted with a double suture, allowing for optimal visualization of the base of tongue down to the vallecula [13]. The FK retractor comes with a wide variety of tongue blades with lateralized cuts specific for laterality of interest [9]. The Crowe-Davis retractor, which is also used for conventional tonsillectomy and transoral laser microsurgeries, is also used in TORS [12].

It is critical to confirm that the exposure allows visualization of the inferior boundary of the tumor. A 0-degree telescope is then used to confirm adequate visualization of the pharyngeal region and the lateral base of tongue. A 30-degree, upward facing endoscope can be used for greater access into the vallecula as in the original description by O'Malley and Weinstein [9]. The da Vinci system is then stationed at the patient's right side, where the semiflexible endoscopes, the dissecting forceps, and the spatula Bovie are placed on the robotic arms. The instruments are then docked within the patient's oral cavity.

With the assistant surgeon positioned at the head of the patient bed for retraction and suction, the operative surgeon is seated at the operative console. A Bovie monopolar electrocautery is used to incise the mucosa surrounding the tongue tumor with at least 5 mm of visualized clean margins peripherally. The procedure begins with a transverse cut anterior to the tumor. The next incision is a lateral cut along the glossotonsillar sulcus or into the tonsillar fossa. A medial cut is made down to the level of the intrinsic tongue muscles, inferior to the pharyngoepiglottic fold.

The tumor is continuously mobilized in the lateral, medial, and superior directions. The dorsal lingual artery can be seen laterally and clipped using surgical clips (two medially; one laterally). The lingual artery is sometimes seen, and its general location is approximately 1.5 cm deep from the musculature and 1.0 cm medial to the border of lateral base of tongue [9]. With the last remaining peripheral attachments resected, the tumor is then delivered through the mouth and inspected closely on the back table.

For tonsillar tumors:

The procedure begins by creating an incision just anterior to the anterior tonsillar pillar down to the palatoglossal muscle (Fig. 14.3a, b). A deep plane of dissection can be carried into the pharyngeal constrictors for endophytic areas of the tonsil. The incision is then carried down onto the posterior pharyngeal wall to the junction between the lateral wall and the posterior pharyngeal wall (Fig. 14.3c, d). If found to have tumor involvement, then the styloglossus muscle within the midportion of the tonsillar fossa can be divided. This will achieve a plane of dissection between the lateral pharyngeal muscles and the parapharyngeal space fat (along with its associated vasculature; Fig. 14.3e, f). This can be traced down the inferior aspect of the deep margin to expose the lingual artery, which may require surgical clipping and then transecting to release this aspect of the cancer. A surgical clip is left along the deepest aspect of the specimen as well as along the stump of the artery within the lateral pharynx. The deep margin is then released (Fig. 14.3g). The specimen is then oriented on the cork board (Fig. 14.3h).

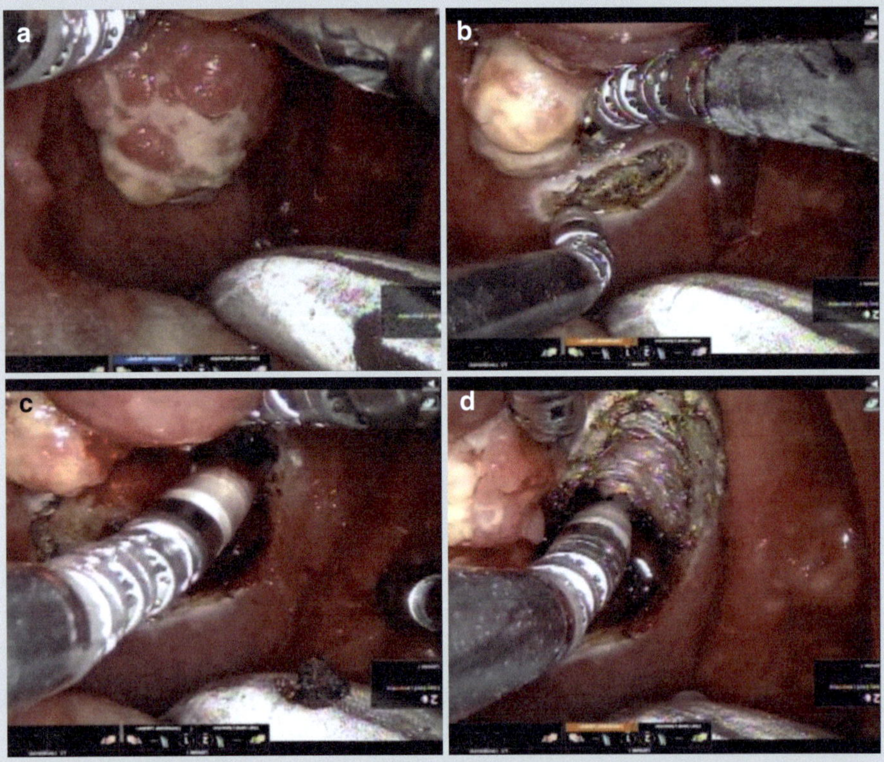

Fig. 14.3 TORS tonsillectomy for squamous cell carcinoma of the tonsil. Tumor identification (**a**). Posterior cut is made first (**b**), and the incision is extended medially (**c**, **d**). The incision is deepened and extended laterally (**e**). The tumor is freed from its deep attachments (**f**) then subsequently removed (**g**). (**h**) shows the specimen in its orientation

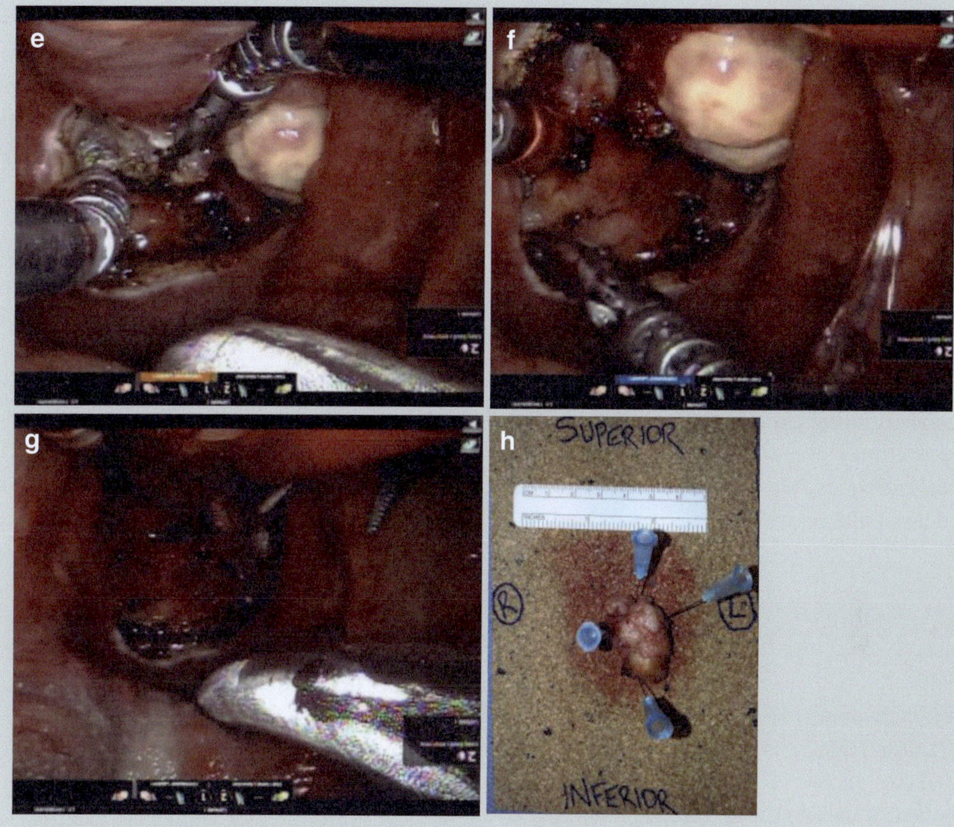

Fig. 14.3 (continued)

The margins are assessed by visual inspection and palpation. Mucosal margins are taken in four quadrants and deep margins from the specimen. The specimens are sent to pathology for intraoperative frozen section analysis. If a positive margin is observed, re-resection must be attempted to clear the disease. This concludes the surgery. All retractors are withdrawn from the patient, and the patient is turned to the anesthesiologist for extubation.

FDA approval of the use of da Vinci Xi for TORS is still pending at the time of writing; making an "off-label" use for pharyngeal and base of tongue resections. The literature supports overall benefit from the use of flexible and versatile robotic arms resulting in shorter operative time and lower postoperative pain [13]. The newer single port (da Vinci SP) system was FDA approved for lateral oropharyngectomy procedures (i.e., radical tonsillectomy) and tongue base resection in 2019.

14.7 TORS for Laryngeal Surgeries

Since the seminal publications of prospective data on TORS partial laryngectomy [14, 15], TORS systems have become more widely available and have been enhanced with improved exposure and visualization. Here we describe an example of TORS-assisted cordectomy for early (T1-T2) glottic cancers (European Laryngological

Society type III [16]). Patient selection is key because the base of tongue anatomy and the size of the robotic arms can result in difficulties when obtaining exposure [17].

After informed consent is obtained, the patient is brought to the operating room where general anesthesia is induced. The patient may receive either nasal (preferred with 5.5 or 6.0 tube for glottic primary) or oral intubation [18]. The patient is then rotated 180 degrees away from the anesthesiologist. An operative distending pharyngolaryngeal retractor system (i.e., LARS) is placed intraorally and advanced to the glottis, with good resulting exposure of the larynx. The authors routinely use LARS retractor for TORS laryngeal surgeries, although FK retractors can be used as an alternative [18].

Optimal exposure is critical for TORS laryngeal surgeries. Similar to De Virgilio et al., the authors recommend anterior traction of the tongue, use of muscle relaxants, and angled scopes [19]. Surgical manipulation of the aerodigestive tract to improve access (partial epiglottectomy, temporary tracheostomy) should be performed only after careful consideration of risks and benefits [20].

The SP robotic surgical system is parked on the patient's right side. Using the robotic endoscope and surgical instruments, the glottis is closely inspected. In this case, the examination demonstrated a vocal fold lesion positioned along the posterior one-third of the right vocal fold, extending up onto the superior surface of the vocal fold and extending anteriorly, but stopping well short of the anterior commissure. Occasionally, a considerable amount of chronic laryngeal irritation and edema can be seen, presumably from poorly controlled laryngopharyngeal reflux disease.

Using both cutting Bovie energy as well as sharp resection with the robotic scissors, the resection begins along the right false vocal fold, and it is carried posteriorly onto the body of the arytenoid and down to resect the vocal process along with the attachment of the vocal ligament (to ensure intramuscular resection of the cancer). CO_2 laser can be used in TORS for glottic cancers, similar to transoral laser microsurgery (TLM) [21]. The posterior cuts are made first because they are often obscured by the pooling of blood. A deep cut is made within the vocal musculature. We then create circumferential incisions of the partial laryngectomy anteriorly directly within the anterior commissure and down to include the infraglottic mucosa. Ultimately, the tumor is removed en bloc with minimal manipulation. The margins of the laryngectomy are assessed from the specimen side (ideal) or the patient side.

TORS supraglottic laryngectomy can be performed in the following manner, similar to the operative techniques of TLM (Fig. 14.4) [22]. The posterior boundary must be cut first for most supraglottic cancers because blood can obscure this area during the dissection. For laryngeal epiglottic cancers, the dissection may proceed from the anterior to the posterior direction starting at the pharyngoepiglottic fold [23]. The dissection continues down laterally on the vallecula and the hyoid bone as well as the inner cortex of the thyroid cartilage. The preepiglottic fat should be contained within the incisions to remove the specimen en bloc. During the dissection deep to the pharyngoepiglottic fold, the superior thyroid artery may be encountered. Surgical clips can be applied by the assistant (Fig. 14.4c).

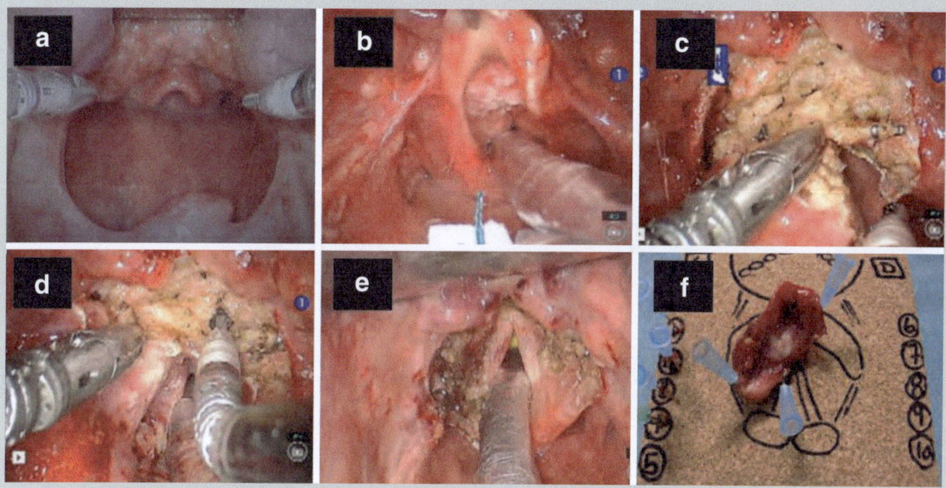

Fig. 14.4 TORS supraglottic laryngectomy. Excellent exposure of the airway is critical for successful surgery (**a**). Retraction of the epiglottis reveals the tumor in the laryngeal epiglottis (**b**). During the dissection superior laryngeal vessels are encountered, which were clipped (**c**), and pre-epiglottic fat were seen (**d**). The surgical wound after supraglottic laryngectomy (**e**) and specimen (**f**) are seen. (Adapted from Mendelsohn et al. Current Opinion in Otolaryngology—Head and Neck Surgery [20], with permission)

14.8 TORS for Hypopharyngectomy

Robotic systems can provide magnified three-dimensional views of the hypopharynx that cannot otherwise be obtained in TLM. For this reason, TORS was utilized for tumors in the hypopharyngectomy early on [24], sometimes with working laser [25]. Although some teams in earlier studies advocated for preventative tracheostomy, authors of later studies have successfully performed TORS for hypopharyngectomy without preventative tracheostomy [26].

After informed consent is obtained, the patient is brought to the operating room. General anesthesia is induced, and the patient is rotated 180 degrees away from the anesthesiologist. For TORS hypopharyngectomy, either a LARS [26] or FK-WO [27] retractor can be introduced into the oral cavity. In general, 30-degree endoscope that is "turned down" can provide adequate view of the hypopharynx [24, 28].

The hypopharyngeal lesion is first assessed and examined visually and by instrumental palpation to determine its extent. In this case, the tumor in question was in the medial wall of the right pyriform sinus (Fig. 14.5a). We recommend the initial cut be the incision in the posterior pharyngeal wall often including part of the inferior constrictor muscle (Fig. 14.5b). This initial pos-

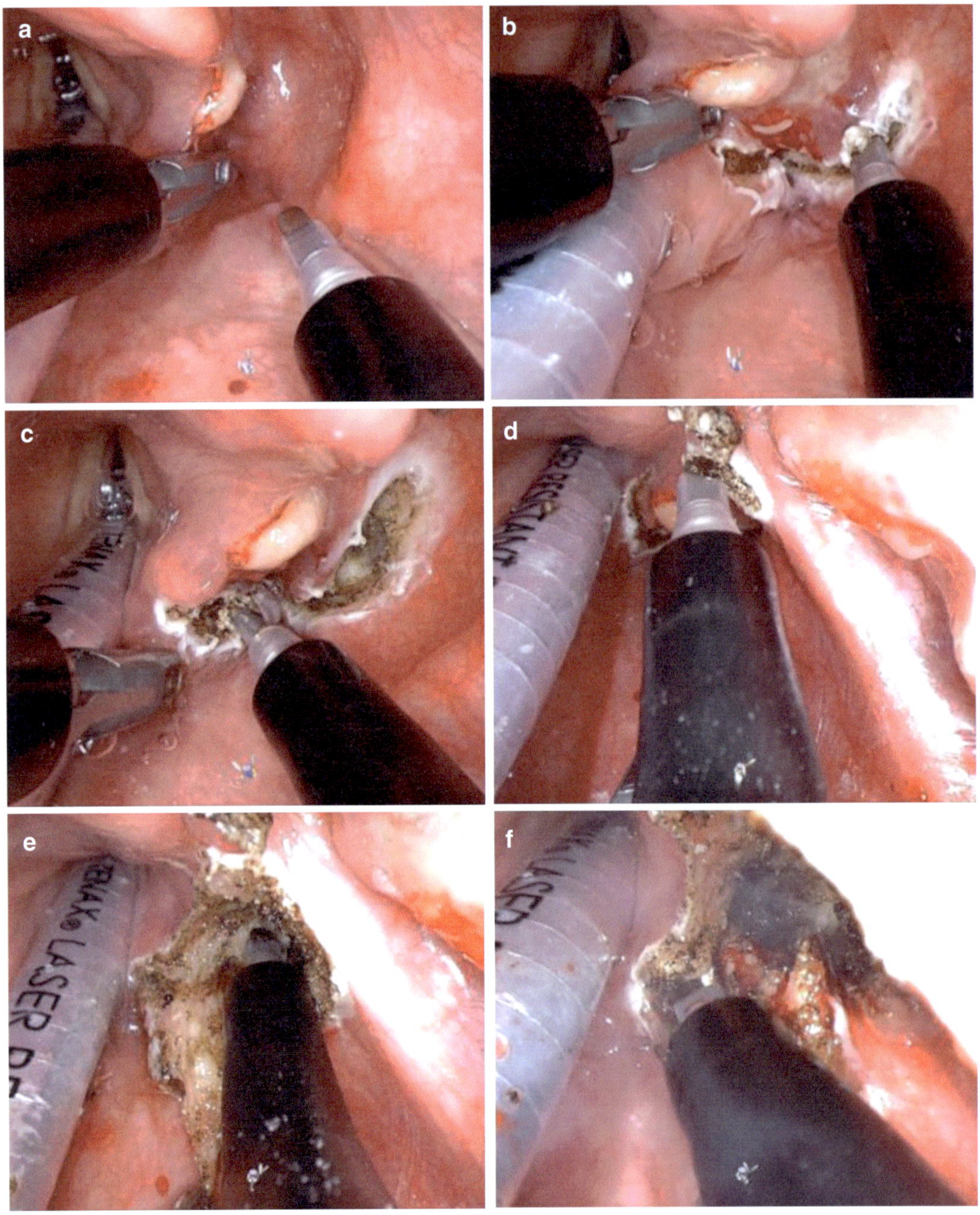

Fig. 14.5 Transoral robotic hypopharyngectomy. The tumor is identified in the medial wall of the right pyriform sinus (**a**). The posterior incision is made first (**b**). The incision is extended medially (**c**) and anteriorly (**d**). The anterior cut is made from lateral to medial direction (**e**, **f**). Deeper attachments are dissected free (**g**). During this time, the superior thyroid artery may be encountered, which is clipped using surgical clips by the surgical assistant (**h**). The surgical defect postresection (**i**). Specimen is displayed in anatomical orientation (**j**). (Adapted from Mendelsohn AM and Lawson G. Head & Neck 2021 [28], with permission)

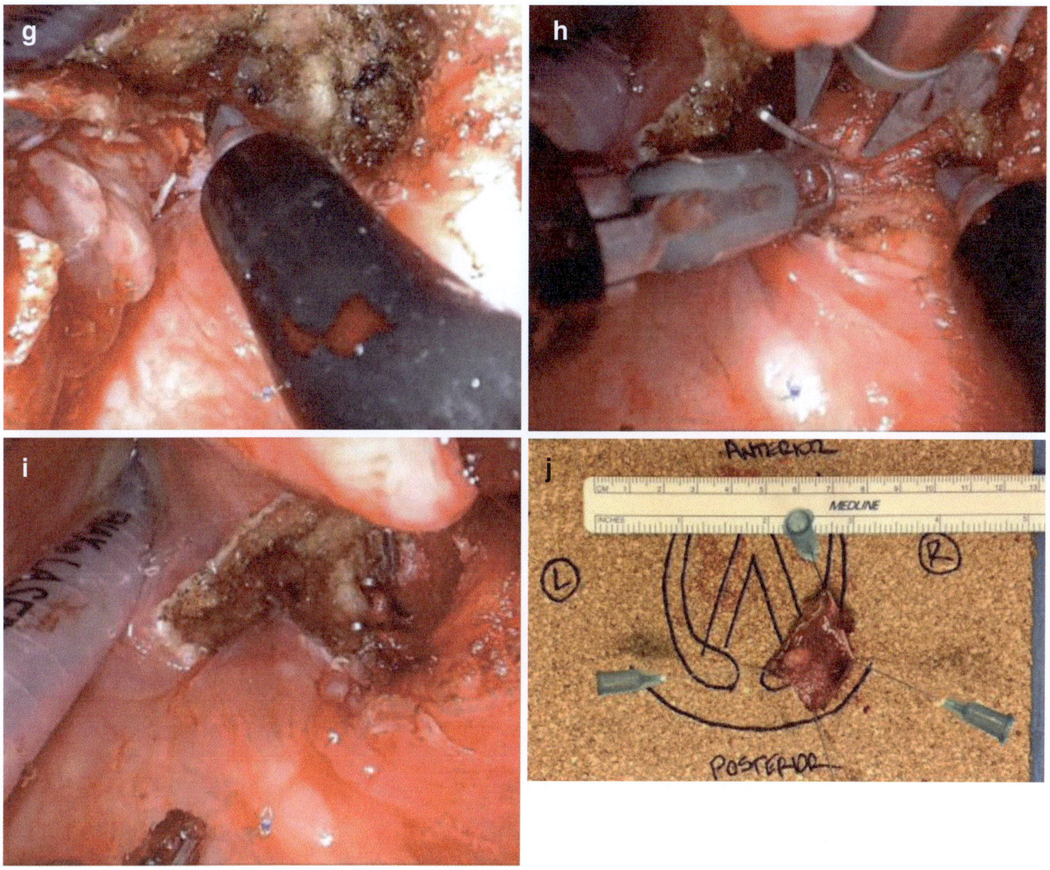

Fig. 14.5 (continued)

terior incision is critical because blood can obscure this location making it difficult to obtain a tumor-free posterior margin. The dissection continues medially and laterally 5–10 mm from the superior edge of the tumor (Fig. 14.5c). The dissection continues along the aryepiglottic fold and anteriorly toward the inner side of the thyroid cartilage (Fig. 14.5d). The exposure can be improved by turning the 30-degree endoscope "face up" [28]. During this time, the hypopharyngeal mucosa is gently grasped to preserve underlying arytenoid structures, if possible. The benefit of TORS in contrast to TLM is the use of manipulators to remove cartilage and perichondrium as needed during the lateral dissection [27]. Continued dissection laterally and inferiorly completes the tumor resection (Fig. 14.5e, f, g). The tumor is removed from the surgical site by the assistant (Fig. 14.5h, i). The tumor margins are obtained from the specimen; this includes the four quadrants as well as the deep margin (Fig. 14.5j). During the dissection, we surgically ligate any blood vessels larger than 3 mm in caliber. In some cases, a thin layer of surgical glue can be used in the wound bed to help with hemostasis.

The surgical retractors are removed from the patient. Subsequently, the patient is turned back to the anesthesiologist for extubation and transport to the recovery area.

14.9 TORS for Parapharyngeal Tumor Resection

First described by O'Malley and colleagues, using TORS for parapharyngeal tumors has become more popular due to its low morbidity in the resection of the tumor [29]. The setup and approach is very similar to TORS for radical tonsillectomy. It is critical to highlight that TORS is reserved for benign neoplasms in the parapharyngeal space that do not displace the internal carotid artery [30].

Exposure is obtained with a Crowe-Davis intraoral retractor, advanced to the base of tongue, held in open retraction, and placed in suspension. The soft palate can be retracted with a soft Red-Robinson catheter delivered via the nasal cavity, similar to the practice in a tonsillectomy. Depending on the patient's anatomy, the LARS pharyngoscope can be used as well [31]. The 0-degree telescope is then used to confirm adequate visualization of the pharyngeal region. The da Vinci robotic surgical system is then parked on the patient's right side with the use of the high-definition endoscope as well as the robotic surgical dissecting instruments and the spatula tip Bovie. The instruments are then docked within the patient's oral cavity. The assistant surgeon is positioned at the head of the patient's bed for retraction and suction, and the operative surgeon is seated at the operative console.

The procedure begins by creating a modified "question mark" incision just anterior to the anterior tonsillar pillar to the depth of the pterygomandibular raphe [30]. This incision is carried up onto the soft palate. Following the mucosal incision, the pharyngeal constrictor and buccopharyngeal fascial layer will be encountered. These must be carefully dissected and transected in the vertical direction. The posterior-lateral dissection exposes the parapharyngeal space fat pad. The parapharyngeal space tumor is likely to be identified deep to this area. The muscular/facial attachments from the medial aspect including pterygoid muscles and tendon are dissected while controlling the small venous plexus with the bipolar forceps. Blunt dissection using the spatula tip is performed to identify the boundaries of the tumor. Finger dissection has also been reported as helpful [29]. It is critical to understand the course of the internal carotid artery and visually inspect for carotid pulsation [32]. The tumor resection can be removed entirely en bloc or in a piecemeal fashion. Grasping the tumor body, the curvature of the tumor to the inferior aspect is followed where vascular attachments are transected. During the dissection from the inferior aspect of the tumor around to the lateral aspect, care must be taken to avoid traction on the arterial structures that are present lateral to this area.

The dissection around the superior aspect of the tumor is continued, and with the release of final attachments the tumor is delivered through the mouth. The cavity is irrigated with copious amount of sterile water. Venous bleeders are controlled with bipolar forceps. The surgeon uses the endoscopic system to reinspect the parapharyngeal space cavity. Normal salivary gland tissue may be visible. If the surgical site is hemostatic, the area is treated with Surgifoam procoagulant. The surgical wound is then closed with the use of multiple 3–0 Vicryl sutures in horizontal mattress fashion. Some studies have described placement of a Penrose drain placed via the mouth [30], but when a drain is necessary, we prefer delivery via the nasal cavity [31]. At this point, the patient is turned to anesthesia, extubated, and transported to the recovery room.

14.10 Postoperative Course and Management

The specific criteria that dictate postoperative management include concerns for airway edema, adequate pain control, and diet intake. Depending on the extent of resection, the patient may be discharged or admitted for observation. In uncomplicated TORS tonsillectomies for non-oncologic indications, the patient follows the usual postoperative course similar to conventional tonsillectomies. Patients undergoing oncologic resections (e.g., radical tonsillectomy, base of tongue resection), especially of the larynx and hypopharynx, may need additional instrumental tests of swallow function. Surgical manipulation of the larynx warrants close observation in a monitored unit because airway edema may require securing of the airway, or rarely, tracheotomy.

14.11 Complications

Understanding potential complications helps with decision making and counseling of patients who elect to undergo TORS.

14.12 Bleeding

Postoperative hemorrhage is the most common complication that results in unplanned visits to the hospital [33]. Bleeding usually occurs between postoperative days 8 and 11 but can occur as late as postoperative day 33 [34]. Several risk factors have been proposed, including perioperative antithrombotic medications [33–36]. Some studies have found that prophylactic arterial ligation [33, 34, 37] reduced the incidence of severe hemorrhage. However, others did not find this to be of significant benefit [33, 38]. The authors of this chapter recommend vigilant monitoring and strict emergency room return precautions for the first 2 weeks after surgery.

14.13 Dysphagia/Aspiration

Surgical manipulation of the upper aerodigestive tract causes inflammation and disruption of the lymphatic flow that result in edema. Dysphagia and concomitant dehydration can occur after TORS, with severe instances resulting in readmission. Alternatively, altered swallowing mechanics due to absence of tissue bulk or changes in the musculature involved in swallowing can lead to aspiration and pneumonia. Patients who receive bilateral neck dissection in addition to TORS are at a greater risk of dehydration [36]. The authors recommend gradual advancement of diet consistency to "re-learn" swallowing and setting a low threshold at which to discuss the case with speech language pathologists. In some patients, gastrostomy tubes may be necessary, with some studies reporting the rate of gastrostomy tube dependence as high as 11% [39].

14.14 A Case Example of p16+ Squamous Cell Carcinoma of the Base of Tongue

A 74-year-old male with hypertension, diabetes mellitus, and history of colon cancer (status post hemicolectomy and chemotherapy in 1990s), presented to our clinic with a right neck mass that had been growing for 6 weeks. A biopsy of the neck mass was performed, which was found to be p16+ squamous cell carcinoma. The clinical exam and PET/CT were suggestive of right base of tongue primary location staged T1 N1 M0. The patient was discussed at the tumor board and given the localized disease with small neck adenopathy (24 × 19 mm), the patient was offered TORS resection.

After informed consent was obtained, the patient was brought to the operating room where general endotracheal anesthesia was administered. The patient was then rotated 180 degrees away from the anesthesiologist and a shoulder roll and tooth guard were placed. The Dedo laryngoscope was placed intraorally and advanced to the glottis and piriform sinuses bilaterally and the bilateral tonsillar fossa. Each of these areas was closely inspected, leading to an identification of a submucosal lesion in the right base of tongue that did not extend into the lateral pharyngeal wall.

A large Crowe-Davis retractor was placed intraorally and advanced to the base of the tongue, and the 30-degree telescope was then used to confirm adequate visualization of the oropharynx and base of tongue lesion. The da Vinci SP robotic system was then parked at the patient's right side with Maryland forceps and Bovie for the robotic arms, and the instruments were docked within the patient's oral cavity, with the assisting surgeon sitting at the head of the patient's bed for retraction and flexion.

The operative surgeon, seated at the operative console, began the procedure by making a posterior incision at least 5 mm away from the tumor, down to the intrinsic tongue muscles. The incision was then extended to the lateral pharyngeal wall, keeping margins greater than 5 mm. We then used the Maryland forceps to palpate the extent of the tumor into the lateral pharyngeal space. Inferiorly, the dissection carried down to the pharyngoepiglottic fold, but included neither the epiglottis nor the larynx. After the surgeon dissected the last peripheral attachments, the surgical assistant delivered the tumor through the mouth and brought it to the back table.

The margins were felt to be clear of tumor by visual inspection and palpation. Frozen section margins were taken from the four quadrants around the tumor from the specimen side. These specimens were sent for fresh frozen pathology and returned negative for carcinoma. Hemostasis was achieved using Maryland bipolar forceps. Intraoral retractors were removed from the patient. The surgery proceeded with ipsilateral neck dissection.

14.15 Conclusions

TORS provides an excellent visualization and instrument control ideal for resection of head and neck cancers. The indications and robotic technologies are expanding to provide minimally invasive options for treating benign and malignant entities. With the single-port systems and flexible endoscope, access is even greater than before. Due to its wide use in routine head and neck resection, we recommend robotic surgical training be included in all head and neck surgery training programs. Furthermore, the safety profile of TORS and its ability to minimize postoperative complications should be further explored in clinical trials.

Conflicts of Interest Dr. Mendelsohn is a paid surgical proctor and has received grant funding from Intuitive Surgical, Inc.

Financial Disclosures: None

References

1. Kim YJ, Kim JH. Increasing incidence and improving survival of oral tongue squamous cell carcinoma. Sci Rep. 2020;10(1):7877.
2. Strohl MP, Wai KC, Ha PK. De-intensification strategies in HPV-related oropharyngeal squamous cell carcinoma-a narrative review. Ann Transl Med. 2020;8(23):1601.
3. Kwoh YS, et al. A robot with improved absolute positioning accuracy for CT guided stereotactic brain surgery. IEEE Trans Biomed Eng. 1988;35(2):153–60.
4. Kalan S, et al. History of robotic surgery. J Robot Surg. 2010;4(3):141–7.
5. Paul HA, et al. Development of a surgical robot for cementless total hip arthroplasty. Clin Orthop Relat Res. 1992;285:57–66.
6. Rininsland HH. Basics of robotics and manipulators in endoscopic surgery. Endosc Surg Allied Technol. 1993;1(3):154–9.
7. Haus BM, et al. Surgical robotic applications in otolaryngology. Laryngoscope. 2003;113(7):1139–44.
8. McLeod IK, Melder PC. Da Vinci robot-assisted excision of a vallecular cyst: a case report. Ear Nose Throat J. 2005;84(3):170–2.
9. O'Malley BW Jr, et al. Transoral robotic surgery (TORS) for base of tongue neoplasms. Laryngoscope. 2006;116(8):1465–72.
10. Chan JYK, et al. Early results of a safety and feasibility clinical trial of a novel single-port flexible robot for transoral robotic surgery. Eur Arch Otorrinolaringol. 2017;274(11):3993–6.
11. Chan JYK, et al. Prospective clinical trial to evaluate safety and feasibility of using a single port flexible robotic system for transoral head and neck surgery. Oral Oncol. 2019;94:101–5.
12. Van Abel KM, Moore EJ. Surgical management of the base of tongue. Oper Tech Otolaryngol Head Neck Surg. 2013;24(2):74–85.
13. Alessandrini M, et al. Transoral robotic surgery for the base of tongue squamous cell carcinoma: a preliminary comparison between da Vinci Xi and Si. J Robot Surg. 2018;12(3):417–23.
14. Mendelsohn AH, et al. Outcomes following transoral robotic surgery: supraglottic laryngectomy. Laryngoscope. 2013;123(1):208–14.
15. O'Malley BW Jr, Weinstein GS, Hockstein NG. Transoral robotic surgery (TORS): glottic microsurgery in a canine model. J Voice. 2006;20(2):263–8.
16. Remacle M, et al. Endoscopic cordectomy. A proposal for a classification by the working committee, European laryngological society. Eur Arch Otorrinolaringol. 2000;257(4):227–31.
17. Hans S, et al. Oncological, surgical and functional outcomes of transoral robotic cordectomy for early glottic carcinoma. J Voice. 2021.
18. Kayhan FT, Kaya KH, Sayin I. Transoral robotic cordectomy for early glottic carcinoma. Ann Otol Rhinol Laryngol. 2012;121(8):497–502.
19. De Virgilio A, et al. How to optimize laryngeal and hypopharyngeal exposure in transoral robotic surgery. Auris Nasus Larynx. 2013;40(3):312–9.
20. Mendelsohn AH, Remacle M. Transoral robotic surgery for laryngeal cancer. Curr Opin Otolaryngol Head Neck Surg. 2015;23(2):148–52.

21. Remacle M, et al. Combining a new CO2 laser wave guide with transoral robotic surgery: a feasibility study on four patients with malignant tumors. Eur Arch Otorrinolaringol. 2012;269(7):1833–7.
22. Remacle M, et al. Endoscopic partial supraglottic laryngectomies: techniques and results. Otolaryngol Head Neck Surg. 2009;141(3):374–81.
23. Park YM, et al. Surgical techniques and treatment outcomes of transoral robotic supraglottic partial laryngectomy. Laryngoscope. 2013;123(3):670–7.
24. Park YM, et al. Transoral robotic surgery (TORS) in laryngeal and hypopharyngeal cancer. J Laparoendosc Adv Surg Tech A. 2009;19(3):361–8.
25. Kucur C, et al. Transoral robot-assisted carbon dioxide laser surgery for hypopharyngeal cancer. Head Neck. 2015;37(5):743–5.
26. Hassid S, et al. Transoral robotic surgery hypopharyngectomy (TORSH): feasibility and outcomes. Eur Arch Otorrinolaringol. 2020;277(10):2883–92.
27. Park YM, et al. Transoral robotic surgery for hypopharyngeal squamous cell carcinoma: 3-year oncologic and functional analysis. Oral Oncol. 2012;48(6):560–6.
28. Mendelsohn AH, Lawson G. Single-port transoral robotic surgery hypopharyngectomy. Head Neck. 2021;43(10):3234–7.
29. O'Malley BW Jr, et al. Transoral robotic surgery for parapharyngeal space tumors. ORL J Otorhinolaryngol Relat Spec. 2010;72(6):332–6.
30. Rassekh CH, et al. Transoral robotic surgery for prestyloid parapharyngeal space masses. Oper Tech Otolaryngol Head Neck Surg. 2013;24(2):99–105.
31. Mendelsohn AH. Transoral robotic assisted resection of the parapharyngeal space. Head Neck. 2015;37(2):273–80.
32. Arshad H, Durmus K, Ozer E. Transoral robotic resection of selected parapharyngeal space tumors. Eur Arch Otorrinolaringol. 2013;270(5): 1737–40.
33. Mandal R, et al. Analysis of post-transoral robotic-assisted surgery hemorrhage: frequency, outcomes, and prevention. Head Neck. 2016;38(Suppl 1):E776–82.
34. Gleysteen J, et al. The impact of prophylactic external carotid artery ligation on postoperative bleeding after transoral robotic surgery (TORS) for oropharyngeal squamous cell carcinoma. Oral Oncol. 2017; 70:1–6.
35. Asher SA, et al. Hemorrhage after transoral robotic-assisted surgery. Otolaryngol Head Neck Surg. 2013;149(1):112–7.
36. Topf MC, et al. Unplanned readmission following transoral robotic surgery. Oral Oncol. 2017;75:127–32.
37. Kubik M, et al. Effect of transcervical arterial ligation on the severity of postoperative hemorrhage after transoral robotic surgery. Head Neck. 2017;39(8): 1510–5.
38. Pollei TR, et al. Analysis of postoperative bleeding and risk factors in transoral surgery of the oropharynx. JAMA Otolaryngol Head Neck Surg. 2013;139(11):1212–8.
39. Hay A, et al. Complications following transoral robotic surgery (TORS): a detailed institutional review of complications. Oral Oncol. 2017;67:160–6.

15 Minimally Invasive Thyroidectomy: Transoral Endoscopic Thyroidectomy by Vestibular Approach (TOETVA)

Lucas Ribeiro Tenório, Marianne Yumi Nakai, Júlio Patrocínio Moraes, Antonio Augusto Tupinambá Bertelli, Marcelo Benedito Menezes, and Antônio José Gonçalves

Abstract

Introduction

To date, TOETVA (transoral endoscopic thyroidectomy by vestibular approach) is the most widely adopted remote access technique for thyroid surgery. The technique consists of making a surgical access to the central neck through the oral vestibule, followed by an endoscope-guided thyroidectomy while running CO_2 insufflation. Besides the technical differences between TOETVA and the open technique, the main steps of the thyroidectomy are the same. TOETVA has similar complication rates regarding the laryngeal nerves and parathyroid glands when compared to open surgery. *Material and Methods:* We recorded this video of TOETVA for treating papillary thyroid cancer in a young woman. The patient involved in the case gave written informed consent to participate in this study. *Results:* This case had a successful development, without complications. *Conclusion:* This video illustrates a typical case of TOETVA for the treatment of PTC.

Keywords

TOETVA · Scarless thyroidectomy · Vestibular approach · Thyroidectomy · Notes · Minimally invasive surgery · Thyroid surgery

15.1 Introduction

To date, TOETVA (transoral endoscopic thyroidectomy by vestibular approach) is the most widely adopted remote access technique for thyroid surgery [1]. It was firstly described in 2011 after an experimental study in human cadavers [2], which was based on another experimental study from 2008 that described an endoscopic access to the central neck through the floor of the mouth in suines [3]. Beyond being described as a minimally invasive surgical technique, it is also a true natural orifice surgery (NOTES™) [1, 4, 5], once the surgical scars stay hidden in the oral mucosa. Seeing that, the better cosmetic results are undoubtedly an

Supplementary Information The online version contains supplementary material available at https://doi.org/10.1007/978-981-97-7059-5_15.

L. R. Tenório (✉) · M. Y. Nakai · J. P. Moraes · A. A. T. Bertelli · M. B. Menezes · A. J. Gonçalves
Santa Casa de São Paulo School of Medical Science, Head and Neck Surgery Division, São Paulo, Brazil
e-mail: lucas.tenorio@aluno.fcmsantacasasp.edu.br

M. Tewari (ed.), *Minimally Invasive Surgery in Cancer*,
https://doi.org/10.1007/978-981-97-7059-5_15

unquestionable feature of this approach [6]. Although strong evidence of other benefits is still pending, TOETVA promotes great magnification of image, which may show other benefits after a wider adoption along the next years, such as more delicate dissection of structures and better preservation of parathyroid glands [4, 7].

The technique consists of making a surgical access to the central neck through the oral vestibule, followed by an endoscope-guided thyroidectomy while running CO_2 insufflation [1, 4, 5]. Before this approach, several other techniques for remote thyroidectomy such as transaxillary and transthoracic were applied, mostly in Asia, but none of them was established in the other continents, mostly due to low reproducibility and new relevant complications [1, 8]. Besides the technical differences between TOETVA and the open technique with Kocher incision, the main steps of the thyroidectomy are the same, performed with a different view and sometimes in a different order [1].

TOETVA has similar complication rates regarding the laryngeal nerves and parathyroid glands when compared to open surgery [4]. It gives good visualization to both thyroid lobes and to the level VI and, despite concerns about infection, once the technique creates a communication between the oral cavity and the central neck, the existing data shows that TOETVA has similar rates of infection when compared to open surgery [8–10].

15.2 Material and Methods

We recorded this video of TOETVA for treating papillary thyroid cancer in a young woman. The patient involved in the case gave written informed consent to participate in this study.

15.3 Case

A 32-year-old woman with no past medical history presented with papillary thyroid cancer. She had no complaints. Clinical examination showed a normal thyroid gland with a small nodule in the right lobe. The patient underwent an ultrasonography that showed a 0.7 cm nodule with central vascularization and microcalcification. Our team indicated a right lobectomy by transoral endoscopic vestibular approach. The surgery began with the confection of three endoscopic portals through the oral vestibule. After that, the working space was made with an ultrasonic scalpel while running CO_2 insufflation. The CO_2 insufflation begins right after placing the central trocar—it is recommended to always use low pressure, around 6 or 7 mmhg, and intermediate to high flow, around 10–20 L/min. At the beginning, a 10 mm/0° endoscope is used to guide the creation of the working space. After inserting the instruments in the portals, the surgeon should find their tips to start dissection of the soft tissue. We start using a Maryland on the left hand and the energy scalpel on the right hand (To make this step faster, it is possible to use a Space Maker. If you don't have this gadget in your hospital, you can improvise using a Foley catheter dressed on the aspirator). To a right-handed surgeon, the left dissector is used to keep the skin flap suspended as a roof. The soft tissue is dissected and some small vessels are ligated, in this case we used the harmonic, keeping the platysma muscle attached to the roof, making it thicker in order to avoid skin burns or tears. When the pocket is ready, we usually see the anterior jugular veins in the center of the screen—marking the rafe. After that the assistant switches the scope to a 10 mm/30° endoscope. It gives a better view of the surgical site. The rafe is opened with the energy scalpel, and the thyroid isthmus is visualized. Some soft tissue is dissected to fully expose the cricothyroid muscle. The Delphian node is dissected and the soft tissue above it is ligated. In this case we choose to remove it, but it can be left attached to the soft tissue around the thyroid gland, in order to remove an en bloc specimen. After that, we delimitate the plane between the thyroid gland and the trachea, creating a tunnel to pass the harmonic. To a right lobectomy the gland should be sectioned on the left side of the midline, using the energy scalpel and the right lobe is detached of the trachea by soft dissection with the energy scalpel from medial to lateral, releasing the lobe. The superior pole ligation began, using the harmonic to embrace the superior pole with a diving movement, respecting the limits of Joll's triangle. The superior parathyroid gland appears right after the progressive ligation of the superior pole and it marks the moment that the surgeon should finish superior pole ligation and start seeking the recurrent laryngeal nerve. We use a Maryland to dissect the nerve. You can note that in this case the inferior parathyroid gland appeared to be escalating the inferior pole, and we had to dissect and release it from medial to lateral, to avoid damaging the gland or its pedicle. After finding the recurrent laryngeal nerve, we use monitoring to confirm its function and start to dissect the soft tissue around it in order to make a path to release the right lobe. Gentle dissection is done around the Berry ligament moving away the recurrent laryngeal nerve from the thyroid gland. Soft tissue dissection is done in order to detach the gland from the trachea and the right lobectomy is finally completed. The specimen is removed using an endobag, which is inserted in the pocket through the central port. Nerve monitoring is done at the end to confirm nerve function again. Portal incisions were closed with vicryl 3.0. Our operative time was 100 min. A pressure dressing was placed overnight. There were no complications during the procedure and the patient was discharged on the first postoperative day. She had amoxicillin-clavulanate for 7 days after surgery and to control pain she took dipyrone 4000 mg/day and ketoprofen 200 mg/day for 5 days. She didn't need any opioids. A soft diet was recommended for 2 days and exercises were restricted for 10 days as we do to open surgery. She was back to consultation after 2 weeks and the oral wounds were healed, and almost imperceptible. She was back to her regular activities and only complained about submental numbness and tenderness. After 3 months the patient was fully recovered and had no complaints.

15.4 Conclusion

This video illustrates a typical case of TOETVA for the treatment of papillary thyroid cancer.

Disclosures No competing financial interests exist.

Video Caption

This is a video record of a transoral endoscopic thyroidectomy by vestibular approach (TOETVA)

TOETVA is already a standardized procedure and it is considered a true natural orifice transluminal endoscopic surgerycal

Several health centers around the world are performing it

The access is made through the oral vestibule, by creating three endoscopic portals

The one in the center to pass the endoscope and the other two create path to the instruments

The CO_2 *insufflation begins right after placing the central trocar—it is recommended to always use low pressure, around 6 or 7 mmhg, and intermediate to high flow, around 10 to 20 L/min.*

At the beginning a 10mm/0° endoscope is used to guide the creation of the working space

After inserting the instruments in the portals, the surgeon should find their tips to start dissection of the soft tissue.

We start using a Maryland on the left hand and the energy scalpel on the right hand

To make this step faster, it is possible to use a Space Maker. If you don't have this gadget in your service, you can improvise using a Foley catheter dressed on the aspirator

To a right-handed surgeon, the left dissector is used to keep the skin flap suspended as a roof

The soft tissue is dissected and some small vessels are ligated, in this case with the harmonic, keeping the platisma muscle attached to the roof, making it thicker in order to avoid skin burns or tears

Note that we use blunt dissection to the fat tissue

When the pocket is ready, we usually see the anterior jugular veins in the center of the screen—marking the rafe

After that the assistant switches the scope to a 10 mm/30° endoscope—it gives a better view of the surgical site

The rafe is opened with the energy scalpel. The Delphian node is dissected and the soft tissue above it is ligated

We choose to remove the Delphian node in this case, but you can leave it attached to the soft tissue around the thyroid gland, in order to remove an en bloc specimen

Some soft tissue is dissected to fully expose the Cricothyroid muscle

The surgeon keeps dissecting to fully expose the strap muscles and the thyroid gland

The midline dissection goes on and the thyroid isthmus is visualized

The pyramidal lobe is identified, after that we dissected and ligated, in order to release it

After that, we delimitate the plane between the thyroid gland and the trachea, creating a tunnel to pass the harmonic

To a right lobectomy, the gland should be sectioned on the left side of the midline, using the energy scalpel and the right lobe is detached of the trachea by soft dissection with the energy scalpel from medial to lateral, releasing the lobe

The plane between the strap muscles and the thyroid gland is dissected in order to release the right thyroid lobe

After that the superior pole ligation began, using the harmonic to embrace the superior pole with a diving movement, respecting the limits of Joll's triangle

In this case during the dissection of the superior pole we visualized the inferior parathyroid

The superior parathyroid gland appears right after the progressive ligation of the superior pole and it marks the moment that the surgeon should finish superior pole ligation and start seeking the recurrent laryngeal nerve

In this frame you can see a beautiful image of both parathyroid glands

Note that in this case the inferior parathyroid gland appeared to be escalating the inferior pole, and we had to dissect and release it from medial to lateral, to avoid damaging the gland or its pedicle

We used a Maryland to dissect the nerve

After finding the recurrent laryngeal nerve we started to dissect the soft tissue around it in order to make a path to release the right lobe

As same as we do in open surgery we use monitoring to confirm the nerve function

Gentle dissection is done around Berry's ligament moving away the recurrent laryngeal nerve from the thyroid gland

Soft tissue dissection is done in order to detach the gland from the trachea and the right lobectomy is finally completed

The specimen is removed using an endobag, which is inserted in the pocket through the central port

References

1. Bertelli AAT, Rangel LG, Lira RB, Tesseroli MAS, Santos IC, Silva GD, et al. Trans oral endoscopic thyroidectomy vestibular approach (TOETVA) in Brazil: safety and complications during learning curve. Arch Endocrinol Metab. 2021;65(3):259–64.
2. Richmon JD, Pattani KM, Benhidjeb T, Tufano RP. Transoral robotic-assisted thyroidectomy: a preclinical feasibility study in 2 cadavers. Head Neck 2011;33(3):330–3.
3. Witzel K, Von Rahden BHA, Kaminski C, Stein HJ. Transoral access for endoscopic thyroid resection. Surg Endosc Other Interv Tech. 2008;22(8):1871–5.
4. Anuwong A. Transoral endoscopic thyroidectomy vestibular approach: a series of the first 60 human cases. World J Surg. 2015;40(3):491–7.
5. Anuwong A, Sasanakietkul T, Jitpratoom P, Ketwong K, Kim HY, Dionigi G, et al. Transoral endoscopic thyroidectomy vestibular approach (TOETVA): indications, techniques and results. Surg Endosc. 2018;32(1):456–65.
6. Chen LW, Razavi CR, Hong H, Fondong A, Ranganath R, Khatri S, et al. Cosmetic outcomes following transoral versus transcervical thyroidectomy. Head Neck. 2020;42(11):3336–44.
7. Dionigi G, Bacuzzi A, Lavazza M, Inversini D, Boni L, Rausei S, et al. Transoral endoscopic thyroidec-

tomy: preliminary experience in Italy. Updat Surg. 2017;69:225–34.
8. Berber E, Bernet V, Fahey TJ III, Kebebew E, Shaha A, Stack BC Jr, et al. American Thyroid Association statement on remote-access thyroid surgery. Thyroid. 2016;26(3):331–7.
9. Russell JO, Clark J, Noureldine SI, Anuwong A, Al Khadem MG, Yub Kim H, et al. Transoral thyroidectomy and parathyroidectomy—a North American series of robotic and endoscopic transoral approaches to the central neck. Oral Oncol. 2017;71:75–80.
10. Karakas E, Klein G, Michlmayr L, Schardey M, Schopf S. Transoral thyroid surgery vestibular approach: is there an increased risk of surgical site infections? Updates Surg. 2021;74:303.

Minimally Invasive Thyroidectomy 16

Nicholas Scott-Wittenborn
and Jonathon O. Russell

Abstract

The evolution of thyroid surgery and its progress toward minimally invasive techniques have changed greatly over the past 30 years, from simple reduction of incision length to the use of robotic and endoscopic remote access approaches. Current innovations aim to decrease neck scarring while maintaining the low complication rates of traditional open surgery. One of the new approaches to thyroid surgery, inspired by the rise of natural orifice endoscopic surgery (NOTES), is the transoral endoscopic thyroidectomy-vestibular approach (TOTEVA). The surgery was first published in 2011 by Richmond et al. Published outcomes with patients were reported in 2016 by Anuwong et al. This new approach is well received by endocrine surgeons and gaining widespread acceptance, with drastically increasing case numbers. This chapter reviews the history of the procedure, its indications, surgical steps, and a discussion on its benefits and safety.

N. Scott-Wittenborn (✉) · J. O. Russell
Department of Otolaryngology—Head and Neck Surgery, Johns Hopkins University, Baltimore, MD, USA
e-mail: info@russell-center.com

Keywords

TOETVA · Thyroid surgery · Minimally invasive surgery

16.1 History of Thyroid Surgery

Surgery of the thyroid gland is a challenging and delicate endeavor; over time, it has evolved from a dangerous surgical endeavor with untenable mortality rates, to an elegant minimally invasive procedure without any cutaneous incision. Early attempts at thyroid surgery were notorious for their poor outcomes. The earliest well-documented Western thyroid surgery was performed by Rogerius in 1170; He used setsons, forceps, and caustic powders to eliminate thyroid tissue to reduce the size of a large goiter [1]. While there were occasional successes during these early attempts, the overall results were so morbid that the procedure was banned in the United States [2]. Because surgical outcomes were inconsistent, alternative techniques were explored to alleviate compressive symptoms caused by large goiters. These less invasive surgical techniques included the release of cervical fascia to allow for ventral protrusion of the mass, as well as injections of caustic or iodine-based compounds to decrease the size of the mass [3]. In a sense, these early attempts at treating large

M. Tewari (ed.), *Minimally Invasive Surgery in Cancer*,
https://doi.org/10.1007/978-981-97-7059-5_16

goiters were a type of minimally invasive surgical treatment for certain thyroid disease.

It was not until the later part of the nineteenth century that surgery on the thyroid gland was performed on a regular basis. This was because of a number of technological innovations: the use of antiseptic techniques, proper anesthesia, and the implementation of hemostatic forceps [4]. With these advances, the dangers of thyroid surgery described by Dr. Samuel Gross gave way to a controlled and meticulous operation [5].

Dr. Emil Kocher was the foremost pioneer of thyroid surgery. He used these technological advancements along with detailed and meticulous extracapsular dissection of the thyroid, in order to prevent bleeding, which helped to decrease the mortality rate of the surgery from 40% to under 1% [6]. Kocher was also the first surgeon to connect the symptoms of hypothyroidism to removal of the entirety of the thyroid gland. His work would eventually lead to the 1909 Noble prize in medicine.

16.2 Minimally Invasive Surgery

Little changed from Kocher's original surgical technique until the 1990s when surgeons focused on decreasing the size of the incision, with some case series limiting their cervical incision to 2.5 cm [7–9]. Having reached the limits of the open cervical approach, technological innovation again changed the practice of thyroid surgery as the development of endoscopes allowed for new surgical techniques to be developed.

The first use of an endoscopic approach for anterior neck surgery was performed by Dr. Gagner in 1996. He completed a four gland parathyroid exploration in roughly 5 h, showing the feasibility of using endoscopic techniques with insufflation [10]. Others eagerly embraced this new technology and the first endoscopic thyroid procedure soon followed, performed by Huscher in 1997 [11]. This approach used a supra-sternal incision and was completed in less than 3 h. A number of different endoscopic techniques arose, though they all still required an incision of at least 2 cm [9, 12].

The next advance in thyroid surgery was when surgeons began to use remote access incision to approach the anterior neck. This was started by Dr. Ohgamhi, who approached the thyroid with endoscopic dissection from the mammary area in 2000 [13]. Other remote access approaches were quickly developed including axillary, areolar, and retro-auricular. Endoscopic techniques were first utilized due to their low cost and simplicity but over time, the use of robotic surgical devices increased.

The first use of a robotic surgical device for remote access thyroid surgery was in 2007 by *Chung* et al. via the axilla [14]. The use of the robot since that time has grown, especially in Asia [15]. There are several advantages to robotic surgery when compared to endocrine surgery including 3-dimensional visualization, higher magnification, and better range of motion with instruments. The oncologic and safety outcomes of these robotic procedures are similar to open surgery [15–17]. However, there are two main drawbacks to any robotic thyroid surgery, the increased cost and the prolonged operating time [16, 18]. While these remote access techniques, both robotic and endoscopic, did not leave the patient with a visible neck scar, they can hardly be termed minimally invasive as they required much more extensive tissue dissection than other approaches, leading to a larger number of complications in Western patients. This increased complication rate precluded widespread adoption [19].

With the advent of natural orifice endoscopic surgery (NOTES) surgery, access to the thyroid and anterior neck spaces was approached via the mouth in both cadaveric and porcine models [20, 21]. However, these approaches were retromandibular and not in the vestibule of the mouth. Accessing the thyroid through the floor of mouth had high complications rates with damage to many of the vulnerable structures in that anatomic region, while also increasing the risks of airway compromise. The transoral endoscopic vestibular approach (TOETVA) was fully codified by Anuwong in 2016 [22, 23]. It combined the promise of the early endoscopic procedures to minimize tissue disruption while still obviating the need for a cutaneous scar. This approach uses three incisions, one at the base of the labial frenulum, and two incisions placed on the edge of the wet lip by the oral commissure. These incisions allowed a safe and effective way to access the bilateral central neck compartments and required less dissection and tissue manipulation than other techniques [24]. Furthermore, the required laparoscopic instrumentation was readily available at most hospitals, which allowed broad adoption. Since that time, thousands of cases have been performed, with hundreds of thyroid surgeons learning this new approach [25].

16.2.1 TransOral Endoscopic Thyroidectomy Vestibular Approach (TOETVA)

The main indication for TOETVA is the patient's desire to avoid an anterior cervical scar. This is especially true for patients with history of keloid formation. High volume surgeons using TOETVA have published their own indications and contraindications for the procedure. Most thyroid surgeons who are proficient with TOETVA advocate for a maximum thyroid size of 8–10 cm in any one dimension, while others focus on thyroid volume [26]. Nodule size and pathology also play a role for determining if a patient is an appropriate candidate for TOETVA. A benign or cytologically indeterminate but low risk nodule (Bethesda II, III, IV) can measure up to 6 cm in greatest dimension and still be considered for removal via TOETVA [27, 28]. For nodules that are at high suspicion or confirmed malignancy (Bethesda V and VI or with suspicious molecular markers), most surgeons will only attempt surgical removal of masses that are 2–4 cm in greatest dimension [29]. Also, suspicious nodules that are at the superior pole of the thyroid or are located posterior/medial to the capsule maybe challenging and require greater experience with the technique.

There is still contention about what other types of thyroid pathology are appropriately treated with this approach. There are now reports that some surgeons are operating on patients with active thyroiditis without significant complciations [30]. In addition, a few surgeons including our group are using TOETVA to cure Graves' disease [26, 30].

In addition to size constraints, contraindications for TOETVA include previous neck surgery or poorly differentiated thyroid carcinoma. Relative contraindications include a history of previous neck surgery or radiation [31]. There was some concern that in Western populations, with a higher rate of obesity, that a larger percentage of individuals would not be appropriate TOETVA candidates due to increased submental adiposity [19]. However, obesity has only been shown to be a relative contraindication [32, 33].

It is hard to estimate what percentage of patients are eligible for this surgical approach, but a recent review found that 50% of patients at three academic institutions met the criteria for TOETVA [34]. However, the appropriateness for TOETVA is often surgeon-specific.

As with any thyroid surgery, imaging is an important part of the preoperative work up for TOETVA. The use of surgeon-directed ultrasound (US) should be viewed as a critical part for determining eligibility for TOETVA as well as a tool for operative planning. US has been shown to alter surgical planning in up to 40% of endocrine cases [35]. US can be used to identify substernal extension of the thyroid, extra thyroid extension for malignancies, and the presence of nodal disease, which would preclude TOETVA [36].

While other minimally invasive surgeries do not require perioperative antibiotics, all TOETVA patients should be given appropriate broad-spectrum coverage for oral flora prior to surgery and after (we prefer amoxicillin-clavulanic acid or, for patients with a penicillin allergy, dual coverage with metronidazole and another such as clindamycin).

16.2.1.1 TOETVA Technique

The patient is placed in a supine position on the operating table in a standardized fashion for optimal retraction (Fig. 16.1). The patient is intubated with a NIMS nerve monitoring endotracheal tube (Medtronic Minneapolis, MN, USA). The

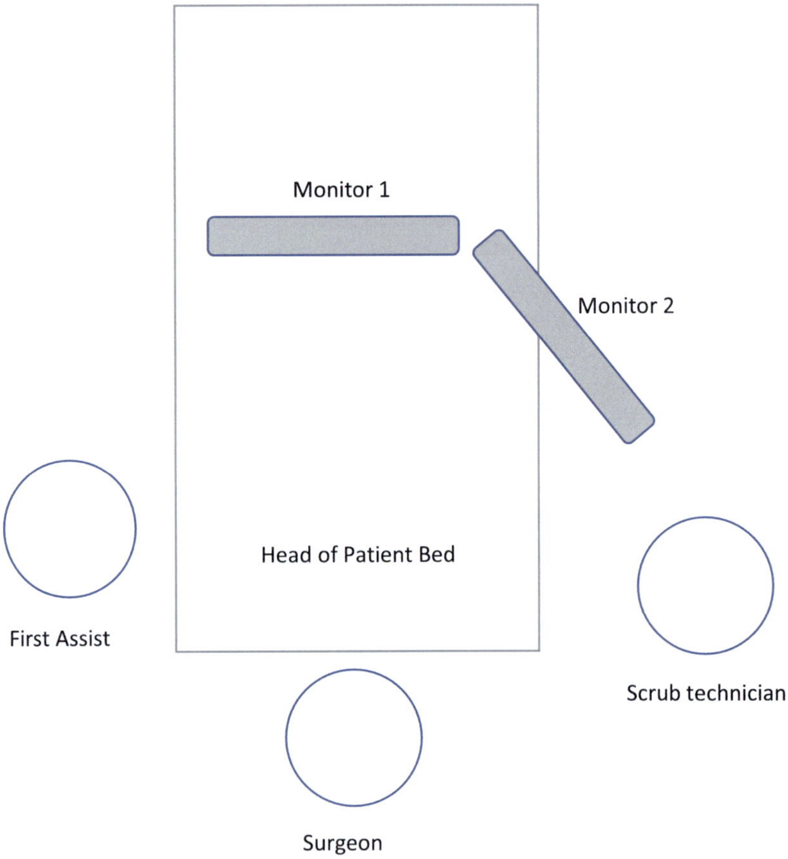

Fig. 16.1 Overhead schematic of operating room layout

tube is secured to the left upper lip, outside the patient's dentition. While ideal depth of tube placement may vary, 21 cm at the lip is the advised depth for men and 20 cm for women. Glycopyrrolate can be administered to reduce salivary gland activity as the tube may move with increased salivation.

1:100,000 lidocaine 1% with epinephrine is injected along the future tracts of the ports, creating hydrodissection over the mentum and facilitating atraumatic port placement. The vestibular incision is placed 2 cm above the labial insertion of the gingivolabial frenulum. To avoid tearing the fragile oral mucosa during closure, a significant amount of tissue should be left on the mandibular side of the incision. The smaller lateral incisions are placed 2 mm anterior to the oral commissure and away from the vermillion border in the mucosa. Port placement that is too close to the vermillion border is less desirable. After the initial incision through the mucosa, the remainder of the dissection for port placement is done bluntly to minimize tissue trauma and the risk of cutaneous injury.

A Crile is first used bluntly to create a tract for the vestibular trochar, over the chin. Leaving more tissue superficial to the dissection decreases the risk of sensory changes but increases the risks of mucosal tears that could injure the gingiva. The surgeon must ensure that there is enough tissue above the instrument to protect the skin from perforation, using a hand to cup the skin over the chin and push upward away from the instrument. After this, a Kelly forceps is used to enlarge the tract. Finally, Hegar dilators are used to dilate the passage. Dilators of at least 10–14 French diameter are used. Smaller 5 mm trocars are inserted into the lateral incisions and a larger 10 mm trocar is inserted into the vestibule.

The endoscopic screen is positioned for optimal surgeon viewing, and, if possible, a second screen is then placed on the patient's right facing toward the assistant who stands on the patient's left side. The assistant inserts the camera into the central port, using the right hand in an overhand grip. The assistant may also use a step to increase their height; both maneuvers help to keep the assistant's arm out of the way of the surgeon. The first instruments the surgeon uses are the Maryland graspers and an electrocautery device or other energy device. The initial step in the surgery is to advance both instruments in the field of view of the camera (Fig. 16.2). This is done blindly at first and without the use of energy until the movement is visible and the proto-pocket is created. After this a subplatysmal pocket may be created. The surgeon must be careful to avoid thermal injury to the skin at all points. The goal of this initial pocket is to see the strap muscles inferiorly and the Sternocleidomastoid muscles laterally.

Next, the sternohyoid and sternothyroid muscles are separated along the raphe with the energy device (Fig. 16.3). While the dividing of the raphe, the most medial heads of the cricothyroid muscles may appear but these heads are often not recognized yet. Once the raphe is opened, a 30-degree endoscope is inserted. The first step in dissecting the thyroid is to free the Delphian node, which is done in a cranial to caudal fashion. The next step in dissection is to split the isthmus (Fig. 16.4). The surgeon should then work laterally and elevate the strap muscles from the thyroid capsule to the lateral edge of the gland. This is best done with endoscopic Kittners, to avoid injury to the thyroid and possible hemorrhage. If the middle thyroid veins are encountered, they should be taken down with advanced energy devices. Dissection of the superior pole is then achieved, cautiously dissecting the blood supply. This dissection will allow for visualization of the posterior portion of the superior thyroid pole and the superior parathyroid gland. The surgeon should identify the recurrent laryngeal nerve (RLN) close to its insertion point near Berry's ligament, and the nerve stimulator may be helpful to expedite the process (Fig. 16.5).

Once the nerve is identified via visualization or stimulation, the surgeon should remove the

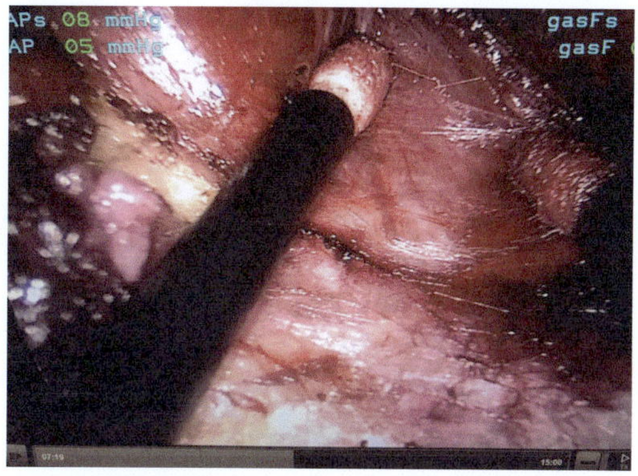

Fig. 16.2 Opening of initial dissection pocket

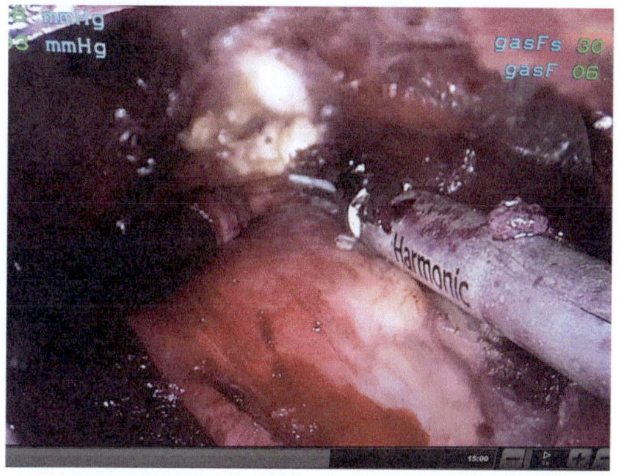

Fig. 16.3 Splitting of strap muscles above thyroid

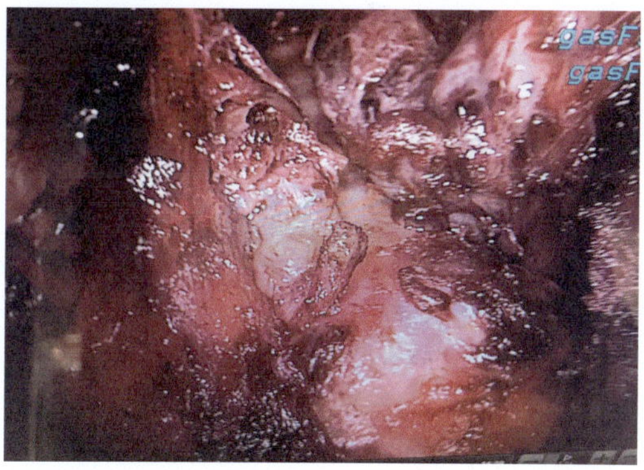

Fig. 16.4 Splitting of Isthmus

medial and later anterior attachments of the nerve to the thyroid capsule. The nerve can then be moved away from the thyroid inferiorly, and the surgeon can address any remaining inferior tissue. If a total thyroidectomy is to be performed, the same procedure is carried out on the

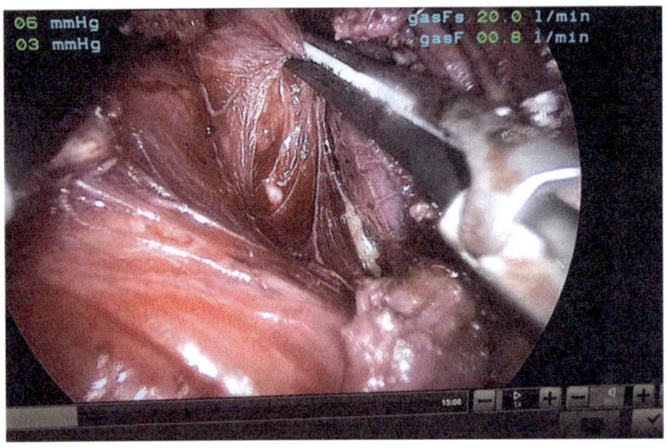

Fig. 16.5 Dissection of recurrent laryngeal nerve

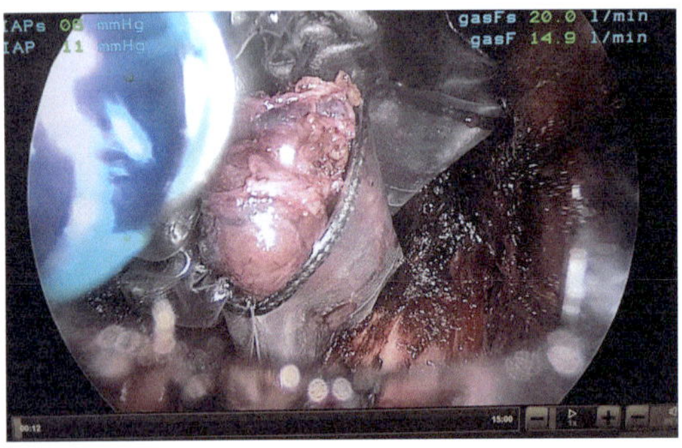

Fig. 16.6 Bagging of specimen

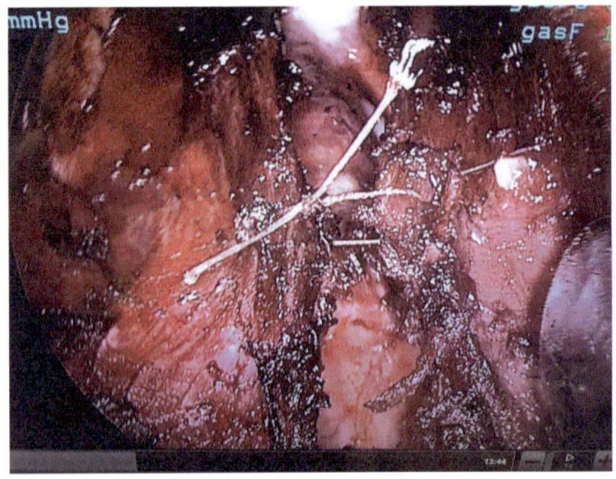

Fig. 16.7 Suturing of strap muscles

contralateral side after ensuring that the first sides' RLN has maintained its conductive integrity.

Once dissection is completed and the specimen removed via a specimen retrieval bag, (Fig. 16.6), application of a hemostatic agent can be considered. In patients with little cervical adiposity, an endoscopic stitch may be used to approximate the strap muscles, ensuring coverage of the cricoid (Fig. 16.7). It is our opinion that this may provide a subtle cosmetic benefit in patients with little cervical adiposity, but does not benefit most Western patients. The placement of a drain is not necessary. A 4–0 chromic suture is used to close the anterior incision in a running interlocking stitch and the lateral incisions with simple stitches. A compressive dressing is placed and then covered with a Jaw Bra (PMT Corporation, Chanhassen, MI, USA); gauze may be placed underneath in order to aide compression of the surgical site. The patient may be sent home the same day if appropriate. The patient should wear the Jaw Bra overnight and may continue to wear it for comfort. The patient should be placed on antibiotic prophylaxis for 5 days. Our preferred antibiotic is Augmentin. Hydration is encouraged, as are neck exercises to improve vertical range of motion beginning on the first postoperative day.

16.2.1.2 TOETVA Outcomes and Complications

The most feared complication from thyroid surgery is injury to the RLN. When an injury to the RLN does occur, the sequelae include dysphagia, dysphonia, and aspiration [37]. Such injuries are a common cause of lawsuits [38–40]. The rate of injury in thyroidectomies using a standard approach is low at around 2% with expert surgeons, which has been found to vary by surgeon volume [41, 42] TOETVA has proven to be non-inferior to RLN [24].

Rates of infection have been low to date, and are similar to rates experienced with open surgery [22]. Contrast to other surgeons, in our center's experience there is no need for oral rinses pre- and post-TOETVA. Another uncommon complication of TOETVA is the possibility for pneumothorax and pneumoperitoneum [43].

The other significant, though rare, complication of TOETVA is CO_2 air embolism. There are only two case reports of it; however there is a risk of it occurring in any procedure with CO_2 insufflation [44, 45]. Initially the patient will have a decreased PaO_2 and $PaCO_2$, and may progress to arrhythmia and hypotension [46]. If a CO_2 embolism is suspected, insufflation should be stopped and pressure should be immediately placed on the neck. Anesthetic gases can exacerbate the pulmonary emboli and need to be discontinued [47]. The patient can then be rolled into the left lateral decubitus position. This positioning limits the emboli's ability to progress into the pulmonary vasculature. If the patient continues to be in extremis, needle aspiration of the gas embolus can be considered [48, 49].

The risk of this occurring is greatest when there is an inadvertent injury to the veins, such as an anterior jugular vein [50]. The surgical and anesthesia teams should be prepared for this complication.

Overall, numerous improvements have been made to minimally invasive thyroid surgery, from decreasing scar length to the use of remote access surgery. However, TOETVA is the only type of surgery that minimizes the disruption of native tissue while also allowing for a non-visible scar. Given TOETVA's equality in outcomes and patient satisfaction it is certainly the preferred minimally invasive technique for thyroid surgery.

However, TOETVA is not the only new approach in treating thyroid pathologies; there is currently an increase in the use of nonsurgical techniques to ablate thyroid nodules. The two most used are radiofrequency ablation (RFA) and percutaneous laser ablation (LA). Both techniques use minimally invasive methods to reduce the volume of thyroid nodules successfully with minimal complications and good efficacy [51]. Recent studies have shown a greater reduction in nodule volume of RFA over LA [52, 53]. RFA has been shown to reduce nodules of all types in size by over 50%, and some types up to 90% [54, 55]. RFA was initially only used for ablation of benign nodules, but recently it has been used for papillary microcarcinoma as well with promising results [56–58]. As surgeons become more familiar with such office-based treatments of thyroid disease, the landscape of thyroid surgery may undergo significant change.

Overall, the future gold standard treatment of thyroid disease will likely be focused on the use of minimally invasive techniques both surgical and nonsurgical.

Disclosures None
Support: None

References

1. Corner GW. The rise of medicine at Salerno in the twelfth century. Ann Med Hist. 1931;3(1):1.
2. Fortuny JV, Guigard S, Karenovics W, Triponez F. Surgery of the thyroid: recent developments and perspective. Swiss Med Wkly. 2015;145:w14144. https://doi.org/10.4414/smw.2015.14144.
3. Rogers-Stevane J, Kauffman GL. A historical perspective on surgery of the thyroid and parathyroid glands. Otolaryngol Clin N Am. 2008;41(6):1059–67. https://doi.org/10.1016/j.otc.2008.08.003.
4. Sarkar S, Banerjee S, Sarkar R, Sikder B. A review on the history of 'Thyroid Surgery'. Indian J Surg. 2016;78(1):32–6. https://doi.org/10.1007/s12262-015-1317-5.
5. Gross S. A system of surgery; pathological, diagnostic, therapeutic, and operative. Philidelphia: Blanchard and Lea; 1882.
6. Becker WF. Presidential address: pioneers in thyroid surgery. Ann Surg. 1977;185(5):493.
7. Ferzli GS, Sayad P, Abdo Z, Cacchione RN. Minimally invasive, nonendoscopic thyroid surgery. J Am Coll Surg. 2001;192(5):665–8. https://doi.org/10.1016/S1072-7515(01)00831-6.
8. Rafferty M, Miller I, Timon C. Minimal incision for open thyroidectomy. Otolaryngol Head Neck Surg. 2006;135(2):295–8. https://doi.org/10.1016/j.otohns.2006.03.013.
9. Miccoli P, Berti P, Conte M, Bendinelli C, Marcocci C. Minimally invasive surgery for thyroid small nodules: preliminary report. J Endocrinol Investig. 1999;22(11):849–51. https://doi.org/10.1007/bf03343657.
10. Gagner M. Endoscopic subtotal parathyroidectomy in patients with primary hyperparathyroidism. Br J Surg. 2005;83(6):875. https://doi.org/10.1002/bjs.1800830656.
11. Huscher C. Endoscopic right thyroid lobectomy. Surg Endosc. 1997;11:877.
12. Yeung GH. Endoscopic surgery of the neck: a new frontier. Surg Laparosc Endosc. 1998;8(3):227–32. http://europepmc.org/abstract/MED/9649050
13. Ohgami M, Ishii S, Arisawa Y, et al. Scarless endoscopic thyroidectomy: breast approach for better cosmesis. Surg Laparosc Endosc Percutan Tech. 2000;10(1):1–4.
14. Lee J, Chung WY. Robotic thyroidectomy and neck dissection: past, present, and future. Cancer J. 2013;19(2):151–61. https://doi.org/10.1097/PPO.0b013e31828aab61.

15. Sephton BM. Extracervical approaches to thyroid surgery: evolution and review: Minim Invasive Surg 2019;2019:5961690–5961690. https://doi.org/10.1155/2019/5961690.
16. Aidan P, Arora A, Lorincz B, Tolley N, Garas G. Robotic thyroid surgery: current perspectives and future considerations. J Oto-rhino-laryngol Related Specialties. 2018;80(3–4):186–94. https://doi.org/10.1159/000488354.
17. Jackson NR, Yao L, Tufano RP, Kandil EH. Safety of robotic thyroidectomy approaches: meta-analysis and systematic review. Head Neck. 2014;36(1):137–43. https://doi.org/10.1002/hed.23223.
18. Cabot JC, Lee CR, Brunaud L, et al. Robotic and endoscopic transaxillary thyroidectomies may be cost prohibitive when compared to standard cervical thyroidectomy: a cost analysis. Surgery. 2012;152(6):1016–24. https://doi.org/10.1016/j.surg.2012.08.029.
19. Berber E, Bernet V, Fahey TJ III, et al. American thyroid association statement on remote-access thyroid surgery. Thyroid. 2016;26(3):331–7.
20. Benhidjeb T, Wilhelm T, Harlaar J, Kleinrensink GJ, Schneider TA, Stark M. Natural orifice surgery on thyroid gland: totally transoral video-assisted thyroidectomy (TOVAT): report of first experimental results of a new surgical method. Surg Endosc. 2009;23(5):1119–20. https://doi.org/10.1007/s00464-009-0347-0.
21. Witzel K, Von Rahden B, Kaminski C, Stein H. Transoral access for endoscopic thyroid resection. Surg Endosc. 2008;22(8):1871–5.
22. Anuwong A. Transoral endoscopic thyroidectomy vestibular approach: a series of the first 60 human cases. World J Surg. 2016;40(3):491–7. https://doi.org/10.1007/s00268-015-3320-1.
23. Wilhelm T, Metzig A. Endoscopic minimally invasive thyroidectomy (eMIT): a prospective proof-of-concept study in humans. World J Surg. 2011;35(3):543–51. https://doi.org/10.1007/s00268-010-0846-0.
24. Anuwong A, Sasanakietkul T, Jitpratoom P, et al. Transoral endoscopic thyroidectomy vestibular approach (TOETVA): indications, techniques and results. Surg Endosc. 2018;32(1):456–65. https://doi.org/10.1007/s00464-017-5705-8.
25. Russell JO, Sahli ZT, Shaear M, Razavi C, Ali K, Tufano RP. Transoral thyroid and parathyroid surgery via the vestibular approach-a 2020 update. Gland Surg. 2020;9(2):409–16. https://doi.org/10.21037/gs.2020.03.05.
26. Jitpratoom P, Ketwong K, Sasanakietkul T, Anuwong A. Transoral endoscopic thyroidectomy vestibular approach (TOETVA) for Graves' disease: a comparison of surgical results with open thyroidectomy. Gland Surg. 2016;5(6):546–52. https://doi.org/10.21037/gs.2016.11.04.
27. Wang C, Zhai H, Liu W, et al. Thyroidectomy: a novel endoscopic oral vestibular approach. Surgery. 2014;155(1):33–8. https://doi.org/10.1016/j.surg.2013.06.010.
28. Russell JO, Clark J, Noureldine SI, et al. Transoral thyroidectomy and parathyroidectomy - a north American series of robotic and endoscopic transoral approaches to the central neck. Oral Oncol. 2017;71:75–80. https://doi.org/10.1016/j.oraloncology.2017.06.001.
29. Richmon JD, Kim HY. Transoral robotic thyroidectomy (TORT): procedures and outcomes. Gland Surg. 2017;6(3):285–9. https://doi.org/10.21037/gs.2017.05.05.
30. Dinc B, Gunduz UR, Belen NH. Transoral endoscopic thyroidectomy vestibular approach (TOETVA) in thyroiditis. Surg Laparosc Endosc Percutan Tech. 2020;31(2):188–92. https://doi.org/10.1097/sle.0000000000000864.
31. Razavi CR, Russell JO. Indications and contraindications to transoral thyroidectomy. Ann Thyroid. 2017;2(5):12.
32. Tanavde VA, Razavi CR, Chen LW, Ranganath R, Tufano RP, Russell JO. Predictive model of operative time in transoral endoscopic thyroidectomy vestibular approach. Head Neck. 2021;43(4):1220–8. https://doi.org/10.1002/hed.26581.
33. Tai DKC, Kim HY, Park D, et al. Obesity may not affect outcomes of transoral robotic thyroidectomy: subset analysis of 304 patients. Laryngoscope. 2020;130(5):1343–8. https://doi.org/10.1002/lary.28239.
34. Grogan RH, Suh I, Chomsky-Higgins K, et al. Patient eligibility for transoral endocrine surgery procedures in the United States. JAMA Netw Open. 2019;2(5):e194829. https://doi.org/10.1001/jamanetworkopen.2019.4829.
35. Milas M, Stephen A, Berber E, Wagner K, Miskulin J, Siperstein A. Ultrasonography for the endocrine surgeon: a valuable clinical tool that enhances diagnostic and therapeutic outcomes. Surgery. 2005;138(6):1193–200.; discussion 1200-1. https://doi.org/10.1016/j.surg.2005.08.032.
36. Razavi CR, Shaear M, Anuwong A, Russell JO. The role of surgeon-performed ultrasound in transoral endoscopic thyroidectomy vestibular approach (TOETVA). World J Otorhinolaryngol Head Neck Surg. 2020;6(3):150–4. https://doi.org/10.1016/j.wjorl.2020.01.009.
37. Caragacianu D, Kamani D, Randolph GW. Intraoperative monitoring: normative range associated with normal postoperative glottic function. Laryngoscope. 2013;123(12):3026–31. https://doi.org/10.1002/lary.24195.
38. Lydiatt DD. Medical malpractice and the thyroid gland. Head Neck. 2003;25(6):429–31. https://doi.org/10.1002/hed.10254.
39. Angelos P. Ethical and medicolegal issues in neuromonitoring during thyroid and parathyroid surgery: a review of the recent literature. Curr Opin Oncol. 2012;24(1):16–21. https://doi.org/10.1097/CCO.0b013e32834cd596.
40. Gartland RM, Bloom JP, Parangi S, et al. A long, unnerving road: malpractice claims involving the surgical management of thyroid and parathyroid dis-

ease. World J Surg. 2019;43(11):2850–5. https://doi.org/10.1007/s00268-019-05102-y.

41. Randolph GW, Dralle H, Abdullah H, et al. Electrophysiologic recurrent laryngeal nerve monitoring during thyroid and parathyroid surgery: international standards guideline statement. Laryngoscope. 2011;121(Suppl 1):S1–16. https://doi.org/10.1002/lary.21119.
42. Shindo M, Chheda NN. Incidence of vocal cord paralysis with and without recurrent laryngeal nerve monitoring during thyroidectomy. Arch Otolaryngol Head Neck Surg. 2007;133(5):481–5. https://doi.org/10.1001/archotol.133.5.481.
43. Kwek JWM, Pang MJ, Heah HHW. Pneumoperitoneum after transoral endoscopic thyroidectomy vestibular approach. Laryngosc Investig Otolaryngol. 2020;5(3):580–3. https://doi.org/10.1002/lio2.393.
44. Rajan S, Paul J, Kumar L. Carbon dioxide embolism during endoscopic thyroidectomy. Indian J Anaesth. 2016;60(1):65–6. https://doi.org/10.4103/0019-5049.174806.
45. Kim KN, Lee DW, Kim JY, Han KH, Tae K. Carbon dioxide embolism during transoral robotic thyroidectomy: a case report. Head Neck. 2018;40(3):E25–e28. https://doi.org/10.1002/hed.25037.
46. Park EY, Kwon JY, Kim KJ. Carbon dioxide embolism during laparoscopic surgery. Yonsei Med J. 2012;53(3):459–66. https://doi.org/10.3349/ymj.2012.53.3.459.
47. Yahagi N, Furuya H, Sai Y, Amakata Y. Effect of halothane, fentanyl, and ketamine on the threshold for transpulmonary passage of venous air emboli in dogs. Anesth Analg. 1992;75(5):720–3. https://doi.org/10.1213/00000539-199211000-00011.
48. Cobb WS, Fleishman HA, Kercher KW, Matthews BD, Heniford BT. Gas embolism during laparoscopic cholecystectomy. J Laparoendosc Adv Surg Tech A. 2005;15(4):387–90. https://doi.org/10.1089/lap.2005.15.387.
49. Herron DM, Vernon JK, Gryska PV, Reines HD. Venous gas embolism during endoscopy. Surg Endosc. 1999;13(3):276–9. https://doi.org/10.1007/s004649900963.
50. Dion YM, Lévesque C, Doillon CJ. Experimental carbon dioxide pulmonary embolization after vena cava laceration under pneumoperitoneum. Surg Endosc. 1995;9(10):1065–9. https://doi.org/10.1007/bf00188988.
51. Muhammad H, Tehreem A, Russell JO. Radiofrequency ablation and thyroid cancer: review of the current literature. Am J Otolaryngol. 2021;43(1):103204. https://doi.org/10.1016/j.amjoto.2021.103204.
52. Cesareo R, Pacella CM, Pasqualini V, et al. Laser ablation versus radiofrequency ablation for benign non-functioning thyroid nodules: six-month results of a randomized, parallel, open-label, trial (LARA trial). Thyroid. 2020;30(6):847–56. https://doi.org/10.1089/thy.2019.0660.
53. Cesareo R, Manfrini S, Pasqualini V, et al. Laser ablation versus radiofrequency ablation for thyroid nodules: 12-month results of a randomized trial (LARA II study). J Clin Endocrinol Metab. 2021;106(6):1692–701. https://doi.org/10.1210/clinem/dgab102.
54. Gharib H, Hegedüs L, Pacella CM, Baek JH, Papini E. Nonsurgical, image-guided, minimally invasive therapy for thyroid nodules. J Clin Endocrinol Metabol. 2013;98(10):3949–57. https://doi.org/10.1210/jc.2013-1806.
55. Baek JH, Kim YS, Lee D, Huh JY, Lee JH. Benign predominantly solid thyroid nodules: prospective study of efficacy of sonographically guided radiofrequency ablation versus control condition. AJR Am J Roentgenol. 2010;194(4):1137–42. https://doi.org/10.2214/ajr.09.3372.
56. Tufano RP, Pace-Asciak P, Russell J, et al. Update of radiofrequency ablation for treating benign and malignant thyroid nodules. The future is now. Front Endocrinol. 2021;12:710.
57. Russell JO, Razavi CR, Shaear M, et al. Transoral thyroidectomy: safety and outcomes of 200 consecutive north American cases. World J Surg. 2021;45(3):774–81. https://doi.org/10.1007/s00268-020-05874-8.
58. Cohen O, Tufano RP, Anuwong A, et al. Transoral endoscopic vestibular approach for thyroidectomy and parathyroidectomy - from promise to practice. Am J Otolaryngol. 2021;42(5):103022. https://doi.org/10.1016/j.amjoto.2021.103022.

Importance of Fluorescence Imaging for Minimally Invasive Cancer Surgery

17

Shreeyash Modak and G. V. Rao

Abstract

Surgery is one of the important modalities of treatment for cancers arising from gastrointestinal tract. With the advent of technology, minimally invasive surgery (MIS) is found to be both feasible and safe. The primary goal of abdominal cancer surgery, whether open or MIS is to achieve adequate radicality at the safe surgery. Also, evidence is emerging that few early-stage malignancies can be treated with organ conservation and limited lymphadenectomy. Limitations in MIS to achieve all this are identification of tumor locations and to differentiate between viable and nonviable tissues. Optical systems that have near infrared (NIR) imaging, have clinical applications like checking perfusion status of different organs (e.g., colonic segment in colectomy, liver segments in hepatectomy, gastric conduit in esophagectomy), to identify vital structures (e.g., bile duct anatomy, thoracic duct, ureters), detect tumor tissue (liver SOLs like secondaries, peritoneal metastases), and to guide lymph node dissection (sentinel lymph node and radical lymphadenectomy). Some of these uses have shown to be clinically important in practice while others are not that clinically relevant. As most of the newer optical systems have integrated NIR technology, it will be widely available. Also, the most commonly used dye is indocyanine green (ICG), which is not very tissue-specific, availability of compounds that can target tissue of interest can widen the practical use of this technology.

Keywords

Minimally invasive surgery (MIS) · Indocyanine green (ICG) · Fluorescence imaging · Cancer surgery

17.1 Introduction

Surgery is often the cornerstone in the treatment of abdominal malignancies, wherein the purpose is to remove as much tumor as possible and prevent damage to residual tissues, thus decreasing complications. Traditionally a good cancer surgery depends on visual and tactile feedback to distinguish between tissues. Additional measures to help are intraoperative ultrasound and gamma probe. Despite all this, chances of R1/R2 resection or incomplete lymphadenectomy remain. Also, many gastrointestinal oncological resections require some form of anastomosis between two structures and one must depend on criteria like, bleeding from cut edge, pulsations in mesentery, color of mucosa, and peristalsis to decide vascularity. Minimally invasive surgery (MIS, both laparoscopy and robotic) lacks tactile feedback, which has led to increased demand of

S. Modak (✉) · G. V. Rao
AIG Hospitals, Hyderabad, India

M. Tewari (ed.), *Minimally Invasive Surgery in Cancer*,
https://doi.org/10.1007/978-981-97-7059-5_17

methods to distinguish different tissues, structures, and assess viability. Newer intraoperative imaging systems that make use of near infrared (NIR) light spectrum have been evaluated for different clinical applications. In this chapter we will discuss the role of fluorescence imaging in MIS cancer surgery.

17.2 Fluorescence Imaging: Technique and Principles

Before clinical application, one must know the concept, pharmacokinetics, and tools of fluorescence imaging. NIR spectrum ranges from 700 nm to 900 nm. Fluorescence imaging has the following advantages:

1. NIR light has the ability to penetrate deeper into tissues, up to 10 mm.
2. NIR spectrum tissues exhibit almost no autofluorescence, hence better contrast between different tissue types.
3. It takes only milliseconds to record a fluorescence signal.
4. Most systems can merge fluorescence signal with RGB signal to give direct anatomical orientation.

NIR—Fluorescence imaging requires (1) Fluorescent agent (i.e., fluorophore) and (2) System that both excites and detects the fluorophore.

Different fluorophores have been evaluated in preclinical setting and two are used clinically: indocyanine green (ICG) and methylene blue (MB). They can be administered by either local injection or systemic intravenous injection. These are nonspecific contrast agents in NIR spectrum. ICG has excitation peak at 800 nm and is solely cleared by liver with half-life of 150–180 s. It is very safe with adverse reactions reported in 1 in 40,000 patients, which are mostly hypersensitivity type. MB has excitation peak at 700 nm, hence less tissue penetration. It is partially cleared by kidneys. At low doses (<2 mg/kg) it is safe, but can induce arrhythmias, hemolytic anemia, and coronary vasoconstriction in renal insufficiency or higher doses [1]. As the two fluorophores have different clearance mechanisms, they have been utilized in different clinical applications. The mode of administration of dye, composition of administered dye (dilution, mixing of other compound, etc.), and the time taken for detection of fluorescence vary between the indications.

Many manufacturers are producing imaging systems that can detect NIR fluorescence. These systems may be integrated in the normal white light laparoscopy or can be used separately whenever the need arises. The color generated by fluorescence may differ between different systems from blue to green.

In minimally invasive cancer surgery, NIR fluorescence imaging is used for four main purposes.

1. Identification of vital structures.
2. Lymph node mapping.
3. Detection of tumor.
4. Assessment of tissue perfusion.

17.3 Identification of Vital Structures

17.3.1 Ureter

Though intraoperative ureteric injury is rare, it is essential to safeguard ureters while doing radical surgeries for colorectal and gynecological malignancies. NIR fluorescence can identify ureters after fluorescent dye is injected either intravenously (methylene blue) or intraurethral (ICG). For ICG, the dose is 25 mg in 10 ml saline in each ureter through a catheter inserted under cystoscopy just before incision. Detection rate has been described to be 100%. For methylene blue, which is cleared by kidneys, 0.25–1 mg/kg intravenous injection is given at the time of incision, detection rate is variable, and fluorescence lasts for a shorter duration than that of ICG. Experimental dyes have been evaluated, which give brighter fluorescence at a low dose; they can be administered intravenously and cleared exclusively by kidney (thus avoiding cystoscopy) and lasts longer. The dye ZW800–1 looks promising in this respect [2].

17.3.2 Bile Ducts

Due to its exclusive hepatic clearance, ICG is being increasingly used to identify extrahepatic biliary anatomy during laparoscopic cholecystectomy. With a dose of 5 mg injected intravenously 3–7 h before surgery, the extrahepatic biliary tract gives good fluorescence signal with minimal background hepatic fluorescence [3]. In MIS radical cholecystectomy, ICG fluorescence can be used as a guide to safeguard common bile duct (Fig. 17.1). In MIS hepatectomies, ICG might be useful in identifying biliary structures in glissonian pedicle after isolating the same and to detect bile leaks from cut surface at the end of the procedure.

17.3.3 Lymphangiography (Thoracic Duct Identification)

Due to small hydrodynamic diameter of ICG molecule and its binding to plasma lipoproteins, it easily flows through lymphatic channels, making it a potential agent to detect thoracic duct in video-assisted thoracoscopic esophagectomy [4]. Also, it can be used during reoperation for chylothorax. There are many animal studies and few human case series, describing its usefulness. ICG can be injected at a dose of 1–2 mg/kg, 2 ml either in bilateral inguinal lymph nodes, in the web space between first and second toes or small bowel mesentery. Fluorescence is seen after 15–20 min and can last up to an hour [5]. Due to limited evidence, the technique is not yet standardized. Also, large, controlled trials are required to see whether ICG fluorescence really helps in decreasing thoracic duct injuries or it just helps in localizing the duct or leak.

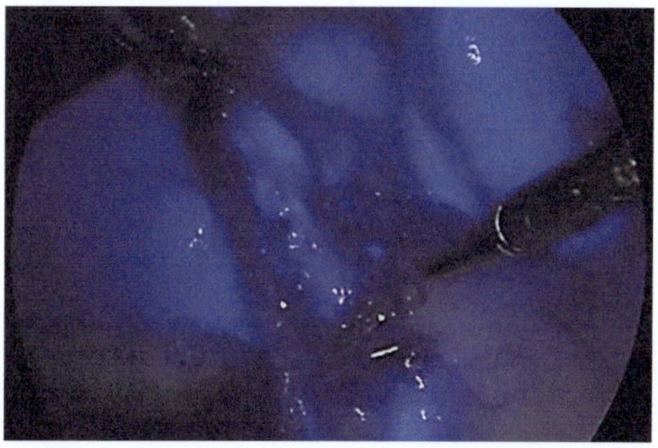

Fig. 17.1 ICG cholangiogram highlighting extrahepatic biliary system

17.3.4 Lymph Node Mapping

Most abdominal malignancies metastasize through lymphatic system and lymphadenectomy is part of any radical cancer surgery. As multimodality treatment options are emerging, trend is seen toward conservative surgery in the form of primary tumor resection with sentinel lymph node sampling in early-stage tumors. Detection of sentinel lymph nodes (SLN) can be achieved by blue dye injection or gamma camera; both techniques are either subjective or hazardous. NIR fluorescence is very safe and can provide objective evidence of SLN. Further it can be used to assess completeness of lymphadenectomy at the end of a radical surgery. These techniques are increasingly being used in gastric and colonic cancers.

D2 lymphadenectomy is the cornerstone of radical gastrectomy and includes lymph node station dissection as described by the Japanese. Similarly, a D3 lymphadenectomy and complete mesocolic excision is becoming standard of care in colonic cancers. Such radical approaches improve overall survival. These dissections are typically done along embryological planes and feeding arteries.

17.3.5 Sentinel Lymph Node Dissection

The technique of sentinel lymph node dissection involves injection of ICG dye mixed with albumin, usually in 1:10 ratio, in submucosal plane in four quadrants of the tumor. Dose and concentration may vary depending on prior experience of the operation team. This ranges from 0.05 mg/ml to 5 mg/ml of ICG in 0.5 to 2 ml injections. Injection of dye is performed after the ports are placed and tumor is localized. It is preferably to be done by an expert endoscopist to avoid extravasation of the dye in surgical field and to reach the most difficult tumor locations. Albumin used to mix the dye allows slow passage of dye through the lymphatic system, thus giving enough time window to detect sentinel lymph nodes (usually 2–5 min).

Sentinel node detection is important in early T stage (T1) cancers of GI tract where there is up to 10% chance of nodal metastases/micrometastases. While detecting metastases is easy by routine histopathology examination, detection of micrometastases requires immunohistochemistry (IHC) or other molecular methods. These are time consuming and costly to apply to each of the node dissected with specimen and found to be negative. Identification of micrometastases in sentinel lymph nodes dissected on table under ICG guidance will upstage a node negative cancer and direct further treatment options (Fig. 17.2).

Limitations of This Technique

- The concentration, dose, and timing of ICG are yet to be standardized and needs a pilot study before application in given setting of immunofluorescence detection systems and set of patients.
- Due to limitations arising from fatty mesentery, bulky tumors, higher BMI patients, and distention of bowels due to intraoperative endoscopy detection and dissection of SLN in given time frame might be difficult.
- Issue of false-negative lymph nodes may occur with application of routine histopathological methods.

17.3.6 Guiding Lymphadenectomy

Though radical lymphadenectomy follows anatomical landmark, sometimes it may be difficult to do a complete lymphadenectomy due to many reasons such as novice surgeon, lack of haptic feedback in MIS, and different anatomical orientation of MIS. ICG-guided lymphadenectomy has the potential to overcome these limitations. Typically, ICG is injected a day prior to surgery in peritumoral submucosal fashion. Again, the dose and concentration may vary as stated before. The operative field can be inspected at the end of surgery for any nodes left behind. Pitfall of this technique is extended lymphadenectomy (which otherwise may not be required). One more use of this technology is lateral pelvic lymph node dissection whenever indicated. ICG-enhanced lymph nodes can be safely dissected away from non-enhanced vital structures (Fig. 17.3).

17.3.7 Identification of Tumors

It is proposed that ICG injected intravenously gets delayed clearance from tumor tissue due to altered vascular environment. Thus, small tumors can be detected with NIR technique using ICG in

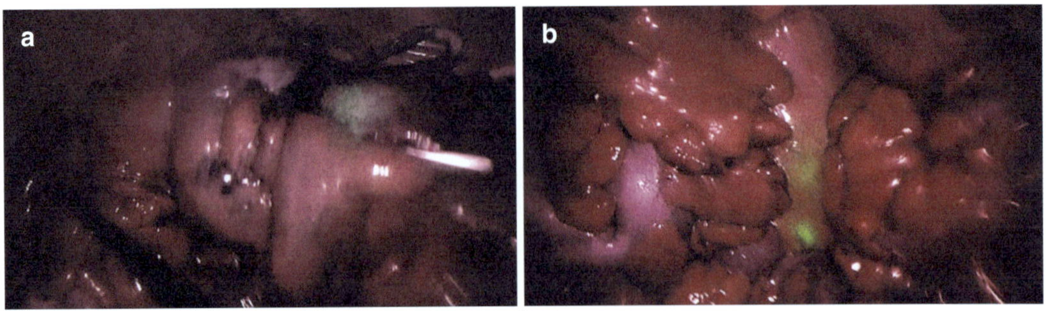

Fig. 17.2 On table detection of sentinel lymph node during sigmoidectomy. (**a**) Colonoscopic peritumoral ICG dye injection (**b**) Lymph node visualization in sigmoid mesocolon

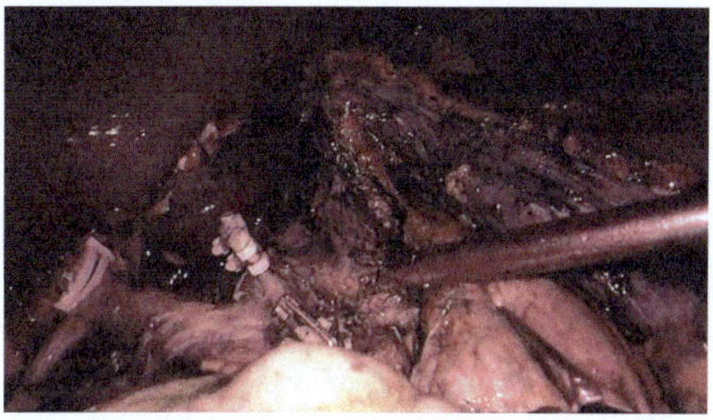

Fig. 17.3 Near fluorescence mode laparoscopic view at the end of D2 lymphadenectomy for carcinoma stomach. Note the absence of fluorescence in areas of interest, confirming complete lymphadenectomy

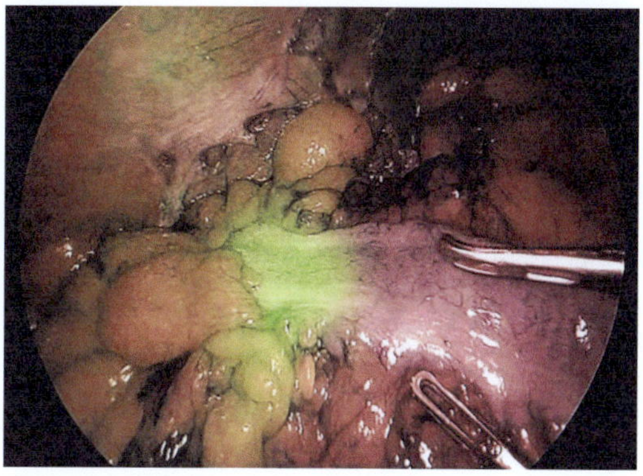

Fig. 17.4 ICG fluorescence imaging demonstrating demarcation line on large bowel before transection

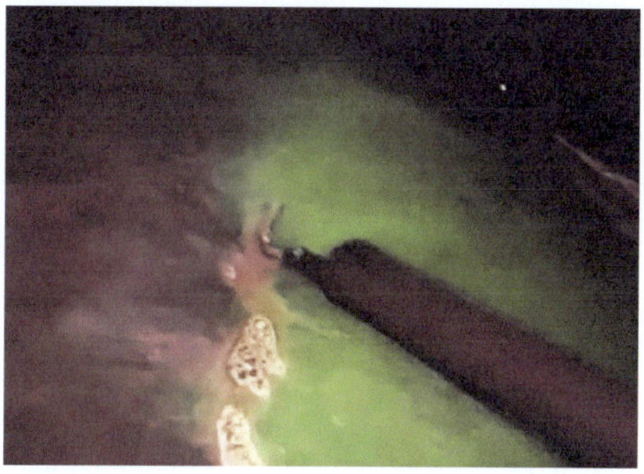

Fig. 17.5 Transection line on liver surface after inflow control well demarcated by ICG fluorescence

liver and peritoneum, which are common sites of metastases. Further improvement can be achieved by making ICG nanoparticle, which are tumor-specific by binding them with antibodies, tumor cell membrane antigen, etc. [6]

Luminal Tumor Localization: Colonic and gastric tumors, which are early T stage, can be localized easily with ICG injected in submucosa around the tumor. Either a tattooing at index endoscopy or on table injection will serve the purpose. This can also help in deciding margins of resection.

Detection of Liver Space Occupying Lesions (SOLs): In cases of liver SOLs, ICG given intravenously is picked up well by hemangiomas, well differentiated hepatocellular carcinomas, and colorectal liver metastases. ICG-guided surgery may help in identifying SOLs and resections of the same.

17.3.8 Assessment of Perfusion

ICG given as intravenous injection has a half-life of 2–3 min and gets cleared very fast. This phenomenon can be used effectively in two areas

I. Visceral surgery involves resection and anastomosis of stomach, intestines, or colon. Though majority of times surgeons depend on visual parameters such as color of mucosa or serosa and bleeding from edge of resected bowel, sometimes such assessment might be in doubt. NIR technology with intravenous ICG can help in differentiating well vascularized from devascularized segment (Fig. 17.4). This may reflect in reducing the leak rates of an anastomosis particularly in low anterior resections. Injection of ICG should be done after complete division of mesentery and vascular ligation, but before bowel transection. Even though meta-analysis of comparative studies [7] has shown that ICG use decreases anastomotic leaks in colorectal surgeries, multicenter RCT [8] has failed to show a conclusive advantage.
II. Liver resections typically involve partition along the intersegmental planes. Due to the segmental blood supply of liver, ICG given intravenously after isolating and clamping the inflow very well shows the demarcation between FLR and specimen (Fig. 17.5).

17.4 Conclusion

This is an overview of the technology, and its potential uses in MIS for abdominal cancers. We have not included the current evidence or published literature, as there are many and most of them are showing the feasibility of ICG technology. The perceived improvement in clinical outcomes (viz., bile leaks or anastomotic leaks) cannot be solely attributed to the use of ICG; this being seen in our day-to-day practice. In our opinion, immunofluorescence technology is still a subjective assessment where the surgeon has to interpret the findings. It helps in supporting our clinical judgment (e.g., if bowel is looking ischemic, ICG also may show low perfusion/dark or dull fluorescence) and in some areas it is not so useful (e.g., to assess extent of lymphadenectomy). Surgical principles and anatomical knowledge cannot be replaced by this technology. As most of the newer laparoscopic and robotic systems now come with integrated ICG/immunofluorescence technology, it might be used routinely henceforth. Systems, which have normal white light background with fluorescence overlay, will help in operating in normal operative milieu with target structures showing fluorescence.

17.5 Takeaway Points

- NIR technology with ICG can be used for many purposes during minimally invasive cancer surgery.
- ICG enhances and shows the surgical field in different color.
- Except few areas, e.g., assessment of perfusion and tumor localization the real practical use of ICG is limited.
- Further advancement in technology making tumor specific ICG particles, simultaneous white light and NIR imaging and development of newer fluorescent dyes might increase its use.

References

1. van Manen L, et al. A practical guide for the use of indocyanine green and methylene blue in fluorescence-guided abdominal surgery. J Surg Oncol. 2018;118(2):283–300. https://doi.org/10.1002/jso.25105.
2. Slooter MD, Janssen A, Bemelman WA, et al. Currently available and experimental dyes for intraoperative near-infrared fluorescence imaging of the ureters: a systematic review. Tech Coloproctol. 2019;23:305–13. https://doi.org/10.1007/s10151-019-01973-4.
3. Boogerd LSF, Handgraaf HJM, Huurman VAL, et al. The best approach for laparoscopic fluorescence cholangiography: overview of the literature and optimization of dose and dosing time. Surg Innov. 2017;24(4):386–96. https://doi.org/10.1177/1553350617702311.
4. Ashitate Y, Tanaka E, Stockdale A, Choi HS, Frangioni JV. Near-infrared fluorescence imaging of thoracic duct anatomy and function in open surgery and video-assisted thoracic surgery. J Thorac Cardiovasc Surg. 2011;142(1):31–8.e82. https://doi.org/10.1016/j.jtcvs.2011.03.004.
5. Matsuura Y, Ichinose J, Nakao M, Okumura S, Mun M. Recent fluorescence imaging technology applications of indocyanine green in general thoracic surgery. Surg Today. 2019;50:1332. https://doi.org/10.1007/s00595-019-01906-6.
6. Egloff-Juras C, et al. NIR fluorescence-guided tumor surgery: new strategies for the use of indocyanine green. Int J Nanomedicine. 2019;14(7823–7838):25. https://doi.org/10.2147/IJN.S207486.
7. Shen R, Zhang Y, Wang T. Indocyanine green fluorescence angiography and the incidence of anastomotic leak after colorectal resection for colorectal cancer: a meta-analysis. Dis Colon Rectum. 2018;61(10):1228–34. https://doi.org/10.1097/DCR.0000000000001123
8. De Nardi P, Elmore U, Maggi G, Maggiore R, Boni L, Cassinotti E, Fumagalli U, Gardani M, De Pascale S, Parise P, Vignali A, Rosati R. Intraoperative angiography with indocyanine green to assess anastomosis perfusion in patients undergoing laparoscopic colorectal resection: results of a multicenter randomized controlled trial. Surg Endosc. 2020;34(1):53–60. https://doi.org/10.1007/s00464-019-06730-0.

Minimally Invasive Surgery in Cancer: Pros and Cons

18

Monish Karunakaran and Savio George Barreto

Abstract

In this chapter the authors provide a broad, overarching view of the current state of play of minimally invasive surgery (MIS) in the management of solid organ cancers. This summary, that draws on the available evidence in literature, aims to provide the reader with answers to some very specific questions that have plagued the protagonists, as well as, sceptics of MIS in visceral cancers. The eventual aim is to reflect on the evidence using a real-world lens so that the reader is empowered to understand where we stand today in terms of MIS in cancer and what work needs to be done, if any, to better utilize the complementary strengths of MIS and open surgery, which can be put to use in a patient requiring surgery for cancer.

Keywords

Cancer · Outcome · Quality · Survival

18.1 Introduction

Minimally invasive surgery (MIS) was pioneered by Prof Dr. Erich Mühe when he presented his findings on laparoscopic cholecystectomy in 1986 [1]. After surviving a few initial years of scepticism, MIS ushered in a new paradigm not only in the surgical management of diseases, but more so in surgical training. There was, and continues to be, a move away from the 'apprenticeship model', towards structured programs of teaching new skills outside the operating room even using simulations. Over the years, an appreciation in the benefits of MIS has heralded its entry into the management of cancers. In this chapter, we examine key issues relating to the use of minimally invasive techniques, pertaining to the surgical management of solid organ cancer using data curated from the most recent, as well as largest meta-analyses for each malignancy.

18.2 MIS in Solid Organ Cancers: Intraoperative Factors

There remains no doubt with regard to the feasibility of MIS in the management of solid organ cancers. One of the most important advantages of

M. Karunakaran
Department of Surgical Gastroenterology, Asian Institute of Gastroenterology, Hyderabad, India

College of Medicine and Public Health, Flinders University, Bedford Park, SA, Australia

S. G. Barreto (✉)
College of Medicine and Public Health, Flinders University, Bedford Park, SA, Australia

Division of Surgery and Perioperative Medicine, Flinders Medical Center,
Bedford Park, Adelaide, South Australia, Australia
e-mail: savio.barreto@sa.gov.au; Savio.barreto@flinders.edu.au

M. Tewari (ed.), *Minimally Invasive Surgery in Cancer*,
https://doi.org/10.1007/978-981-97-7059-5_18

MIS is improved visibility. The development of a vast armamentarium of instruments to facilitate the replication of nearly every movement conceivable in open surgery, as well as, provide the surgeon with safe and adequate retraction to enable the safe surgery has further helped enhance the aspect of feasibility. However, when it comes to cancer, there is more to surgery than mere feasibility, or the ability to safely complete an operation. Survival in cancer is determined by other factors, including blood loss, surgical duration, margins of resection, lymph node yield, morbidity, etc. We will now address each of these factors comparing MIS with open surgery.

MIS requires a clear field of vision. Blood, by absorbing light not only reduces visibility, but also obscures planes of dissection. Studies comparing blood loss in MIS versus open surgeries have demonstrated variable results with some studies noting lower intraoperative operative blood loss, while others reporting no difference (Table 18.1). Blood loss has been shown to be less with MIS in oesophageal [2] gastric [3], colonic [4], rectal [5, 6] cancer resections as well as in distal pancreatectomies (DP) [7, 8]. Pressure exerted by pneumoperitoneum might play a bigger role in reducing venous bleeding during parenchymal transection in liver resections [9]. Among the three published RCTs on pancreatoduodenectomy (PD), Palanivelu et al. [10] reported a significantly lesser intra-operative bleeding in the laparoscopic arm, while the other two trials reported no difference [11, 12]. The hypothesized reasons to support lower blood loss in MIS are better vision, meticulous surgical manoeuvres and haemostasis, and reduced trauma to the abdominal wall and pressure of pneumoperitoneum compressing capillary and venous bleeding [13, 14]. As much as these findings appear to support a superiority, or non-inferiority, of the laparoscopic approach, the results are not uniform across studies for a given organ system. Even in open surgery there exists a significant variability in blood loss between surgeons, as well as between institutes. One of the reasons for this could simply be the inconsistencies in methods to estimate blood loss. Thus, from the available evidence it is reasonable to infer that intraoperative blood loss is lower in MIS compared to open surgery although there remains a lack of consistency across studies.

The duration of surgery is believed to be an independent, and potentially modifiable, risk factor for complications. MIS has consistently been associated with increased operative duration in oesophagectomies [2, 15], gastrectomies [3, 16], colectomies [17], rectal resections [5, 6], liver [18] and pancreatic [19] resections (Table 18.1). This may largely be attributed to the increased technical expertise required, not only during the long learning curve, but even after its negotiation. Additional time requirement in robotic surgery in comparison to laparoscopic technique may be due to a multitude of factors including port placement and angulation, adequate insufflation, robot positioning, and docking. Proficient docking involves a learning curve and additional time owing to the variability in port placement and robot positioning for multiple procedures further [20]. Thus, it can be inferred that the operative

Table 18.1 Intra-operative factors

Cancer type	Operative time	Blood loss	*R0* resection	Lymph nodal harvest
Oesophagus [15, 23, 54]	Longer	Lower	Similar	Similar
Stomach [3]	Longer	Lower	Similar	Similar
Colon [55]	Longer	Lower	Similar	Similar
Rectum [41]	Longer	Lower	Lower[a]	Similar
Liver [56, 57]	Longer	Similar	Similar	Lower
Pancreas [19]	Longer	Lower	Higher	Higher
Ovary [51]	Longer	Lower	–	Higher
Endometrium [58]	Longer	Lower	–	Similar

[a] Higher rates of CRM positivity and incomplete mesorectal excisions in laparoscopic arm, though statistically insignificant

duration in MIS is prolonged when compared to open surgery. While this certainly does not preclude the performance of MIS in solid organ cancer surgery, it is important to consider if the prolonged operative duration has arisen from *preventable operative disruptions* which may force surgeons and patients to endure unnecessary delays [21]. The main sources of this disruption arise from incoordination in teamwork, operating table/patient positioning and arrangement of instruments. Teams involved in MIS for solid organ cancers must be mindful of such disruptions and consider auditing their processes with a view to improving remediable aspects of their processes.

Radicality remains the litmus test for any approach in cancer surgery and it cannot be overemphasized that a (*R0*) resection with minimal morbidity is a surgeon's best contribution towards treatment in a patient affected by cancer [22]. In terms of completeness of resection, there doesn't seem to be a significant difference between open (OE) and minimally invasive oesophagectomy (MIE), as evidenced by similar rates of *R0* resection [23] and lymph nodal harvest [24, 25]. Innovations such as MIE in prone position has translated into higher average number of harvested lymph nodes compared to lateral decubitus position [26]. Recent studies in gastric cancer [3, 27] also found no significant difference in the nodal harvest between laparoscopic (LG) and open gastrectomy (OG) ($p = 0.16$), though the quality of evidence was low on account of moderate heterogeneity ($I^2 = 40\%$). Furthermore, one needs to understand that many of the trials [28–30] on LG versus OG dealt with distal gastrectomies for early gastric cancer [31], which was accompanied by less than D2 lymphadenectomy in many patients. KLASS 01 trial [32], which included D1+ lymphadenectomy, reported a significant difference in lymph-node yield, though a difference between 40.5 and 43.7 nodes in a real clinical scenario is debatable. Similarly, in the COACT 1001 trial [33], wherein adherence to D2 lymphadenectomy was the primary outcome, there was no difference between the laparoscopic and the open approach, though compliance was lower in the laparoscopic group in the subgroup of patients with stage III disease. The reasons for this observation might be twofold, including increased technical difficulty in laparoscopic lymphadenectomy, or more aggressive lymphadenectomy in open surgery or a combination of both.

Laparoscopic surgery for colon cancer has been demonstrated to be equivalent to open surgery in terms of adequacy of margins and lymphadenectomy [34, 35]. Laparoscopic colectomy with complete mesocolic excision (CME) has been found to be technically feasible with similar oncological appropriacy and lesser blood loss in elective as well as emergency presentations [36]. In comparison to colonic surgery, the results with laparoscopic rectal cancer surgery have been less flattering. It has been hypothesized that the challenges are afforded by the deep and narrow pelvis, limited angulation of laparoscopic instruments and stapling devices and the assist-dependent procedure [37], though it provides a better appreciation of the total mesorectal excision plane (TME) by the virtue of its magnified and clean vision. The rate of conversion to open surgery has varied widely between trials (34%, 11.3%, 9% and 1.2% in CLASSIC [38], ACOSOG Z6051 [39], ALaCaRT [6] and COREAN [40] trials, respectively), which may be a reflection of differences in inclusion criteria, local extent of the disease, patient body habitus and surgeon expertise. While most of the studies [5, 40] demonstrated no significant differences in completeness of meso-rectal excision, circumferential resection margin (CRM) positivity, nodal harvest, or tumour recurrence rates between the two surgical approaches in patients with rectal cancer, laparoscopic technique failed to meet the non-inferiority criteria in ACOSOG Z6051 [39] and ALaCaRT [6] trials, especially in those with large T3 tumours, which questions its suitability in lower rectal cancers and locally advanced disease. The meta-analysis by Conticchio et al. [41] confirmed higher rates of CRM positivity and incomplete mesorectal excisions in the MIS arm, albeit statistically insignificant. Again, though the role of lateral lymph node dissection continues to be debated, MIS has not been shown to confer a disadvantage in terms of lateral lymph node harvest [42]. It is postulated that the robotic approach may help in circumventing many of the technical difficulties of laparoscopic rectal cancer dissection as evidenced by the lower conversion rates [43], especially in obese males [44], a particularly difficult group of patients.

Despite ample evidence in literature to support MIS in liver surgery, the retrospective nature of the studies and a likely treatment allocation bias reduces the generalizability of the findings. For example, liver tumours close to vascular structures [45] and large sub-capsular tumour or previous history of abdominal surgeries [46] might have been preferentially included in the open group. It is important to understand that [47], patients undergoing minimally invasive DP were found to have early stage tumours in the meta-analysis by van Hilst et al. Data on technical feasibility of laparoscopic pancreatic resection [7, 8, 10, 11] comes high volume centres and surgeons with advanced laparoscopic skills, precluding its immediate reproducibility to other centres. Zhang et al. [19] found a higher nodal yield and R0 resection rates with laparoscopic PD, though one needs to factor in the retrospective nature of the studies and that patients who underwent laparoscopic PD had significantly smaller tumours. Again, the meta-analysis by Nickel et al. [48] on randomized controlled trials (RCTs) alone failed to find a difference in nodal harvest or *R0* resection rates between MIS and open surgery. Although the decision to opt for open or MIS largely depends on surgical expertise and institutional preferences, careful patient selection using predictive models [49, 50] to anticipate intra-operative difficulty may offer a more pragmatic approach to patient selection for minimally invasive hepato-pancreato-biliary (HPB) surgeries.

While Bogani et al. [51] found no difference in tumour spillage and upstaging rates between open and laparoscopic approach in early-stage ovarian cancers, intraoperative tumour capsule rupture resulting in tumour seeding of the abdominal cavity has been shown to negatively affect survival in ovarian cancer in more recent studies [52]. Increased adoption of MIS might have led to an alarming trend of concomitant increase in tumour rupture rates (23.9% vs. 20.2%, $p = 0.02$), with resultant decrease in survival [53].

In summary, while the feasibility of the performance of MIS in solid organ cancers is undisputed and estimated blood loss may be less than in open surgery, looking beyond the longer operative times, the evidence to support the oncological radicality of MIS in solid organ cancers is not consistent across organ sub-sites. The radicality of MIS in terms of distal gastric resections, oesophageal and colonic resections appear to be comparable to open surgery. However, the findings in rectal and ovarian cancers remain concerning. For HPB cancers, the evidence to support the radicality of MIS is evolving.

18.3 MIS in Solid Organ Cancers: Post-Operative Outcomes

Reduced post-operative pain is not only a benefit, but has majorly endorsed MIS over open surgery in benign disease. Reduced pain translates into lesser analgesic (opiate) requirements, earlier mobilization and greater patient satisfaction. The reasons for lesser pain are broadly twofold, namely, smaller abdominal wounds and lesser trauma to musculoaponeurotic structures resulting in an attenuated inflammatory/immunological response to surgical stress. Rat models have shown that CO_2 pneumoperitoneum decreases the inflammatory response based on decreased levels of Interleukin (IL)-2 [59], α-2 macroglobulin messenger ribonucleic acid (mRNA) and β-fibrinogen [60]. MIS may also result in a faster return of inflammatory markers to baseline, compared to open surgery [61]. However, one needs to be sceptical over this generalization as laparoscopic PD was not shown to be associated with a decrease in the post-operative inflammatory markers (IL-6, IL-8 and CRP) when compared to open PD, in quite contradistinction to minimally invasive colectomy or esophagectomy [62–64]. This lends strength to the belief that minimally invasive approach alone may not be sufficient to assuage the stress of PD nor minimize its morbidity [65]. Again, although the differences may be small and short-lived, MIS may have a significantly better-preserved immune function than equivalent open procedures, which in turn might have implications on occurrence and pattern of recurrences following cancer surgery [66].

MIE gained popularity in the 1990s when it was shown to be associated with a reduction in respiratory complications [15, 67] and overall morbidity [67, 68]. Studies have shown no difference in the rates of anastomotic leak [15, 23, 67] and recurrent laryngeal nerve injury [68, 69] between OE and MIE. Zhou et al. [70] noted that while gastrointestinal complications including gastric tube necrosis, anastomotic strictures and delayed gastric emptying were similar between MIE and OE groups, cardiovascular complications, and thromboembolic events were less common in the MIE group ($p < 0.05$). Although Yibulayin et al. [67] reported a significant decrease in mortality (OR 0.668; $p < 0.05$) following MIE, this has not been replicated in other studies [15, 23] despite lesser blood loss, pulmonary complications and shorter hospitalization. In gastric cancer, overall post-operative complications were found to be significantly less in the laparoscopic gastrectomy group in the meta-analysis by Zeng et al. [3] while Cochrane review published in 2016 [27] and Beyer et al. [16] reported no significant difference between the two groups in terms of severe post-operative complications. Majority of the included studies were from Japan, China and South Korea on early gastric cancer patients with favourable body habitus, potentially limiting its global applicability.

Similar findings have been noted in colorectal surgery, where functional recovery with respect to time to first bowel movement ($p < 0.001$), overall complication rate ($p < 0.001$), readmission rate ($p < 0.001$), and mortality ($p < 0.001$) were significantly reduced in the laparoscopic surgery group compared to open group in the meta-analysis by Zhao et al. [71] that included four RCTs and six clinical controlled trials. In early-stage ovarian [51] as well as endometrial [58] malignancies, MIS was associated with a decrease in immediate post-operative morbidity.

Compared to open liver resections, patients who underwent laparoscopic liver resection had lower overall complications rates with no differences in post-operative mortality [18, 56, 72]. An individual patient data meta-analysis [73] of two RCTs [7, 8] on DP revealed reduced rates of delayed gastric emptying ($p = 0.049$) and no difference in major complications ($p = 0.148$) in MIS arm, though there was a trend towards higher rates of post-operative pancreatic fistula (POPF) following MIDP ($p = 0.067$). Again, in PD, recent meta-analyses [19, 48] found no difference between short-term outcomes including overall morbidity, mortality and re-admission rates. Besides, the results of Dutch multi-centric LEOPARD-2 trial [12], wherein there was greater complication-related 90-day mortality (10% vs. 2%) in the laparoscopic arm leading to its premature termination, sound a strong word of caution.. This 'real world' study has provided a much-needed tempering of the concerning enthusiasm that may accompany the willingness to undertake laparoscopic pancreatic and HPB resections without adequate training. Though post-operative outcomes in robotic and laparoscopic approaches have been more or less similar, robotic approach may gain greater traction in future in view of its lower incidence of intraoperative conversions [74].

In summary, while MIE and laparoscopic colonic and segmental liver resections have helped to significantly improve post-operative outcomes compared to open surgery when performed by adequately trained surgeons, MIS for gastric and ovarian cancer has a morbidity rate comparable to open surgery. Although reported together with colonic surgeries under the broad, and often imprecise, umbrella of colorectal surgery, the technical successes of MIS rectal surgery need to be balanced with the not so impressive determinants of oncological outcomes noted in the preceding section, especially with large T3 tumours, lower rectal cancers and locally advanced disease. While laparoscopic DP is feasible, the POPF rates are higher than open surgery. Laparoscopic PD remains an area that warrants more evidence.

Length of post-operative hospitalization, despite its inherent flaws, has often been used as a metric to audit an intervention intended to

Table 18.2 Post-operative outcomes

Cancer type	Morbidity	Mortality	Reoperations	Hospital stay (WMD[a] (days)/p-value/I^2)
Oesophagus [54]	Lesser[a]	Similar	Similar	Shorter (−0.51/<0.001/92%)
Stomach [3]	Lower	Similar	–	Shorter (−1.37/<0.001/93%)
Colon [55]	Lower	Lower	Similar	Shorter (−1.65 days/p < 0.001/75%)
Rectum [41, 80]	Similar	Similar	–	Shorter (−1.71/p < 0.003/90%)
Liver [56]	Lower	Similar	–	Shorter (−3.09/p = 0.001/72.4%)
Pancreas [19, 48]	Similar	Similar	Similar	Similar (−2.51/0.37/62%)
Ovary [51]	Lower	–	–	Shorter (−3.92/0.00001/87%)
Endometrium [58]	Lower	–	–	Shorter (−0.23/0.00001/82%)

[a] Lesser pulmonary complications; no difference in anastomotic leak and cardiac complications

Table 18.3 Oncological outcomes

Cancer type	Disease-free survival	Overall survival
Oesophagus [24, 25, 81]	Similar	Similar
Stomach [83]	Similar	Similar
Colon [55]	Better	Better
Rectum [102]	Similar	Similar
Liver [56]	–	Similar (both CRLM and HCC)
Pancreas [92]	–	Similar
Ovary [97]	Lower	Similar
Endometrium [101]	–	Similar

(Abbreviations: *CRLM* Colorectal liver metastases; *HCC* Hepatocellular carcinoma)

improve patient outcomes. In comparison to open surgery, MIS has been instrumental in significantly reducing post-operative length of stay (LoS) in almost all surgical sub-specialities (Table 18.2) [3, 41, 51, 54–56, 58]. Although, the most recent meta-analysis in PD fails to highlight any difference in the length of stay [48]. In gastric cancer, Best et al. [27] and Zeng et al. [3] found a significant reduction in LoS, though there was considerable heterogeneity (I^2 = 76%) in both the studies, whereas hospital stay tended to be lower in the minimally invasive group but not in a manner that reached statistical significance in the study by Beyer et al. [16]. A closer look at available data (Table 18.2) makes one ponder over the actual significance of the improvement of 1–2 days for an individual patient who has just undergone a major surgery for malignancy and brings to mind the thought, '*Just because one can measure something, doesn't mean it amounts to anything*'. Again, there is substantial heterogeneity in the results, which might be accounted by the difference in sociocultural practices and health regulations impacting discharge decisions. Uniform adoption of ERAS protocols, a great leveller, has been shown to improve patient outcomes, irrespective of the surgical approach [75–79].

18.4 Oncological Outcomes

In terms of survival and recurrence rates, MIS is believed to be equivalent to open surgery in colon cancer, though the same cannot be yet inferred about other intra-abdominal malignancies where currently available literature doesn't confirm or refute the oncological equivalence of MIS (Table 18.3). In oesophageal cancer, Osugi et al. [24, 25] described comparable 3-year survival rates following hybrid MIE and OE in patients who underwent 3-field and 2-field lymphadenectomy, respectively. Chen et al. [81] noted that in patients who underwent neoadjuvant chemoradiotherapy, overall survival (OS) was significantly better in the MIE group (log rank = 6.197; p = 0.013), although there was no difference in disease-free-survival (DFS). Data in gastric cancer, too, seems encouraging with no difference in OS rates [82]. In the meta-analysis by Zhu et al. [83], in studies published in 2010–2015, there was no significant difference in terms of 5-year OS. However, LG was associated with better survival in studies published between 2016 and 2020. The CLASS-01 trial [84] did not report inferior disease-free survival at 3 years with LG, compared with OG.

The non-inferiority of laparoscopic versus open techniques has already been established in colon cancer [55]. One of the more contentious areas have been the role of laparoscopy in bulky advanced tumours. In the study by Park et al. [85] *R0* resection rates were similar for both laparoscopic and open approaches. While the 5-year OS was similar (72.0% vs. 71.8%, $p = 0.611$) in left-sided tumours, the laparoscopic approach was associated with decreased, although non-significant, 5 year-OS in comparison to open surgery (60.0% vs. 70.0%, $p = 0.284$) in right colonic cancers. In rectal cancer, COLOR II [86] CLASICC [87, 88], and COREAN [89] trials demonstrated non-inferior outcomes to open surgery. The long-term results of the ACOSOG Z6051 and ALaCaRT trials have further strengthened the safety belief which reported no difference in 2-year DFS or loco-regional recurrence rates [90], though short-term pathological outcomes had failed to meet the non-inferiority criteria in both of these trials. Currently, there are no compelling long-term data to suggest that robotic rectal cancer surgery is clearly advantageous over open, or the laparoscopic, approaches [44, 91].

In pancreatic head cancer, the meta-analysis by Chen et al. [92] revealed equivalent survival between MIS and open groups, and a possible tendency towards increased survival in the laparoscopic group by the fifth year (OR 2.11; $p = 0.001$). It is important to highlight that this analysis was based on the findings of single-institution, retrospective series. It would appear prudent to revisit this after the availability of the long-term outcomes of RCTs [10–12]. In left pancreatic tumours, Røsok et al. [93] found no difference in the OS between Minimally Invasive Distal Pancreatectomy (MIDP) and Open Distal Pancreatectomy (ODP) cohorts, though they acknowledge the retrospective nature of the included studies and possible risk-minimization allocation as patients in the ODP cohort had larger tumours and higher margin positivity rates. Recently, MIDP received a shot in the arm with the publication of the results of the DIPLOMA trial, which testifies its feasibility and oncological adequacy [94]. Xie et al. [72] compared oncological outcomes of open versus laparoscopic liver resection in colorectal liver metastases alone, and found no significant differences in disease recurrence, 3- or 5-year OS and DFS between the two approaches, despite higher rates of clear surgical margins (OR: 1.64, 95%CI: 1.32 to 2.05, $p < 0.00001$) in the laparoscopic group. One must appreciate that the cohort lacked aggressive tumours. These were either not attempted laparoscopically, or converted to open surgery.

MIS has historically been viewed unfavourably in gall bladder cancer (GBC) on account of concerns regarding port site/peritoneal metastasis after laparoscopic surgery. With increasing detection of incidental GBC, it has been realized that laparoscopic surgery is not associated with decreased survival, if definite resection is performed during, or soon after, laparoscopic cholecystectomy [95]. However, the outcome of laparoscopic surgery is concerning in GBC with preoperative evidence of liver invasion or acute cholecystitis [96] and therefore, the role of MIS in GBC needs to be better clarified. Though laparoscopic extended cholecystectomy has shown acceptable post-operative outcomes [97], the published experience comes from small, retrospective studies from few expert centres, and is currently not generalizable.

Laparoscopic approach has yielded similar 4–5-year OS, progression-free survival and post-operative upstaging rate for early-stage ovarian epithelial neoplasms [98]. The same study reported lower recurrence rates with laparoscopic surgery, which might be attributed to larger tumour size and increased utilization of fertility sparing surgery in the open arm. Uterine cancer with cervical involvement presents an interesting scenario. Unlike retrospective studies [99, 100] wherein there was no difference between MIS and open hysterectomy for cervical cancer in terms of mortality or recurrence rates, Ramirez et al. [101] in a prospective RCT, found lower rate of DFS and OS with laparoscopic and robotic approaches in early-stage cervical cancer. In contrast, there was no survival disadvantage with MIS in stage II uterine cancer with cervical involvement [102]. Possible explanation to this observation would be that uterine tumours generally remain confined to the corpus without an involvement of ectocervix, while exophytic nature of cervical malignancies may render them susceptible to local spread from vagina into the peritoneal cavity, upon CO_2 insufflation in a minimally invasive approach.

In summary, the oncological outcomes (OS and DFS) are improved with MIS in oesophageal and gastric cancer and even with colon and some rectal cancers. There is a definite benefit of MIS in segmental and non-anatomical liver resections, although the role in larger tumours remains uncertain. Evidence on the role of MIS in pancreatic cancer surgery is evolving.

18.5 Port-Site Metastases (PSM)

Earlier reports of a prohibitive PSM rate of 21% in colorectal cancer [103], possibly attributed to the direct manipulation of the tumour, extraction of the tumour through the small wound without adequate wound protection, contamination of the laparoscopic instruments with cancer cells and technical inadequacy, tempered the enthusiasm for the MIS approach [104]. Similarly, in ovarian cancer, studies reported PSM in 2–3% of patients [105, 106], though most of these occurred in the setting of advanced disease. The possible reasons [104] were direct manipulation of the tumour, direct transmission along the port device (chimney stack effect) [107], extraction of the tumour through the small wound without adequate wound protection, inflammation induced by pneumoperitoneum and technical inadequacy. Evidently, as surgeons gained more experience with this approach, the rate of PSM declined to less than 1%, comparable to wound recurrences reported for open procedures [108, 109]. A meta-analysis by Zhangi et al. [110] failed to determine any significant difference in the wound, or port-site, metastasis and peritoneal seeding between the laparoscopic and open surgery in patients with colorectal cancer. In GBC, notorious for PSM [111], Berger-Richardson et al. [112] found that PSM were more common at extraction ports than non-extraction ports and the incidence decreased from 18.6% to 10.3%, when studies between 2000 and 2014 were compared to those from 1991–1999. Also, PSM is often associated with diffuse peritoneal disease [113].

In summary, it is not possible to suggest with absolute certainty whether PSM represents aggressive disease biology or is reflective of the surgical approach.

18.6 Receipt of Adjuvant Therapy

Geest et al. [114] reported that complicated post-operative recovery increases omission, delay and / or discontinuation of adjuvant chemotherapy in patients with Stage III colon cancer and highlighted that MIS, though not statistically significant, was associated with an increased probability of receiving adjuvant chemotherapy ($p = 0.09$). This benefit of MIS in the earlier initiation of chemotherapy was again underlined by Jung et al. [115]. Gantt Jr. et al. [116] noted that delay in the initiation of adjuvant chemotherapy adversely affected DFS and OS in the open surgery group, but not in the MIS group, though there was no difference in proportions of patients who received adjuvant chemotherapy more than 8 weeks after surgery between the two groups. Laparoscopic approach was associated with improved compliance to adjuvant therapy in gastric cancer as well, which was cited one of the factors for favourable survival in laparoscopic arm in the study by Bao et al. [117]. Similarly, Anderson et al. [118] reported that patients undergoing MIDP were more likely to receive adjuvant chemotherapy after adjusting for clinical and demographic variables ($p = 0.03$).

In summary, MIS, by its inherent ability to enhance recovery, provides an additional benefit in terms of commencement of adjuvant therapy in those patients who require it.

18.7 Quality of Life and Functional Outcomes

Laparoscopic rectal cancer surgery is associated with better autonomic nerve preservation and consequently genitourinary function, possibly by the virtue of better image magnification. While open rectal resection with TME is associated with significant deterioration in post-operative genitourinary function [119], laparoscopic TME has been shown to be associated with low urinary (6%) and sexual (6%) dysfunction, when performed by experienced surgeons [120]. Asoglu et al. [121] showed significantly lesser sexual dysfunction (5% vs. 29% impotence in males (p = 0.03) and 7% vs. 50% decreased sexual activity in females (p = 0.03)) following laparoscopic TME, but Morino et al. reported no difference [122]. In comparison to laparoscopy, robotic TME is associated with lower rates of urinary symptoms including retention and ileus, and a better quality of life and no significant differences in sexual function [123], possibly due to improved visualization and more precise dissection. However, these results need to be interpreted with the understanding that most of it comes from non-randomized studies with functional outcomes reported as secondary endpoints.

Additionally, following radical oesophagectomy, patients reported better global quality of life scores for physical function, fatigue and pain 3 months after MIS compared with open surgery. However, these differences ceased to exist at 6- and 12-months follow-up [124]. These results may indicate that current evidence is not sufficient to recommend minimally invasive oesophagectomy as standard of care. Similarly, long-term quality of life analysis of the patients in LEOPARD trial at 3 years found no improvement in QALYs (Quality Adjusted Life Years) or overall quality of life scores with MIDP, whereas cosmetic satisfaction was higher in MIDP [125].

18.8 Training in Laparoscopic Cancer Surgery

Surgical learning curves are long on account of increased complexity of oncological operations. There is an increasing need to implement safe programs to diminish learning-associated patient morbidity. It might take years to negotiate the learning curves of technically challenging procedures with a possibility of suboptimal results during the learning phase (Table 18.4) [126]. Surgeon experience was found to be an indepen-

Table 18.4 Learning curves associated with various minimal access oncological procedures

Minimally invasive procedure	Method of analysis	Minimum number of cases	Outcome parameter used
McKeown MIE [132]	CUSUM	175	Operative time, blood loss
Ivor Lewis MIE [133]	CUSUM	119	Anastomotic leakage
Total Gastrectomy [134]	Moving average method	100	Operative time, blood loss
Distal Gastrectomy [135]	Not clearly mentioned	60	Operative time, blood loss
Right colectomy [127]	CUSUM	55	Operation time, conversion rate, and readmission and post-operative complications
Left colectomy [127]	CUSUM	62	
Distal pancreatectomy [136]	Not clearly mentioned	30	Not clearly mentioned
Pancreatoduodenectomy [137]	CUSUM	40	Operative time
Major hepatectomy [138]	CUSUM	45–75	Operative time
Radical hysterectomy [139]	CUSUM	40	Operative time

(Abbreviations: MIE: Minimally invasive oesophagectomy)

[a] CUSUM: Cumulative sum control chart is a sequential analysis technique used for monitoring change detection

dent risk factor for conversion of laparoscopic to open surgery in colorectal (OR 0.9 per 10 additional cases performed [127]) cancer.

The implications of the learning curve have been difficult to interpret as the currently available literature suffers from significant methodological diversity among the studies, outcomes of interest, curve evaluation and interpretation methods and corrections for case mix. The Cumulative Sum Control Chart (CUSUM) analysis is the preferred form of analysis as it helps in establishing proof of technical competence for the purpose of accreditation [128]. CUSUM avoids arbitrary splitting of patients into groups by authors, which results in a lower risk of bias and identifies the length of the learning curve for a given patient instead of analysing groups of patients, resulting in more precise estimates. Again, correction for case mix is very important for learning curve analysis, since it is commonly noticed that experienced surgeons, with mounting experience, go on to expand indications to more complex cases. Some of these limitations might be overcome by deducing the length of the learning curve by analysing pooled data from multi-centre datasets.

Novel procedures ought to be sieved through the Idea, Development, Exploration, Assessment, Long-term monitoring (IDEAL) framework [129] prior to its widespread adoption. First stage (Stage I {Idea}) involves assessment of the proof of concept and feasibility, following which the procedure is refined (Stage IIa {Development} and Stage IIb {Exploration}). Next stage involves comparison of the newer innovative technique to older ones (Stage III {Assessment}) and studies regarding its short and long-term outcomes (Stage IV {Long-term}). Stages III and IV are marked by evolution of a stable surgical technique which can be incorporated into standardized training programs. For individual surgeons the training process may be divided into phases [130]. Implementation of complex minimally invasive oncological surgery should entail technical training, evaluation of outcomes including assessment of learning curves, and evaluation of the program including volume and institution's capabilities [131].

18.9 Specific Advantages of Robotics

Conventional laparoscopic surgery is limited in complex operations, on account of loss of depth perception and need for dextrous hand–eye coordination, fulcrum effect of rigid instruments, limited degrees of freedom, and suboptimal surgeon ergonomics [140]. Robotic assistance in surgery facilitates fine intra-corporeal dissections and multiple or delicate reconstructions with increasing reproducibility by different surgeons. Robotic assistance can train newer generations of surgeons, thanks to the availability of the dual console and the immediate restoration of hand–eye coordination. The major deterrent is the cost, though it is expected to come down in the near future as the market becomes more competitive [141].

18.10 Economic Impact and Viability of MIS

There remain uncertainties regarding the financial implications in the use of MIS in the care of a cancer patient. This is an important factor for consideration as surgery is an important contributor to health care expenditure [142] and represents 30% of the global burden of disease [143]. In colorectal cancer, Ribeiro et al. [144] demonstrated that laparoscopic surgery was not costlier than open surgery, perceivably due to the 17% reduction in the LOS in the former, which likely compensated for the increased intraoperative costs. Furthermore, laparoscopic resection resulted in more QALYs and lower costs in colon cancer surgery [145]. In the cost analysis of COLOR-II trial [146], though there were no differences in long-term costs to society between laparoscopic and open surgery at 3 years (mean difference \$684, $p = 0.84$), laparoscopic surgery incurred higher costs to the health care sector, both at 28 days (mean difference \$1910, $p < 0.002$) and 3 years (mean difference \$3854, 95%, $p < 0.001$). Interestingly, King et al. [147] highlighted mean cost savings of £354 favouring laparoscopic surgery when utilized within an enhanced-recovery protocol.

Similarly, MIE was estimated to cost $1641 less than OE, with an incremental gain of 0.022 QALYs, making it dominant (less costly and more effective) in comparison [148]. In the study by Tardiff et al. [149], though costs of LG were $935 greater than those of OG, an incremental gain of 0.05 QALYs resulted in an incremental cost–effectiveness ratio of $18,846 per additional QALY gained from laparoscopic approach. Though the data in pancreatic cancer is not as robust, Kowalsky et al. [150] demonstrated that implementation of robotic PD within an enhanced recovery framework led to optimal cost outcomes.

18.11 Current Status of MIS in Cancer and Conclusions

In the current era of evidence-based medicine, clinical guidelines contribute towards improving the quality of care and treatment outcomes. However, it is disturbing to note that, in guidelines pertaining to laparoscopic surgery, there appears to be a systematic aggrandizement of the strength of recommendation in approximately a third of the guideline statements by the corresponding authors in comparison to an independent assessment based on the same evidence [151]. It is thus important to be mindful of such biases when planning to adopt practices prescribed by guideline documents. It also calls for organizations preparing Guideline documents to be inclusive and widen the representation of individuals on these teams to be practitioners of open as well as MIS. This may help reduce the incidence of personal biases creeping into guidelines, which are documents, perceived by the medical fraternity as well as the public, to be truly representative of the evidence.

In resource-rich health care systems, where trained surgeons and facilities are available, MIS is as good as open surgery for staging of cancers, as well as in the management of early, resectable cancers affecting organs such as the oesophagus, stomach, endometrium and ovary, and liver and those affecting the pancreatic body and tail. It is advantageous in some cancers on account of its potential to reduce immediate post-operative morbidity and post-operative hospitalization, which may in turn facilitate better resource utilization. The health care system, however, needs to factor in the longer operating times associated with MIS and balance this with waiting lists–that in some countries extend to years for benign disease (thereby affecting the quality of life of these patients). In locally advanced cancers and/or cancers needing multi-visceral resections, open surgery is preferred at present, unless evidence to the contrary emerges. For organs such as the pancreas, open surgery remains the standard of care. In resource-poor countries and resource-rich countries where basic access to cancer remains a problem, in the least, open surgery must be made available. There is a need for a concerted effort to improve the overall care and uptake of medical services to patients with the overarching aim of improving survival and meaningful quality of life [152, 153].

Sources of Funding Nil

References

1. Ndungu BM. The evolution of minimal access surgery and the laparoscopic cholecystectomy. Ann Afr Surg. 2014;11(1)
2. Biere SS, van Berge Henegouwen MI, Maas KW, Bonavina L, Rosman C, Garcia JR, Gisbertz SS, Klinkenbijl JH, Hollmann MW, De Lange ES, Bonjer HJ. Minimally invasive versus open oesophagectomy for patients with oesophageal cancer: a multicentre, open-label, randomised controlled trial. Lancet. 2012;379(9829):1887–92.
3. Zeng F, Chen L, Liao M, Chen B, Long J, Wu W, Deng G. Laparoscopic versus open gastrectomy for gastric cancer. World J Surg Oncol. 2020;18(1):1–2.
4. Kiran RP, Delaney CP, Senagore AJ, Millward BL, Fazio VW. Operative blood loss and use of blood products after laparoscopic and conventional open colorectal operations. Arch Surg. 2004;139(1):39–42.
5. van der Pas MH, Haglind E, Cuesta MA, Fürst A, Lacy AM, Hop WC, Bonjer HJ. COlorectal cancer laparoscopic or open resection II (COLOR II) study group. Laparoscopic versus open surgery for

rectal cancer (COLOR II): short-term outcomes of a randomised, phase 3 trial. Lancet Oncol. 2013;14(3):210–8.
6. Stevenson AR, Solomon MJ, Lumley JW, Hewett P, Clouston AD, Gebski VJ, Davies L, Wilson K, Hague W, Simes J. ALaCaRT investigators. Effect of laparoscopic-assisted resection vs open resection on pathological outcomes in rectal cancer: the ALaCaRT randomized clinical trial. JAMA. 2015;314(13):1356–63.
7. de Rooij T, van Hilst J, van Santvoort H, Boerma D, van den Boezem P, Daams F, van Dam R, Dejong C, van Duyn E, Dijkgraaf M, van Eijck C. Minimally invasive versus open distal pancreatectomy (LEOPARD): a multicenter patient-blinded randomized controlled trial. Ann Surg. 2019;269(1):2–9.
8. Björnsson B, Larsson AL, Hjalmarsson C, Gasslander T, Sandström P. Comparison of the duration of hospital stay after laparoscopic or open distal pancreatectomy: randomized controlled trial. J Br Surg. 2020;107(10):1281–8.
9. Elmahi E, Salama Y, Cadden F. A literature review to assess blood loss in minimally invasive liver surgery versus in open liver resection. Cureus. 2021;13(6)
10. Palanivelu C, Senthilnathan P, Sabnis SC, Babu NS, Srivatsan Gurumurthy S, Anand Vijai N, Nalankilli VP, Praveen Raj P, Parthasarathy R, Rajapandian S. Randomized clinical trial of laparoscopic versus open pancreatoduodenectomy for periampullary tumours. J Br Surg. 2017;104(11):1443–50.
11. Poves I, Burdío F, Morató O, Iglesias M, Radosevic A, Ilzarbe L, Visa L, Grande L. Comparison of perioperative outcomes between laparoscopic and open approach for pancreatoduodenectomy: the PADULAP randomized controlled trial. Ann Surg. 2018;268(5):731–9.
12. Van Hilst J, de Rooij T, Bosscha K, Brinkman DJ, van Dieren S, Dijkgraaf MG, Gerhards MF, de Hingh IH, Karsten TM, Lips DJ, Luyer MD. Laparoscopic versus open pancreatoduodenectomy for pancreatic or periampullary tumours (LEOPARD-2): a multicentre, patient-blinded, randomised controlled phase 2/3 trial. Lancet Gastroenterol Hepatol. 2019;4(3):199–207.
13. Kobayashi S, Honda G, Kurata M, Tadano S, Sakamoto K, Okuda Y, Abe K. An experimental study on the relationship among airway pressure, pneumoperitoneum pressure, and central venous pressure in pure laparoscopic hepatectomy. Ann Surg. 2016;263(6):1159–63.
14. Eiriksson K, Fors D, Rubertsson S, Arvidsson D. High intra-abdominal pressure during experimental laparoscopic liver resection reduces bleeding but increases the risk of gas embolism. J Br Surg. 2011;98(6):845–52.
15. Xiong WL, Li R, Lei HK, Jiang ZY. Comparison of outcomes between minimally invasive oesophagectomy and open oesophagectomy for oesophageal cancer. ANZ J Surg. 2017;87(3):165–70.
16. Beyer K, Baukloh AK, Kamphues C, Seeliger H, Heidecke CD, Kreis ME, Patrzyk M. Laparoscopic versus open gastrectomy for locally advanced gastric cancer: a systematic review and meta-analysis of randomized controlled studies. World J Surg Oncol. 2019;17(1):1–9.
17. Hewett PJ, Allardyce RA, Bagshaw PF, Frampton CM, Frizelle FA, Rieger NA, Smith JS, Solomon MJ, Stephens JH, Stevenson AR. Short-term outcomes of the Australasian randomized clinical study comparing laparoscopic and conventional open surgical treatments for colon cancer: the ALCCaS trial. Ann Surg. 2008;248(5):728–38.
18. Hong Q, Wang J, Wang Y, Fu B, Fang Y, Tong Q, Liu T, Wu Z, Zhou J. Clinical outcomes of laparoscopic versus open right hepatectomy for liver tumors: a meta-analysis. Medicine. 2020;99(1):e18667.
19. Zhang H, Lan X, Peng B, Li B. Is total laparoscopic pancreaticoduodenectomy superior to open procedure? A meta-analysis. World J Gastroenterol. 2019;25(37):5711.
20. Ashraf J, Krishnan J, Turner A, Subramaniam R. Robot docking time: cumulative summation analysis of a procedure-independent learning curve in pediatric urology. J Laparoendosc Adv Surg Techniq. 2018;28(9):1139–41.
21. Al-Hakim L. The impact of preventable disruption on the operative time for minimally invasive surgery. Surg Endosc. 2011;25(10):3385–92.
22. Howard TJ, Krug JE, Yu J, Zyromski NJ, Schmidt CM, Jacobson LE, Madura JA, Wiebke EA, Lillemoe KD. A margin-negative R0 resection accomplished with minimal postoperative complications is the surgeon's contribution to long-term survival in pancreatic cancer. J Gastrointest Surg. 2006;10:1338–46.
23. Lv L, Hu W, Ren Y, Wei X. Minimally invasive esophagectomy versus open esophagectomy for esophageal cancer: a meta-analysis. Onco Targets Ther. 2016;9:6751.
24. Osugi H, Takemura M, Higashino M, Takada N, Lee S, Kinoshita H. A comparison of video-assisted thoracoscopic oesophagectomy and radical lymph node dissection for squamous cell cancer of the oesophagus with open operation. J Br Surg. 2003;90(1):108–13.
25. Smithers BM, Gotley DC, Martin I, Thomas JM. Comparison of the outcomes between open and minimally invasive esophagectomy. Ann Surg. 2007;245(2):232.
26. Koyanagi K, Ozawa S, Tachimori Y. Minimally invasive esophagectomy performed with the patient in a prone position: a systematic review. Surg Today. 2016;46(3):275–84.
27. Best LM, Mughal M, Gurusamy KS. Laparoscopic versus open gastrectomy for gastric cancer. Cochrane Database Syst Rev. 2016;3
28. Kitano S, Shiraishi N, Fujii K, Yasuda K, Inomata M, Adachi Y. A randomized controlled trial comparing open vs laparoscopy-assisted distal gastrectomy

for the treatment of early gastric cancer: an interim report. Surgery. 2002;131(1):S306–11.
29. Hayashi H, Ochiai T, Shimada H, Gunji Y. Prospective randomized study of open versus laparoscopy-assisted distal gastrectomy with extraperigastric lymph node dissection for early gastric cancer. Surg Endosc Other Interv Tech. 2005;19(9):1172–6.
30. Hu J, Jiang L, Cai L, Zheng H, Hu S, Chen H, Wu G, Zhang Y, Lv Z. Preliminary experience of fast-track surgery combined with laparoscopy-assisted radical distal gastrectomy for gastric cancer. J Gastrointest Surg. 2012;16(10):1830.
31. Barreto SG, Windsor JA. Redefining early gastric cancer. Surg Endosc. 2016;30(1):24–37.
32. Kim W, Kim HH, Han SU, Kim MC, Hyung WJ, Ryu SW, Cho GS, Kim CY, Yang HK, Park DJ, Song KY. Decreased morbidity of laparoscopic distal gastrectomy compared with open distal gastrectomy for stage I gastric cancer. Ann Surg. 2016;263(1):28–35.
33. Park YK, Yoon HM, Kim YW, Park JY, Ryu KW, Lee YJ, Jeong O, Yoon KY, Lee JH, Lee SE, Yu W. Laparoscopy-assisted versus open D2 distal gastrectomy for advanced gastric cancer: results from a randomized phase II multicenter clinical trial (COACT 1001). Ann Surg. 2018;267(4):638–45.
34. Nelson H. Laparoscopically assisted colectomy is as safe and effective as open colectomy in people with colon cancer. Cancer Treat Rev. 2004;30(8):707–9.
35. Colon Cancer Laparoscopic or Open Resection Study Group. Laparoscopic surgery versus open surgery for colon cancer: short-term outcomes of a randomised trial. Lancet Oncol. 2005;6(7):477–84.
36. Birindelli A, Segalini E, Kwan S, Biscardi A, Tonini V, Di Saverio S. Challenging emergency laparoscopic right colectomy for completely obstructing caecal carcinoma–a video vignette. Color Dis. 2017;19(5):504–6.
37. Cima RR, Pattana-Arun J, Larson DW, Dozois EJ, Wolff BG, Pemberton JH. Experience with 969 minimal access colectomies: the role of hand-assisted laparoscopy in expanding minimally invasive surgery for complex colectomies. J Am Coll Surg. 2008;206(5):946–50.
38. Guillou PJ, Quirke P, Thorpe H, Walker J, Jayne DG, Smith AM, Heath RM, Brown JM, MRC CLASICC trial group. Short-term endpoints of conventional versus laparoscopic-assisted surgery in patients with colorectal cancer (MRC CLASICC trial): multicentre, randomised controlled trial. Lancet. 2005;365(9472):1718–26.
39. Fleshman J, Branda M, Sargent DJ, Boller AM, George V, Abbas M, Peters WR, Maun D, Chang G, Herline A, Fichera A. Effect of laparoscopic-assisted resection vs open resection of stage II or III rectal cancer on pathologic outcomes: the ACOSOG Z6051 randomized clinical trial. JAMA. 2015;314(13):1346–55.
40. Kang SB, Park JW, Jeong SY, Nam BH, Choi HS, Kim DW, Lim SB, Lee TG, Kim DY, Kim JS, Chang HJ. Open versus laparoscopic surgery for mid or low rectal cancer after neoadjuvant chemoradiotherapy (COREAN trial): short-term outcomes of an open-label randomised controlled trial. Lancet Oncol. 2010;11(7):637–45.
41. Conticchio M, Papagni V, Notarnicola M, Delvecchio A, Riccelli U, Ammendola M, Currò G, Pessaux P, Silvestris N, Memeo R. Laparoscopic vs. open mesorectal excision for rectal cancer: are these approaches still comparable? A systematic review and meta-analysis. PLoS One. 2020;15(7):e0235887.
42. Ouyang M, Liao T, Lu Y, Deng L, Luo Z, Wu J, Ju Y, Yao X. Laparoscopic versus open surgery in lateral lymph node dissection for advanced rectal cancer: a meta-analysis. Gastroenterol Res Pract. 2019;2019.
43. Memon S, Heriot AG, Murphy DG, Bressel M, Lynch AC. Robotic versus laparoscopic proctectomy for rectal cancer: a meta-analysis. Ann Surg Oncol. 2012;19(7):2095–101.
44. Jayne D, Pigazzi A, Marshall H, Croft J, Corrigan N, Copeland J, Quirke P, West N, Rautio T, Thomassen N, Tilney H. Effect of robotic-assisted vs conventional laparoscopic surgery on risk of conversion to open laparotomy among patients undergoing resection for rectal cancer: the ROLARR randomized clinical trial. JAMA. 2017;318(16):1569–80.
45. Otto G, Heise M, Hoppe-Lotichius M, Pitton M, Hansen T. Hilar cholangiocarcinoma: right versus left hepatectomy. Zentralblatt fur Chirurgie. 2012;137(6):535–40.
46. Amikura K, Sakamoto H, Takahashi A, Ogura T, Omichi K, Ehara K, Fukuda T, Yatsuoka T, Kawashima Y, Tanaka Y. Useful device for hepatectomy in patients with a surgical history of bile duct-GI tract anastomosis at the porta hepatis. Gan to kagaku ryoho. Cancer Chemotherapy. 2014;41(12):1497–9.
47. van Hilst J, Korrel M, de Rooij T, Lof S, Busch OR, Koerkamp BG, Kooby DA, Van Dieren S, Hilal MA, Besselink MG, DIPLOMA study group. Oncologic outcomes of minimally invasive versus open distal pancreatectomy for pancreatic ductal adenocarcinoma: a systematic review and meta-analysis. Eur J Surg Oncol. 2019;45(5):719–27.
48. Nickel F, Haney CM, Kowalewski KF, Probst P, Limen EF, Kalkum E, Diener MK, Strobel O, Müller-Stich BP, Hackert T. Laparoscopic versus open pancreaticoduodenectomy: a systematic review and meta-analysis of randomized controlled trials. Ann Surg. 2020;271(1):54–66.
49. Hasegawa Y, Wakabayashi G, Nitta H, Takahara T, Katagiri H, Umemura A, Makabe K, Sasaki A. A novel model for prediction of pure laparoscopic liver resection surgical difficulty. Surg Endosc. 2017;31(12):5356–63.
50. Chong JU, Kim SH, Hwang HK, Kang CM, Lee WJ. Yonsei criteria: a clinical reflection of stage I left-sided pancreatic cancer. Oncotarget. 2017;8(67):110830.

51. Bogani G, Cromi A, Serati M, Di Naro E, Casarin J, Pinelli C, Ghezzi F. Laparoscopic and open abdominal staging for early-stage ovarian cancer: our experience, systematic review, and meta-analysis of comparative studies. Int J Gynecol Cancer. 2014;24(7)
52. Machida H, Matsuo K, Yamagami W, Ebina Y, Kobayashi Y, Tabata T, Kaneuchi M, Nagase S, Enomoto T, Mikami M. Intraoperative capsule rupture, postoperative chemotherapy, and survival of women with stage I epithelial ovarian cancer: a JSOG-JSGO joint study. Gynecol Oncol. 2020;159:61.
53. Matsuo K, Huang Y, Matsuzaki S, Klar M, Roman LD, Sood AK, Wright JD. Minimally invasive surgery and risk of capsule rupture for women with early-stage ovarian cancer. JAMA Oncol. 2020;6(7):1110–3.
54. Akhtar NM, Chen D, Zhao Y, Dane D, Xue Y, Wang W, Zhang J, Sang Y, Chen C, Chen Y. Postoperative short-term outcomes of minimally invasive versus open esophagectomy for patients with esophageal cancer: an updated systematic review and meta-analysis. Thoracic Cancer. 2020;11(6):1465–75.
55. Gavriilidis P, Davies RJ, Biondi A, Wheeler J, Testini M, Carcano G, Di Saverio S. Laparoscopic versus open complete mesocolic excision: a systematic review by updated meta-analysis. Updat Surg. 2020;72:639–48.
56. Kasai M, Cipriani F, Gayet B, Aldrighetti L, Ratti F, Sarmiento JM, Scatton O, Kim KH, Dagher I, Topal B, Primrose J. Laparoscopic versus open major hepatectomy: a systematic review and meta-analysis of individual patient data. Surgery. 2018;163(5):985–95.
57. Machairas N, Kostakis ID, Schizas D, Kykalos S, Nikiteas N, Sotiropoulos GC. Meta-analysis of laparoscopic versus open liver resection for intrahepatic cholangiocarcinoma. Updat Surg. 2021;73(1):59–68.
58. Ran L, Jin J, Xu Y, Bu Y, Song F. Comparison of robotic surgery with laparoscopy and laparotomy for treatment of endometrial cancer: a meta-analysis. PLoS One. 2014;9(9):e108361.
59. Fuentes JM, Hanly EJ, Aurora AR, De Maio A, Shih SP, Marohn MR, Talamini MA. CO_2 abdominal insufflation pretreatment increases survival after a lipopolysaccharide-contaminated laparotomy. J Gastrointest Surg. 2006;10(1):32–8.
60. Bachman SL, Hanly EJ, Nwanko JI, Lamb J, Herring AE, Marohn MR, De Maio A, Talamini MA. The effect of timing of pneumoperitoneum on the inflammatory response. Surg Endosc Other Interv Tech. 2004;18(11):1640–4.
61. Lundin ES, Wodlin NB, Nilsson L, Theodorsson E, Ernerudh J, Kjølhede P. Markers of tissue damage and inflammation after robotic and abdominal hysterectomy in early endometrial cancer: a randomised controlled trial. Sci Rep. 2020;10(1):1.
62. Pascual M, Alonso S, Parés D, Courtier R, Gil MJ, Grande L, Pera M. Randomized clinical trial comparing inflammatory and angiogenic response after open versus laparoscopic curative resection for colonic cancer. J Br Surg. 2011;98(1):50–9.
63. Okamura A, Takeuchi H, Matsuda S, Ogura M, Miyasho T, Nakamura R, Takahashi T, Wada N, Kawakubo H, Saikawa Y, Kitagawa Y. Factors affecting cytokine change after esophagectomy for esophageal cancer. Ann Surg Oncol. 2015;22(9):3130–5.
64. van Hilst J, Brinkman DJ, de Rooij T, van Dieren S, Gerhards MF, de Hingh IH, Luyer MD, Marsman HA, Karsten TM, Busch OR, Festen S. The inflammatory response after laparoscopic and open pancreatoduodenectomy and the association with complications in a multicenter randomized controlled trial. HPB. 2019;21(11):1453–61.
65. Shrikhande SV, Barreto SG, Shukla PJ. Laparoscopy in pancreatic tumors. J Minimal Access Surg. 2007;3(2):47.
66. Goldfarb M, Brower S, Schwaitzberg SD. Minimally invasive surgery and cancer: controversies part 1. Surg Endosc. 2010;24(2):304–34.
67. Yibulayin W, Abulizi S, Lv H, Sun W. Minimally invasive oesophagectomy versus open esophagectomy for resectable esophageal cancer: a meta-analysis. World J Surg Oncol. 2016;14(1):1–7.
68. Nagpal K, Ahmed K, Vats A, Yakoub D, James D, Ashrafian H, Darzi A, Moorthy K, Athanasiou T. Is minimally invasive surgery beneficial in the management of esophageal cancer? A meta-analysis. Surg Endoscopy. 2010;24(7):1621–9.
69. Guo W, Ma X, Yang S, Zhu X, Qin W, Xiang J, Lerut T, Li H. Combined thoracoscopic-laparoscopic esophagectomy versus open esophagectomy: a meta-analysis of outcomes. Surg Endosc. 2016;30(9):3873–81.
70. Zhou C, Ma G, Li X, Li J, Yan Y, Liu P, He J, Ren Y. Is minimally invasive esophagectomy effective for preventing anastomotic leakages after esophagectomy for cancer? A systematic review and meta-analysis. World J Surg Oncol 2015;13(1):1–0.
71. Zhao JH, Sun JX, Huang XZ, Gao P, Chen XW, Song YX, Liu J, Cai CZ, Xu HM, Wang ZN. Meta-analysis of the laparoscopic versus open colorectal surgery within fast track surgery. Int J Color Dis. 2016;31(3):613–22.
72. Xie SM, Xiong JJ, Liu XT, Chen HY, Iglesia-Garcia D, Altaf K, Bharucha S, Huang W, Nunes QM, Szatmary P, Liu XB. Laparoscopic versus open liver resection for colorectal liver metastases: a comprehensive systematic review and meta-analysis. Sci Rep. 2017;7(1):1.
73. Korrel M, Vissers FL, van Hilst J, de Rooij T, Dijkgraaf MG, Festen S, Koerkamp BG, Busch OR, Luyer MD, Sandström P, Hilal MA. Minimally invasive versus open distal pancreatectomy: an individual patient data meta-analysis of two randomized controlled trials. HPB. 2020;20:S186.
74. Kamarajah SK, Bundred J, Saint Marc O, Jiao LR, Manas D, Hilal MA, White SA. Robotic versus conventional laparoscopic pancreaticoduodenectomy

a systematic review and meta-analysis. Eur J Surg Oncol. 2020;46(1):6–14.
75. Ni X, Jia D, Chen Y, Wang L, Suo J. Is the enhanced recovery after surgery (ERAS) program effective and safe in laparoscopic colorectal cancer surgery? A meta-analysis of randomized controlled trials. J Gastrointest Surg. 2019;23(7):1502–12.
76. Pisarska M, Małczak P, Major P, Wysocki M, Budzyński A, Pędziwiatr M. Enhanced recovery after surgery protocol in oesophageal cancer surgery: systematic review and meta-analysis. PLoS One. 2017;12(3):e0174382.
77. Lee Y, Yu J, Doumouras AG, Li J, Hong D. Enhanced recovery after surgery (ERAS) versus standard recovery for elective gastric cancer surgery: a meta-analysis of randomized controlled trials. Surg Oncol. 2020;32:75–87.
78. Nelson G, Kalogera E, Dowdy SC. Enhanced recovery pathways in gynecologic oncology. Gynecol Oncol. 2014;135(3):586–94.
79. Karunakaran M, Barreto SG. Is enhancing recovery after pancreatic cancer surgery even possible? Chin Clin Oncol. 2021;10:49.
80. Martínez-Pérez A, Carra MC, Brunetti F, de'Angelis N. Short-term clinical outcomes of laparoscopic vs open rectal excision for rectal cancer: a systematic review and meta-analysis. World J Gastroenterol. 201728;23(44):7906.
81. Chen D, Wang W, Mo J, Ren Q, Miao H, Chen Y, Wen Z. Minimal invasive versus open esophagectomy for patients with esophageal squamous cell carcinoma after neoadjuvant treatments. BMC Cancer 2021;21(1):1–0.
82. Lu J, Yoon C, Xu B, Xie J, Li P, Zheng C, Huang C, Yoon SS. Long-term survival after minimally invasive versus open gastrectomy for gastric adenocarcinoma: a propensity score-matched analysis of patients in the United States and China. Ann Surg Oncol. 2020;27(3):802–11.
83. Zhu Z, Li L, Xu J, Ye W, Zeng J, Chen B, Huang Z. Laparoscopic versus open approach in gastrectomy for advanced gastric cancer: a systematic review. World J Surg Oncol. 2020;18(1):1–24.
84. Yu J, Huang C, Sun Y, Su X, Cao H, Hu J, Wang K, Suo J, Tao K, He X, Wei H. Effect of laparoscopic vs open distal gastrectomy on 3-year disease-free survival in patients with locally advanced gastric cancer: the CLASS-01 randomized clinical trial. JAMA. 2019;321(20):1983–92.
85. Park JH, Park HC, Park SC, Sohn DK, Oh JH, Kang SB, Heo SC, Kim MJ, Park JW, Jeong SY, Park KJ. Laparoscopic approach for left-sided T4 colon cancer is a safe and feasible procedure, compared to open surgery. Surg Endosc. 2019;33(9):2843–9.
86. Bonjer HJ, Deijen CL, Abis GA, Cuesta MA, Van Der Pas MH, De Lange-De Klerk ES, Lacy AM, Bemelman WA, Andersson J, Angenete E, Rosenberg J. A randomized trial of laparoscopic versus open surgery for rectal cancer. N Engl J Med. 2015;372(14):1324–32.
87. Jayne DG, Guillou PJ, Thorpe H, Quirke P, Copeland J, Smith AM, Heath RM, Brown JM. Randomized trial of laparoscopic-assisted resection of colorectal carcinoma: 3-year results of the UK MRC CLASICC trial group. J Clin Oncol. 2007;25(21):3061–8.
88. Jayne DG, Thorpe HC, Copeland J, Quirke P, Brown JM, Guillou PJ. Five-year follow-up of the Medical Research Council CLASICC trial of laparoscopically assisted versus open surgery for colorectal cancer. J Br Surg. 2010;97(11):1638–45.
89. Jeong SY, Park JW, Nam BH, Kim S, Kang SB, Lim SB, Choi HS, Kim DW, Chang HJ, Kim DY, Jung KH. Open versus laparoscopic surgery for mid-rectal or low-rectal cancer after neoadjuvant chemoradiotherapy (COREAN trial): survival outcomes of an open-label, non-inferiority, randomised controlled trial. Lancet Oncol. 2014;15(7):767–74.
90. Branda ME, Sargent DJ, Boller AM, George VV, Abbas MA, Peters WR Jr, Maun DC, Chang GJ, Herline A, Fichera A, Mutch MG. Disease free survival and local recurrence for laparoscopic resection compared to open resection of stage II-III rectal cancer: follow up results of the ACOSOG Z6051 randomized controlled trial. Ann Surg. 2019;269(4):589.
91. Park EJ, Cho MS, Baek SJ, Hur H, Min BS, Baik SH, Lee KY, Kim NK. Long-term oncologic outcomes of robotic low anterior resection for rectal cancer: a comparative study with laparoscopic surgery. Ann Surg. 2015;261(1):129–37.
92. Chen K, Pan Y, Huang CJ, Chen QL, Zhang RC, Zhang MZ, Wang GY, Wang XF, Mou YP, Yan JF. Laparoscopic versus open pancreatic resection for ductal adenocarcinoma: separate propensity score matching analyses of distal pancreatectomy and pancreaticoduodenectomy. BMC Cancer. 2021;21(1):1–2.
93. Røsok BI, de Rooij T, van Hilst J, Diener MK, Allen PJ, Vollmer CM, Kooby DA, Shrikhande SV, Asbun HJ, Barkun J, Besselink MG. Minimally invasive distal pancreatectomy. HPB. 2017;19(3):205–14.
94. Korrel M, Jones LR, van Hilst J, Balzano G, Björnsson B, Boggi U, Bratlie SO, Busch OR, Butturini G, Capretti G, Casadei R. Minimally invasive versus open distal pancreatectomy for resectable pancreatic cancer (DIPLOMA): an international randomised non-inferiority trial. The Lancet Regional Health–Europe. 2023;31.
95. Han HS, Yoon YS, Agarwal AK, Belli G, Itano O, Gumbs AA, Yoon DS, Kang CM, Lee SE, Wakai T, Troisi RI. Laparoscopic surgery for gallbladder cancer: an expert consensus statement. Dig Surg. 2019;36(1):1–6.
96. Clemente G, Nuzzo G, De Rose AM, Giovannini I, La Torre G, Ardito F, Giuliante F. Unexpected gallbladder cancer after laparoscopic cholecystectomy for acute cholecystitis: a worrisome picture. J Gastrointest Surg. 2012;16(8):1462–8.
97. Yoon YS, Han HS, Cho JY, Choi Y, Lee W, Jang JY, Choi H. Is laparoscopy contraindicated for gallblad-

der cancer? A 10-year prospective cohort study. J Am Coll Surg. 2015;221(4):847–53.
98. Kong Q, Wei H, Zhang J, Li Y, Wang Y. Comparison of the survival outcomes of laparoscopy versus laparotomy in treatment of early-stage ovarian cancer: a systematic review and meta-analysis. J Ovarian Res. 2021;14(1):1–1.
99. Sert BM, Boggess JF, Ahmad S, Jackson AL, Stavitzski NM, Dahl AA, Holloway RW. Robot-assisted versus open radical hysterectomy: a multi-institutional experience for early-stage cervical cancer. Eur J Surg Oncol (EJSO). 2016;42(4):513–22.
100. Shah CA, Beck T, Liao JB, Giannakopoulos NV, Veljovich D, Paley P. Surgical and oncologic outcomes after robotic radical hysterectomy as compared to open radical hysterectomy in the treatment of early cervical cancer. J Gynecol Oncol. 2017;28(6)
101. Ramirez PT, Frumovitz M, Pareja R, Lopez A, Vieira M, Ribeiro R, Buda A, Yan X, Shuzhong Y, Chetty N, Isla D. Minimally invasive versus abdominal radical hysterectomy for cervical cancer. N Engl J Med. 2018;379(20):1895–904.
102. Abel MK, Chan JK, Chow S, Darcy K, Tian C, Kapp DS, Mann AK, Liao CI. Trends and survival outcomes of robotic, laparoscopic, and open surgery for stage II uterine cancer. Int J Gynecol Cancer. 2020;30(9):1347.
103. Hsieh C, Cologne KG. Laparoscopic approach to rectal cancer—the new standard? Front Oncol. 2020;10:1239.
104. Berends F, Kazemier G, Bonjer H, Lange J. Subcutaneous metastases after laparoscopic colectomy. Lancet. 1994;344(8914):58.
105. Are C, Talamini MA. Laparoscopy and malignancy. J Laparoendosc Adv Surg Techniq. 2005;15(1):38–47.
106. Zivanovic O, Sonoda Y, Diaz JP, Levine DA, Brown CL, Chi DS, Barakat RR, Abu-Rustum NR. The rate of port-site metastases after 2251 laparoscopic procedures in women with underlying malignant disease. Gynecol Oncol. 2008;111(3):431–7.
107. Rutten MJ, Van Meurs HS, Van De Vrie R, Naaktgeboren CA, Fons G, Opmeer BC, Spijkerboer A, Bossuyt PM, Kenter GG, Buist MR, Gaarenstroom KN. Laparoscopy to predict the result of primary cytoreductive surgery in patients with advanced ovarian cancer: a randomized controlled trial. J Clin Oncol. 2017;35(6):613–21.
108. Ramirez PT, Wolf JK, Levenback C. Laparoscopic port-site metastases: etiology and prevention. Gynecol Oncol. 2003;91(1):179–89.
109. Clinical Outcomes of Surgical Therapy Study Group. A comparison of laparoscopically assisted and open colectomy for colon cancer. N Engl J Med. 2004;350(20):2050–9.
110. Guerrieri M, Campagnacci R, De Sanctis A, Lezoche G, Massucco P, Summa M, Gesuita R, Capussotti L, Spinoglio G, Lezoche E. Laparoscopic versus open colectomy for TNM stage III colon cancer: results of a prospective multicenter study in Italy. Surg Today. 2012;42(11):1071–7.
111. Zanghi A, Cavallaro A, Piccolo G, Fisichella R, Di Vita M, Spartà D, Zanghì G, Berretta S, Palermo F, Cappellani A. Dissemination metastasis after laparoscopic colorectal surgery versus conventional open surgery for colorectal cancer: a metanalysis. Eur Rev Med Pharmacol Sci. 2013;17(9):1174–84.
112. Shukla PJ, Barreto SG, Shrikhande SV, Mohandas KM, Purandare N, Rangarajan V. Detection of gall bladder cancer metastases in rare sites by PET scan. Indian J Gastroenterol. 2007;26(6):303–4.
113. Berger-Richardson D, Chesney TR, Englesakis M, Govindarajan A, Cleary SP, Swallow CJ. Trends in port-site metastasis after laparoscopic resection of incidental gallbladder cancer: a systematic review. Surgery. 2017;161(3):618–27.
114. Suzuki K, Kimura T, Ogawa H. Long-term prognosis of gallbladder cancer diagnosed after laparoscopic cholecystectomy. Surg Endosc. 2000;14(8):712–6.
115. Van der Geest LG, Portielje JE, Wouters MW, Weijl NI, Tanis BC, Tollenaar RA, Struikmans H, Nortier JW. All nine hospitals in the Leiden region of the comprehensive cancer Centre The Netherlands (CCCNL). Complicated postoperative recovery increases omission, delay and discontinuation of adjuvant chemotherapy in patients with Stage III colon cancer. Color Dis. 2013;15(10):e582–91.
116. Jung YB, Kang J, Park EJ, Baik SH, Lee KY. Time to initiation of adjuvant chemotherapy in colon cancer: comparison of open, laparoscopic, and robotic surgery. J Laparoendosc Adv Surg Techniq. 2016;26(10):799–805.
117. Gantt GA, Ashburn J, Kiran RP, Khorana AA, Kalady MF. Laparoscopy mitigates adverse oncological effects of delayed adjuvant chemotherapy for colon cancer. Surg Endosc. 2015;29(2):493–9.
118. Bao H, Xu N, Li Z, Ren H, Xia H, Li N, Yu H, Wei J, Jiang C, Liu L. Effect of laparoscopic gastrectomy on compliance with adjuvant chemotherapy in patients with gastric cancer. Medicine. 2017;96(21):e6839.
119. Anderson KL Jr, Adam MA, Thomas S, Roman SA, Sosa JA. Impact of minimally invasive vs. open distal pancreatectomy on use of adjuvant chemoradiation for pancreatic adenocarcinoma. Am J Surg. 2017;213(4):601–5.
120. Kim NK, Aahn TW, Park JK, Lee KY, Lee WH, Sohn SK, Min JS. Assessment of sexual and voiding function after total mesorectal excision with pelvic autonomic nerve preservation in males with rectal cancer. Dis Colon Rectum. 2002;45(9):1178–85.
121. Jones OM, Stevenson AR, Stitz RW, Lumley JW. Preservation of sexual and bladder function after laparoscopic rectal surgery. Color Dis. 2009;11(5):489–95.
122. Asoglu O, Matlim T, Karanlik H, Atar M, Muslumanoglu M, Kapran Y, Igci A, Ozmen V, Kecer M, Parlak M. Impact of laparoscopic surgery on bladder and sexual function after total

mesorectal excision for rectal cancer. Surg Endosc. 2009;23(2):296–303.
123. Morino M, Parini U, Allaix ME, Monasterolo G, Contul RB, Garrone C. Male sexual and urinary function after laparoscopic total mesorectal excision. Surg Endosc. 2009;23(6):1233–40.
124. Kowalewski KF, Seifert L, Ali S, Schmidt MW, Seide S, Haney C, Tapking C, Shamiyeh A, Kulu Y, Hackert T, Müller-Stich BP. Functional outcomes after laparoscopic versus robotic-assisted rectal resection: a systematic review and meta-analysis. Surg Endosc. 2021;35(1):81–95.
125. Kauppila JH, Xie S, Johar A, Markar SR, Lagergren P. Meta-analysis of health-related quality of life after minimally invasive versus open oesophagectomy for oesophageal cancer. J Br Surg. 2017;104(9):1131–40.
126. Korrel M, Roelofs A, van Hilst J, Busch OR, Daams F, Festen S, Koerkamp BG, Klaase J, Luyer MD, van Oijen MG, Verdonck-de Leeuw IM. Long-term quality of life after minimally invasive vs open distal pancreatectomy in the LEOPARD randomized trial. J Am Coll Surg. 2021;233:730.
127. Mackenzie H, Markar SR, Askari A, Ni M, Faiz O, Hanna GB. National proficiency-gain curves for minimally invasive gastrointestinal cancer surgery. J Br Surg. 2016;103(1):88–96.
128. Tekkis PP, Senagore AJ, Delaney CP, Fazio VW. Evaluation of the learning curve in laparoscopic colorectal surgery: comparison of right-sided and left-sided resections. Ann Surg. 2005;242(1):83.
129. Lim TO, Soraya A, Ding LM, Morad Z. Assessing doctors' competence: application of CUSUM technique in monitoring doctors' performance. Int J Qual Health Care. 2002;14(3):251–8.
130. McCulloch P, Altman DG, Campbell WB, Flum DR, Glasziou P, Marshall JC, Nicholl J, Balliol Collaboration. No surgical innovation without evaluation: the IDEAL recommendations. Lancet. 2009;374(9695):1105–12.
131. Haney CM, Karadza E, Limen EF, de Santibanes M, Kinny-Köster B, Müller PC, Bintintan VV, Kulu Y, Hackert T, Müller-Stich BP, Nickel F. Training and learning curves in minimally invasive pancreatic surgery: from simulation to mastery. J Pancreatol. 2020;3(2):101–10.
132. Moekotte AL, Rawashdeh A, Asbun HJ, Coimbra FJ, Edil BH, Jarufe N, Jeyarajah DR, Kendrick ML, Pessaux P, Zeh HJ, Besselink MG. Safe implementation of minimally invasive pancreas resection: a systematic review. HPB. 2020;22(5):637–48.
133. Okamura A, Watanabe M, Fukudome I, Yamashita K, Yuda M, Hayami M, Imamura Y, Mine S. Surgical team proficiency in minimally invasive esophagectomy is related to case volume and improves patient outcomes. Esophagus. 2018;15(2):115–21.
134. van Workum F, Stenstra MH, Berkelmans GH, Slaman AE, van Berge Henegouwen MI, Gisbertz SS, van den Wildenberg FJ, Polat F, Irino T, Nilsson M, Nieuwenhuijzen GA. Learning curve and associated morbidity of minimally invasive esophagectomy: a retrospective multicenter study. Ann Surg. 2019;269(1):88–94.
135. Jung DH, Son SY, Park YS, Shin DJ, Ahn HS, Ahn SH, Park DJ, Kim HH. The learning curve associated with laparoscopic total gastrectomy. Gastric Cancer. 2016;19(1):264–72.
136. Kunisaki C, Makino H, Yamamoto N, Sato T, Oshima T, Nagano Y, Fujii S, Akiyama H, Otsuka Y, Ono HA, Kosaka T. Learning curve for laparoscopy-assisted distal gastrectomy with regional lymph node dissection for early gastric cancer. Surg Laparosc Endosc Percutan Tech. 2008;18(3):236–41.
137. de Rooij T, Cipriani F, Rawashdeh M, van Dieren S, Barbaro S, Abuawwad M, van Hilst J, Fontana M, Besselink MG, Hilal MA. Single-surgeon learning curve in 111 laparoscopic distal pancreatectomies: does operative time tell the whole story? J Am Coll Surg. 2017;224(5):826–32.
138. Wang M, Meng L, Cai Y, Li Y, Wang X, Zhang Z, Peng B. Learning curve for laparoscopic pancreaticoduodenectomy: a CUSUM analysis. J Gastrointest Surg. 2016;20(5):924–35.
139. Nomi T, Fuks D, Kawaguchi Y, Mal F, Nakajima Y, Gayet B. Learning curve for laparoscopic major hepatectomy. J Br Surg. 2015;102(7):796–804.
140. Hwang JH, Yoo HJ, Joo J, Kim S, Lim MC, Song YJ, Park SY. Learning curve analysis of laparoscopic radical hysterectomy and lymph node dissection in early cervical cancer. Eur J Obstet Gynecol Reprod Biol. 2012;163(2):219–23.
141. Ghezzi TL, Corleta OC. 30 years of robotic surgery. World J Surg. 2016;40(10):2550–7.
142. Boggi U, Vistoli F, Amorese G. Twenty years of robotic surgery: a challenge for human limits. Updat Surg. 2021;73(3):789–93.
143. Shrime MG, Dare AJ, Alkire BC, O'Neill K, Meara JG. Catastrophic expenditure to pay for surgery worldwide: a modelling study. Lancet Glob Health. 2015;(3):S38–44.
144. Shrime MG, Bickler SW, Alkire BC, Mock C. Global burden of surgical disease: an estimation from the provider perspective. Lancet Glob Health. 2015;(3):S8–9.
145. Ribeiro U Jr, Tayar DO, Ribeiro RA, Andrade P, Junqueira SM Jr. Laparoscopic vs open colorectal surgery: economic and clinical outcomes in the Brazilian healthcare. Medicine. 2020;99(42):e22718.
146. Mar J, Anton-Ladislao A, Ibarrondo O, Arrospide A, Lázaro S, Gonzalez N, Bare M, Callejo D, Redondo M, Quintana JM. Cost-effectiveness analysis of laparoscopic versus open surgery in colon cancer. Surg Endosc. 2018;32(12):4912–22.
147. Gehrman J, Björholt I, Angenete E, Andersson J, Bonjer J, Haglind E. Health economic analysis of costs of laparoscopic and open surgery for rectal cancer within a randomized trial (COLOR II). Surg Endosc. 2017;31(3):1225–34.
148. King PM, Blazeby JM, Ewings P, Franks PJ, Longman RJ, Kendrick AH, Kipling RM, Kennedy RH. Randomized clinical trial comparing lapa-

roscopic and open surgery for colorectal cancer within an enhanced recovery programme. J Br Surg. 2006;93(3):300–8.
149. Lee L, Sudarshan M, Li C, Latimer E, Fried GM, Mulder DS, Feldman LS, Ferri LE. Cost-effectiveness of minimally invasive versus open esophagectomy for esophageal cancer. Ann Surg Oncol. 2013;20(12):3732–9.
150. Gosselin-Tardif A, Abou-Khalil M, Mata J, Guigui A, Cools-Lartigue J, Ferri L, Lee L, Mueller C. Laparoscopic versus open subtotal gastrectomy for gastric adenocarcinoma: cost-effectiveness analysis. BJS Open. 2020;4(5):830–9.
151. Kowalsky SJ, Zenati MS, Steve J, Esper SA, Lee KK, Hogg ME, Zeh HJ III, Zureikat AH. A combination of robotic approach and ERAS pathway optimizes outcomes and cost for pancreatoduodenectomy. Ann Surg. 2019;269(6):1138–45.
152. Leung J, Leong J, Au Yeung K, Hao BZ, McCluskey A, Kayani Y, Davidson BR, Gurusamy KS. Can you trust clinical practice guidelines for laparoscopic surgery? A systematic review of clinical practice guidelines for laparoscopic surgery. Updat Surg. 2021;14:1–1.
153. Barreto SG. Pancreatic cancer in Australia: is not it time we address the inequitable resource problem? Future Oncol. 2020;16(19):1385–92.

MIX
Papier aus verantwortungsvollen Quellen
Paper from responsible sources
FSC® C105338

FSC
www.fsc.org

If you have any concerns about our products,
you can contact us on
ProductSafety@springernature.com

In case Publisher is established outside the EU,
the EU authorized representative is:
Springer Nature Customer Service Center GmbH
Europaplatz 3, 69115 Heidelberg, Germany

Printed by Libri Plureos GmbH
in Hamburg, Germany